Habilitation of the Handicapped

Authors' Note

The term 'rehabilitation' usually connotes the restoration of a former capacity. However, training of the developmentally disabled is geared toward teaching new skills rather than restoring skills lost by illness or injury. The term 'habilitation' is gaining increasing acceptance as a better word for describing this endeavor, and we have therefore preferred to use it in this volume.

In current usage the term 'developmental disability' is being applied to a wide range of disabilities, including mental retardation, cerebral palsy, epilepsy, sensory impairment, and autism. While many of the generalizations drawn in this book are applicable to other forms of developmental disability, the major focus of both the theory and application discussed in this text has been on mental retardation.

Habilitation of the Handicapped

New Dimensions in Programs for the Developmentally Disabled

by

Marvin Rosen, Ph.D.
Director of Psychology
Elwyn Institute

Gerald R. Clark, M.D.
Professor of Psychiatry and of Pediatrics
The University of Pennsylvania Medical School;
President, Elwyn Institute

Marvin S. Kivitz, Ph.D.
Director of Programs
Elwyn Institute

With a Foreword by

H. C. Gunzburg, Ph.D.
Consultant Psychologist
Director of Psychological Services
Monyhull Hospital
Birmingham, England

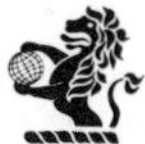

University Park Press
Baltimore · London · Tokyo

UNIVERSITY PARK PRESS
International Publishers in Science and Medicine
Chamber of Commerce Building
Baltimore, Maryland 21202

Typeset by The Composing Room of Michigan, Inc.
Manufactured in the United States of America
by Universal Lithographers, Inc., and The Maple Press Co.

Library of Congress Cataloging in Publication Data

Rosen, Marvin.
Habilitation of the handicapped.

1. Mentally handicapped—Rehabilitation.
I. Clark, Gerald Robert, 1918– joint author.
II. Kivitz, Marvin S., joint author. III. Title.
[DNLM: 1. Mental retardation—Rehabilitation.
2. Mental health services. WM300 R813h]
RC570.R67 362.3 77-5379
ISBN 0-8391-1137-1

Contents

Foreword

Any survey of the literature on mental retardation over the hundred-odd years since the first specialist contributions were published would come to the conclusion that the most important aspects of mental retardation are intellectual inferiority and social incompetence. Indeed, these are the two factors that must be assessed to establish mental retardation in a person, and they are the two aspects that have been studied most consistently and diligently in the research literature. The emphasis on the cognitive deficit, which is so easily observable and nearly as easily measurable, can be easily understood, since it seems to provide the most convincing explanations for the problems caused by the mentally retarded person and his comparative lack of responsiveness to education and training. The continuing exploration of differences in test patterns and of the consistently low test performances indicates that the conspicuous intellectual shortcomings of the mentally retarded continue to fascinate investigators.

Our civilization sets great store by intelligence and intellectual achievement, and it is, therefore, not really surprising that the other diagnostic criterion—social competence—is less readily tackled. Of course, it can also be argued that any improvement in intellectual functioning would automatically raise the level of social functioning, and attention to the cognitive factor is, therefore, supremely important. Only in recent years has there been an increased emphasis on direct teaching and training of social skills without regard to the disheartening influence of a low IQ.

Those who emphasize teaching and training of those behaviors that are relevant and important for living with a reasonable degree of independence in the open community, have, of course, not overlooked the fact that adverse environmental conditions, as well as low intellectual ability, impose a ceiling on possible achievements. It has also become clear that the systematic and consistent practical teaching of vocational and social skills in normal, supportive, and demanding environments has some surprising and encouraging effects on social efficiency. Yet, there is still a very important conglomeration of factors that seems to put a limit to the effectiveness of skilled teaching, highly favorable environments, and most sympathetic human relationships.

Thus, at long last, attention focuses more steadily on that one area, which is responsible for the driving force necessary to make a person *want* to use his limited intelligence, to overcome difficulties, to direct his actions, to make a deliberate choice, and to take responsibility for himself.

Some workers in this field have repeatedly drawn attention to the "inadequate personality" of the mentally retarded and "explained" his social incompetence and low intellectual functioning in these terms. Most workers have fought shy of dealing with something as diffuse and only vaguely definable as personality, particularly because the mentally retarded person's verbal limitations added considerable difficulties to the task of exploring his personal problems. However, there is no doubt in this writer's mind that the real reasons for the mentally retarded person's social inadequacy lie in the field of "personalization," and it is there that the key for maximizing his meager mental resources and achieving his "personal adequacy" will be found.

It was, therefore, with an increasing sense of excitement that this writer followed the theme of this book, as it was developed in the manuscript sent to him for a preview. Having pursued for over 35 years the elusive task of designing more effective social training and assessment methods and having always been foiled—or nearly always—by the "weak drive," the shortsightedness, the "immaturity," the impulsiveness, and many other equally frustrating attributes of the mentally retarded, this writer has found it only too painfully obvious that all our sophisticated approaches dealt only indirectly with the problems caused by the "inadequate personality." The very fact that no serious attempt had been made by the scientific workers in the field (as apart from the theoretical researchers) to face the issues squarely and to come to grips with them has been very discouraging, particularly when studying the proliferation of rather irrelevant and paltry research investigations.

Here, in this work, I found at last scientific workers, alive to the realities of day-to-day work, who attempted to expand practical knowledge in the very area that matters most. Here, too, I found people developing an operational philosophy for an institution that takes into account that dimension that many "perfect" training schemes do not even mention—the mentally retarded individual seen as a "person" and helped as a person, whilst not overlooking the need for support provided by carefully developed and applied training programs.

Mental retardation literature has avalanched in recent years. The purely scientific texts have succeeded in presenting an increasing amount of knowledge, accumulated from a mass of research, but seem to have overlooked the fact that we deal with persons. There are other publications—warm, humane, slightly muddled accounts of what is actually done and experienced by less scientific workers in the field. As human interest stories they are immensely moving, but they fail to push forward the frontiers of our knowledge, even though they add humanity to our outlook.

This volume combines both approaches successfully—and provides practical detail of habilitation work within an institutional environment. The exploration of the difficult areas in the treatment of personal shortcomings could initiate effective ways of reducing the handicap that is the result of a probably permanent defect and could make the inadequate person function more adequately.

The authors discuss certain personality aspects relating to the functioning of the mentally retarded and provide tentative experimental evidence of their possible significance. Opening up this avenue for research is extremely important, but even more important is the fact that this team of workers has adopted a philosophy of remediation. This is based on the belief that much of the inadequate personality make-up of the mentally retarded may have been acquired in the course of "growing up," and is not necessarily a constituent part of the syndrome itself.

I have never had the pleasure of visiting the Elwyn Institute and I have only met one of the authors once for a few hours some years ago. I am really sorry that I did not have opportunities to meet the members of a team that has so purposefully given direction to rehabilitation work of a more relevant and substantial type than usual. I think I would have been immensely stimulated and encouraged to see people developing an operational philosophy and putting their theory into practice, although they were fully aware of the frustrating realities of the situation, but nevertheless maintaining a consistent course in pursuing those rehabilitation targets that have been avoided by most of us as being too vague and too difficult.

The brave effort of this book to push forward our professional aspirations of venturing out into the all-important field of remediating the mentally retarded's personal shortcomings, instead of confining ourselves to improving the relatively easy techniques of vocational and social competence training, deserves not only wide attention, but should, nay must, stimulate people to experiment further in this unknown territory. I think my feelings will be shared by many who have had to confess to themselves that what has been aimed for and what has been achieved so far have been and still are too much like teaching a great number of "circus tricks"—attracting some admiring attention in the arena of the big wide world but not really satisfying the performer himself. All those workers in the field who share this dissatisfaction will find here a door opening up to an intriguing new practical approach that promises well to introduce the mentally retarded person to a fuller life than we have been able to give him so far.

H. C. Gunzburg, M.A., Ph.D., F.B.Ps.S.

Preface

Never before has public concern about the plight of the mentally retarded been coupled so clearly with both the zeal for reform and the resources for innovation. In every era there are pivotal periods—times when new directions can be undertaken and the lessons of previous generations used to guide the way. It is during such periods that history sits in the balance. A critical decision can set succeeding decades on a course that may remain unchecked for years. An alternative choice and other sequences unfold.

Such have been the vicissitudes of thought and action in the treatment of the mentally retarded. In retrospect, the times of choice were clear. When Seguin walked the halls of the Bicêtre and, following the charge of Itard, his mentor, set about teaching those whom he labeled idiots and fools, the world might then have mocked so radical a thought: for who was he to tamper with the products of intemperance and sin? When the exiled Seguin sought solace on American soil and converted the righteous God-fearing men of Boston and Philadelphia to his methods, he might have been called charlatan and fraud instead of teacher. When Goddard stood in front of an august mental retardation group and said, "It's all untrue that retardation can be changed and idiots will learn with proper training; my tests have proved it false," they might have challenged him or listened to the calmer heads who pointed out his measures were too young to be reliable; however, they called him a scientist and accepted what he said about inheritance. It justified their institutions and the segregation and sterilizations that were then imposed upon the retarded.

Now we sit upon the crossroads once again. As institutions empty out their wards, and learned men call out for "normalization," and communities at last take up responsibility for the handicapped, and research seeks out the effects of chromosomes and nucleic acids, and bold new technologies offer promise for socializing those who only yesterday were said to be untrainable, then perhaps we now sit again upon the balance beam and need to make the right decisions.

This volume deals with what the field of rehabilitation has accomplished for the mentally retarded and suggests what is still left to do. The book places the methods and goals of rehabilitation within their proper place in its historical development as a helping and humanitarian concern. More important than its antecedents, however, is the promise that rehabilitation holds. In the succeeding chapters we espouse a research utilization model and illustrate it with efforts of rehabilitation workers. The new dimensions we envision derive from faith in relevant research honestly applied, intelligently interpreted, and diligently translated into programs and services. The new dimensions encompass an acceptance of the empirical method without preconceptions or bias. They require a faith that professionals working with the retarded will correctly read the lessons of the past and will have the courage to follow research results wherever they may lead, regardless of whatever attitudes or trends are currently popular. The new dimensions include the assumption that many of the answers we are seeking are almost within our grasp—they are discoverable in the records of our predecessors and through the technologies we have already developed.

An underlying philosophy of this book was most clearly described in a recent position statement of the National Association of Private Residential Facilities for the Mentally Retarded. This statement defines the developmental model as: "based upon the premise that *all* persons, regardless of their type or degree of disability, are capable of growth. Instead of focusing on the treatment of handicapping conditions, the emphasis is placed upon maximizing an individual's potential for learning and development, and for happiness in a life that approximates, as closely as possible, that enjoyed by the average American. For some persons a continuing effort must be made to maintain the maximum level of development once it has been attained."

This book is intended primarily for the rehabilitation specialist, the rehabilitation student, and others working with the mentally retarded. The process and outcome of rehabilitation are described from the perspective of those who have been deeply immersed in both areas over the past decade and a half. As professionals working with the handicapped, we have attempted to build programs based upon sound theoretical principles and empirical findings. As authors, we have endeavored to integrate theoretical issues with a descriptive account of how these issues affected the implementation of programs and research. If the balance tips in any direction, it is toward the applied rather than the theoretical, toward the specific rather than the general. Elwyn Institute occupies a unique historical position, epitomizing changes that have occurred on a national basis since Seguin's pioneering efforts. It is our direct experience with, and concerns about, these changes that we wish to convey.

The book is organized into seven sections. Section I places the philosophy of rehabilitation within a historical context. Changing concepts of mental retardation affect both the ways in which education and training are applied and the manner in which the mentally retarded are evaluated. Chapter 3 presents the overall research utilization model upon which the major concepts of this book are predicated. In Section II the process of habilitation is examined, and its application at a residential institution is described. Section III explores the effects of institutions upon the development and personality of its residents and considers the goal of "normalization" as an habilitative strategy. Section IV deals with the outcomes of habilitation programs, first by a general review of follow-up studies of mentally retarded persons in the community and then by the results of a specific follow-up study. Chapter 11 considers the predictability of successful and unsuccessful community adjustment from measurable characteristics of rehabilitation clients. Section V, the most lengthy part of the book, suggests a number of personality dimensions that appear significant in evaluating mentally retarded individuals. Section VI deals with the treatment of social and emotional problems of the mentally retarded by psychotherapy, counseling, and behavior modification methods. Finally, the last chapter suggests the need for renewed community-oriented research efforts and calls for a new breed of rehabilitation specialist.

Two books inspired the present effort: Robert B. Edgerton's *The Cloak of Competence* and H. C. Gunzburg's *Social Competence and Mental Handicap.*

Both focus on the need for greater understanding of the social and emotional factors affecting the habilitation and community adjustment of the developmentally disabled. Both books suggest new directions of exploration for research and program development. We hope this volume will also suggest new directions, or instigate others to do so.

Acknowledgments

Many persons contributed to the completion of this book. The authors wish to acknowledge their debt to the teachers, rehabilitation specialists, residential programs staff, and other dedicated individuals at Elwyn Institute whose names usually do not appear on reports and publications, but whose daily commitment to the mentally handicapped makes such projects possible. We are also grateful to the Rehabilitation Services Administration for their guidance and financial support, which were instrumental in initiating the programs described in this book. Mrs. Lucretia Floor was research associate over a seven-year period and was a close collaborator on most of the Elwyn follow-up research reported in this volume. Many of the chapters reflect insights that she contributed during this time, and Chapters 9 and 11 were largely her responsibility. Mr. Albert Bussone and Mr. Earl Wilkie were extremely helpful in compiling material presented in Chapter 5. Ms. Laura Zisfein implemented much of the research and counseling described in Chapters 13, 14, 15, and 19. Typing and editing were competently provided by Ms. Dianne Mruk and Mrs. Carolyn Mitchell. Finally, we are indebted to Mrs. Bonnie Rosen for proofreading the entire manuscript and for translating many convoluted grammatical constructions into basic English.

In memory of Armin Loeb,
who believed in the process of rehabilitation and found ways to measure it.

Habilitation of the Handicapped

Section I

History and Overview

Chapter 1

The Concept of Habilitation

Historical Perspective

Habilitation is usually defined as a process by which various professional services are utilized to help a disabled individual make maximal use of his capacities in order that he might learn to function more effectively. The application of habilitation goals to the developmentally disabled is a relatively recent phenomenon, first appearing in the mid-nineteenth century. It was seriously challenged at the close of that century, tentatively resurrected a few decades later, then given unqualified endorsement by some during the 1960s and 1970s.

Before the work of the physicians Seguin (in Paris in the 1840s) and Guggenbühl (in Switzerland at roughly the same time), attitudes toward the mentally retarded ranged from pity to derision and scorn. Perhaps the most prevalent attitude, dating from antiquity, has been indifference.

Although periods of concern for the mentally retarded occurred throughout the ages, there is little indication, as Kanner (1967) points out, that they were regarded by physicians as part of their medical responsibility. The same may be said of educators. In the wake of eighteenth and nineteenth century humanitarianism, the alienist Pinel cast the chains from the insane in Paris, and the reformer Dorothea L. Dix made her impassioned plea to the Massachusetts Legislature on behalf of the mentally defective and mentally deranged. In the aftermath of such concern over the poor, the insane, and the criminal, the idea of teaching the mentally retarded was germinated.

It is of interest that the earliest teachers of the retarded clung tenaciously to moralistic conceptions of the nature of the disorder they were striving to remediate. Both Luther and Calvin are alleged to have denounced the mentally retarded as "filled with Satan" (Barr, 1904).

The early teachers of the mentally retarded were as convinced of the basic degeneracy of their charges as they were of their potential for improvement with appropriate training. Both Seguin and S. G. Howe thought the causes of mental retardation to be violations of the natural laws, with intemperance, intermarriage of relatives, "self-abuse," and greed occupying positions high on the list of violations. L. P. Brockett (1856), a well-known writer of the time, summarizes these beliefs:

> In short, humiliating as the thought may be, we are driven to the conclusion that the vast amount of idiocy, in our world, is the direct result of violation of the physical and moral laws which govern our being; that oft times the sins of the fathers are thus visited upon their children; and that the parent, for the sake of momentary gratification of his depraved appetite, inflicts upon his helpless offspring a life of utter vacuity (p. 79).

Seguin himself makes it clear that his new treatment of the mentally retarded derives from the highest religious principles, that his treatment is a *moral treatment,* which can only be thought of as God's work:

> That which most essentially constitutes idiocy, is the absence of *moral volition,* superseded by a negative will; that in which the treatment of an idiot essentially consists is, in changing his *negative will* into an affirmative one, his *will* of loneliness into a will of sociability and usefulness; such is the object of the *moral training*....
>
> Thus, thanks to the idiots, that which was, in the hands of the monks of Spain, a divine mystery, is become a fundamental principle of anthropological science. Such is the origin, partly divine and partly human, of the treatment and education of idiots, though we can clearly see that God is at the bottom of this and of all our great discoveries (Seguin, 1864).

It is clear then that whatever the physiological understanding of the causes and treatment of mental retardation, whatever pedagogical justification for the training provided, the early workers with the retarded, whom we cannot help but admire for the strength of their missionary zeal, maintained a totally Christian view of their labors. They were saving idiots—who, according to Seguin, "know(s) nothing, can do nothing, cannot even desire to do anything," and according to Howe represented the lowest classes of human organisms, "breathing masses of flesh, fashioned in the shape of men, but shorn of all other human attributes."

This then was the spirit of habilitation in the mid-nineteenth century, both in Europe and the United States. The attitude was positive, and optimism prevailed. Mentally retarded persons could be trained sufficiently to permit them to function in a normal community. If the concept of cure was not a part of the new spirit, it did not detract from the ardor of the effort. Hervey B. Wilbur, who started the first American private school at Barre, Massachusetts, and later became superintendent of the experimental school at Albany, New York, stated a most reasonable goal for the rehabilitation programs:

> We do not propose to create or supply faculties absolutely wanting (in the retarded) nor to bring all grades of idiocy to the same standard of development or discipline; nor to make them all capable of sustaining, creditably, all the relations of a social and moral life; but rather to give to dormant faculties the greatest practicable development, and to apply those awakened faculties to a useful purpose under the control of an aroused and disciplined will. At the basis of all our efforts lies the principle that the human attributes of intelligence, sensibility and will are not absolutely wanting in an idiot, but dormant and undeveloped (Wilbur, 1852).

It was unfortunate that the proselytizing of Seguin, Howe, and others was not more conservative, for when the mentally retarded students at the first schools failed to live up to expectations for cure and community functioning, a wave of pessimism was generated that was to last many decades.

The rehabilitation philosophy regarding the mentally retarded has been described by White and Wolfensberger (1969) as a shift from the *desire,* between 1850 and 1880, to "make the deviant undeviant," to a *concern,* from 1870 to 1890, to "shelter the deviant from society," to *alarm,* between 1880 and 1900, over "protection of society from the deviant." Like all generalizations, this is probably an overstatement of the actual facts. It is an injustice to the dedicated efforts of many teachers of the mentally retarded, who undoubtedly maintained the fervor of Seguin and the quiet, almost religious dedication to their task.

Nevertheless, as institutions grew in size the tone of the reports and papers emanating from them changed radically from the laudatory case histories of success with the physiological method of instruction. Now there was a fresh concern about economy of operation and a reluctant acknowledgment that many mentally retarded would require life-long care. In 1893, Walter E. Fernald, Superintendent of the Massachusetts School for the Feeble-minded, described the typical American institution as divided into two sections: the school, or educational department, and the custodial department.

The educational department appeared to perpetuate the same programs of sensory, manual, physical, and moral training developed by Seguin and his contemporaries. Children were expected to learn to read and write, to know something about numbers, to learn correct social habits and behavior, and to acquire simple principles of morality. As adults they received instruction in industrial occupations and manual labor. Carpentry, brick-making, gardening, farming, domestic work, printing, painting, and the manufacture of clothing, boots, and shoes, brooms, and mattresses were successfully taught. It is important to read Fernald's own words concerning the potential of students receiving such training for community living, since it is often assumed that community release programs did not originate until the last decade.

> Each year a certain number of persons of this (educable) class go out from these institutions and lead useful, harmless lives. Some of the institutions where only the brightest class of imbeciles are received, and where the system of industrial training has been very carefully carried out, report that from 20 to 30 per cent of the pupils are discharged as absolutely self-supporting. In other institutions, where the lower-grade cases are received, the percentage of cases so discharged is considerably less. It is safe to say that not over 10 to 15 per cent of our inmates can be made self-supporting in the sense of going out into the community and securing and retaining a situation and prudently spending their earnings. With all our training we cannot give our pupils that indispensable something known as good, plain 'common sense.' The amount and value of their labor depend upon the amount of oversight and supervision practicable. But it is safe to say that over 50% of the adults of the higher grade who have been under training from childhood are capable, under intelligent supervision, of doing a sufficient amount of work to pay for the actual cost of their support, whether in an institution or at home (p. 324).

The second, or custodial, section of the institution was designed to deal with "lower grades of idiots," "juvenile insane," and "epileptics." Many of these children and adults were described as completely helpless, lacking in self-help skills, and unable to make their wants known. The habilitation goals for these persons were confined to the teaching of basic habits of self-care, cleanliness, and obedience, "to see that their wants are attended to, and to make them comfortable and happy as long as they live."

Also included in the custodial departments were graduates of the school department who were classified as "moral imbeciles" and who, it was felt, could not be trusted "either for their own good or the good of the community" without the strict surveillance of the institution.

By the turn of the century the commitment to habilitation seemed in danger of total extinction, with the rising popular and professional concern about the "menace" of the mentally retarded. The burgeoning science of genetics naively applied to the inheritance of mental retardation had significant repercussions. Henry H. Goddard, director of the newly founded research department at the Vineland Training School, had a decided impact on popular and professional opinion when he concluded in his family study of the Kallikaks that mental retardation had a genetic basis. The influence of heredity on mental deficiency was described in terms of "bad blood" perpetuating the tainted traits of ancestral stock. Goddard believed his study had demonstrated a strong relationship between feeble-mindedness and criminality, and he estimated that as many as 50 percent of the inmates of penal institutions were mentally deficient.

> Such facts as those revealed by the Kallikak family drive us almost irresistibly to the conclusion that before we can settle our problems of criminality and pauperism and all the rest of the social problems that are taxing our time and our money, the first and fundamental step should be to decide upon the mental capacity of the persons who make up these groups. We must separate, as sharply as possible, those persons who are weak-minded, and therefore irresponsible, from intelligent criminals. But our method of treatment and our attitude towards crime will be changed when we discover what part of this delinquency is due to irresponsibility (Goddard, 1914).

Goddard found his method of separation in the Binet-Simon intelligence scales, which he had translated and used to classify mentally retarded residents at Vineland. Using the new procedure, he concluded that few of the feeble-minded children at Vineland were making any significant mental development, despite their enrollment in special education programs, a conclusion that seemed to reinforce his emphasis on the genetic bases of mental retardation. The notion of irreversibility of intellectual capacity, widely accepted by Fernald and other influential leaders in the field, rang the final death knell to Seguin's optimism and to the idea that mental retardation could be cured (Goddard, 1913).

The vehemence with which policies toward the retarded that were based upon the assumption that they were, indeed, a menace were adopted has been well documented (see Wolfensberger, 1969). Laws forbidding marriage were enacted in several states. Similarly, legislation permitting or mandating sterilization was passed, and permanent custodial care of the retarded was advocated. The mood of cautious concern seems, in retrospect, akin to the hysteria of the McCarthy era a half-century later. Here was the religious fervor of habilitation turned outward toward society in general. The healers of the mid-nineteenth century gave way to the moral guardians of the early twentieth century. Some lived to see the pendulum swing back again and regretted their earlier words. In 1912 Fernald generalized about the moral insensibilities of imbeciles (mildly retarded) and thought them all to be potential criminals:

> The feeble-minded are a parasitic predatory class never capable of self-support or of managing their own affairs. They cause unutterable sorrow at home and are a menace and danger to the community. Feeble-minded women are almost invariably immoral and if at large usually become carriers of veneral *(sic)* disease or give birth to children who are as defective as them-

> selves.... Every feeble-minded person, especially the high grade, is a potential criminal needing only the proper environment and opportunity for the development and expression of his criminal tendencies (p. 90).

The habilitation ideals of Itard and Seguin seemed all but forgotten. Rather than prepare the mentally retarded to adjust to society, the order of the day was to prevent, at all costs, their contamination of the race. In the first American textbook of mental deficiency since Seguin's, Barr (1904) wrote:

> ...(there is) a dangerous element in our midst, an element unprotected and unprovided for, this is our heritage from the last century. The safety of society, therefore, demands its speedy recognition and separation in order to arrest a rapid and appalling increase, and furthermore its permanent detention lest it permeate the whole body socialistic.... (p. 326).

The swing back toward an habilitation philosophy did not occur rapidly. The period between 1920 and 1960 was one of contradictory developments. In general the climate became more optimistic. In many quarters there was a reawakening of the original habilitation and education principles, a re-affirmation that retarded persons could be trained, some sufficiently to permit their functioning within a community setting. Yet the large institutions continued their domination as the treatment of choice for many retarded individuals, and, in many instances, conditions within these institutions were directly antithetical to the idea of habilitation. In examining the origin of our institutional models, Wolfensberger (1969) describes the role perceptions about the mental retardate that must have determined the design, architecture, and operation of many institutions for the retarded. These include a perception of the retardate as a sick person, as subhuman, as a menace, as a burden of charity, and as a "holy innocent." In contrast, he suggests a model of the mentally retarded person as a developing individual but finds little evidence that this influenced the design of institutions.

The seeds of change can be found in certain broad developments occurring during the first part of the twentieth century and in the work and writings of a few progressive-thinking individuals who are fully appreciated by their peers only through the wisdom of historical perspective.

The eugenics alarm reached its peak by the 1920s and then abated. With increased understanding of nongenetic determinants of retardation, such as organic causation, and the influence of environmental factors, the eugenics arguments lost much of their original vehemence. Furthermore, the fallibility of intellectual tests like the Stanford-Binet test began to be appreciated. During World War 1 nearly half of the men drafted for service in the armed forces were found to be functioning with a mental age of twelve years or less. If these figures were applied to the general population, nearly half of the country was mentally retarded! Furthermore, pioneering studies of the effects of stimulation upon intellectual functioning were being performed. The myth of IQ constancy was dispelled with data clearly indicating increases in tested intelligence with programs of stimulation (Kirk, 1958; Skeels and Dye, 1939). More sophisticated studies of the inmates of penal institutions also challenged earlier claims of an association between crime and mental retardation (see Davies, 1930; Wallin, 1956).

Continuing evidence of the satisfactory adjustment of persons leaving institutions for the mentally retarded, often against medical advice, and of mentally retarded students in special classes in the public schools (Baller, 1936; Charles, 1953; Fairbanks, 1933; Kennedy, 1966) all seemed to contradict prevailing attitudes concerning the inability of mentally retarded persons to lead productive lives without the structure of an institutional setting.

Fernald is credited with starting the first farm colony as a satellite of the institution around 1900. Although the experiment was justified in terms of the work training provided in healthy outdoor settings, economics of operation and savings to the parent institution may have been the predominant motivation. Nevertheless, these colonies provide the first evidence of a deinstitutionalization concept and may be considered precursors of later halfway houses and more recent group homes.

A major step forward occurred during World War II, when manpower needs provided a means for many persons to leave institutions for the retarded to serve in the armed forces or as defense workers in factories. The good showing of these persons laid the groundwork for deinstitutionalization trends in the 1960s and 1970s.

The acceptance of financial responsibility for the disabled was a long time in coming to the United States. Dorothea Lynde Dix crusaded not only for the establishment of state asylums for the mentally ill but also for federal assistance for humanitarian and welfare programs for all disabled persons. She was unsuccessful when a bill she sponsored that would have made possible land grants to the states for use in habilitation of the mentally ill and the deaf was vetoed by President Franklin Pierce as an infringement of states' rights. However, in 1862 the Morrill Land Grant Act ceded over 100,000,000 acres of federal land to the states for the founding of educational facilities with a vocational emphasis.

The desire to help disabled war veterans supplied a major impetus in the development of federal programs for the disabled. The passage of Public Law 178 in 1918 by the 65th Congress provided for education and training as fundamental aspects of the vocational habilitation of veterans of World War I. However, Congress refused to include disabled civilians in the program.

The passage of Public Law 236 by the 66th Congress in June, 1920, was a landmark for vocational habilitation in this country. The Civilian Vocational Rehabilitation Act, as it was called, provided for the vocational habilitation of persons disabled in industry or in any legitimate occupation and for their return to civil employment. The Vocational Rehabilitation Act Amendments of 1943 (Public Law 113) expanded the concept of vocational habilitation to include "any services necessary to render a disabled individual fit to engage in a remunerative occupation." For the first time, mentally ill and mentally retarded persons, as well as the physically disabled, could be accepted as habilitation clients. The Office of Vocational Rehabilitation was established to prepare disabled workers to engage in war production, essential industry, and other peacetime pursuits.

In August, 1954, under the Eisenhower administration, the 83rd Congress voted into law the vocational habilitation bill designated Public Law 565. This new law strengthened the existing state-federal program and provided special grants to states that enabled them to enter into new fields of habilitation. Special project grants were made available to states or to public or private nonprofit organizations for the conduct of research and demonstration studies to assist in the solution of vocational habilitation problems. The acts were again amended in 1965, extending services to people with "socially handicapping conditions." A National Advisory Council on Vocational Rehabilitation, chaired by Miss Mary E. Switzer, Director of the Office of Vocational Rehabilitation, evaluated almost five hundred applications for Research and Demonstration grants. These grants were extremely effective in funneling federal funds into long-neglected areas of habilitation of the mentally retarded.

The 1960s witnessed further growth in the habilitation movement. In 1967 the Department of Health, Education, and Welfare was reorganized, and, under the leadership of Miss Switzer, the Social and Rehabilitation Service was established. The Vocational Rehabilitation Amendments of 1968 again increased financial support to the states and provided for state construction of work adjustment centers for physically and mentally handicapped and for those labeled "disadvantaged" by age, education, ethnic, cultural, or other factors detrimental to employment.

The social unrest of the 1960s brought demands from minority groups for equal opportunity. Like others who had achieved less than their full share of rights and recognition, the mentally retarded emerged as a group with militant advocates and with spokesmen voicing demands for an expansion of services, for availability of public school and community programs, for the improvement or complete abolition of institutions, and for the civil rights available to the ordinary citizen. The banding together of interest and lobby groups, as in the National Association for Retarded Children, resulted in a powerful and effective means of producing change. Long-cherished legal principles, such as due process, equal protection under the law, and protection from cruel and unusual punishment, were applied in historic class action decisions. These decisions produced changes in many states, such as the improvement of institutions and the end of institutional peonage systems of unpaid labor by mentally retarded residents and of the exclusion of mentally retarded children from a free public education. Acknowledgment that injustices still exist is seen in the proliferation of legal advocacy groups for the mentally retarded. A recent declaration of the *Rights of Mentally Retarded Persons,* published as an official policy statement of the American Association on Mental Deficiency, specifies the rights to exert freedom of choice in making decisions; to live in the least restrictive environment; to obtain gainful employment and fair pay; to be part of a family; to marry and have a family; to be free to move about without deprivation of liberty by institutionalization; to speak openly; to maintain privacy; to practice a religion; to interact with peers; and to receive public-supported education, vocational training, and habilitation programs.

Thus, habilitation took on an added dimension in the 1960s and 1970s, a direction that represented a departure even from the optimism of the early educators of the retarded. The concept of normalization expressed by Nirje (1969) and others demanded that the mentally retarded be provided their full rights and benefits as citizens:

> ...this principle is given in the formula 'to let the mentally retarded obtain an existence as close to the normal as possible.' Thus, as I see it, the normalization principle means making available to the mentally retarded patterns and conditions of everyday life which are as close as possible to the norms and patterns of the mainstream of society (p. 363).

Efforts to apply this principle have resulted in assiduous attempts on a nation-wide basis to deinstitutionalize the mentally retarded and to find alternative programs for the mentally retarded in group homes, halfway houses, foster homes, and citizen advocacy programs.

Yet, changing the goal of habilitation efforts to include the normalization principle has introduced a contradiction that has invited criticism. Throne (1975) has pointed out that the normalization principle ignores the fact that mentally retarded persons do not develop normally in response to normal procedures: "While specialized procedures may or may not succeed in helping the retarded to become more normal, they always are the prescription of choice over normative procedures if more normal lives for the retarded are indeed the ends sought'' (p. 23). Everyone desires that the retarded live as normal lives as possible. The end is not in question, as Throne explains, only the means.

It should be clear that concern about habilitating the mentally retarded did not originate in the present generation. Nor are our current methods and philosophies drastically different from those of the previous century. Progress has occurred, but change is not a straight line function but rather a sinusoidal wave. The same issues wax and wane. The same problems remain largely unresolved—reversibility and remediation, physical versus environmental factors, classification and measurement, criteria of adjustment, prediction, segregation and control, potential social threat, prevention, and the safeguarding of basic human rights.

Each generation painfully confronts and somehow copes with the same dilemmas. Previous solutions no longer seem acceptable in retrospect. The concept of habilitation is relatively new in the history of man. The desire to help disabled persons reach vocational and economic goals and social potential commensurate with their residual abilities, to reduce their dependence on institutions, nursing homes, and the family, to give them independent lives free of custodial care, and to afford them a degree of happiness available to the ordinary citizen was a revolutionary idea in the mid-nineteenth century. At a national conference dealing with the vocational habilitation of the mentally retarded in 1960, one of the keynote speakers quoted the eminent historian Arnold Toynbee, who wrote in the *New York Times:* ''The Twentieth Century will be chiefly remembered...as an age in which human society dared to think of the welfare of the whole human race as a practicable objective.'' Certainly this conclusion is warranted in light of the dollar expenditures for the rehabilitation of various disability groups. Another contribution of this century is the trust that was placed in research as a guidepost for uncovering areas of habilitation need, for testing the effectiveness of habilitation programs, and for advancing basic knowledge about the laws of behavior. Miss Mary E. Switzer, more than any other person, recognized and gained the acceptance of the research and demonstration project as a means for promoting the field of habilitation. Recent cutbacks in federal spending as a result of recessionary trends in the 1970s have no doubt hampered habilitation programs, so that now, more than ever, the need is felt for sound research utilization in the development of social policy and in the implementation of service delivery systems.

LITERATURE CITED

Baller, W. R. 1936. A study of the present social status of a group of adults who, when they were in elementary schools, were classified as mentally deficient. Genet. Psychol. Monogr. 18:165–244.

Barr, M. 1904. Mental Defectives: Their History, Treatment and Training. Blakiston's Sons & Co., Philadelphia.

Brockett, L. P. 1856. Idiots and the efforts for their improvement. *In* M. Rosen, G. R. Clark and M. S. Kivitz (eds.), The History of Mental Retardation: Collected Papers, pp. 69–86. Vol. 1. University Park Press, Baltimore, 1976.

Charles, D. C. 1953. Ability and accomplishment of persons earlier judged mentally deficient. Genet. Psychol. Monogr. 47:3–71.

Davies, S. P. 1930. Social Control of the Mentally Deficient. Thomas Y. Crowell Company, New York.

Fairbanks, R. 1933. The subnormal child: Seventeen years after. Ment. Hyg. 17:177–208.

Fernald, W. E. 1893. The history of the treatment of the feeble-minded. *In* M. Rosen, G. R. Clark, and M. S. Kivitz (eds.), The History of Mental Retardation: Collected Papers, pp. 321–325. Vol. 1. University Park Press, Baltimore, 1976.

Fernald, W. E. 1912. The burden of feeble-mindedness. Journal of Psycho-Asthenics 17:87–111.

Goddard, H. H. 1913. The improvability of feeble-minded children. *In* M. Rosen, G. R. Clark, and M. S. Kivitz (eds.), The History of Mental Retardation: Collected Papers, pp. 367–376. Vol. 1. University Park Press, Baltimore, 1976.

Goddard, H. H. 1914. The Kallikak Family: A Study in the Heredity of Feeble-mindedness, ch. 3. The Macmillan Company, New York.

Kanner, L. 1967. A History of the Care and Study of the Mentally Retarded. Charles C Thomas, Springfield, Ill.

Kennedy, R. J. R. 1966. A Connecticut community revisited: A study of the social adjustment of a group of mentally deficient adults in 1948 and 1960. Project No. 655, Office of Vocational Rehabilitation, U. S. Department of Health, Education, and Welfare, Washington, D.C.

Kirk, S. A. 1958. Early Education of the Mentally Retarded: An Experimental Study. University of Illinois Press, Urbana.

Nirje, B. 1969. The normalization principle and its human management implications. *In* M. Rosen, G. R. Clark, and M. S. Kivitz (eds.), The History of Mental Retardation: Collected Papers, pp. 361–376. Vol. 2. University Park Press, Baltimore, 1976.

Seguin, E. 1864. Origin of treatment and training of idiots. *In* M. Rosen, G. R. Clark, and M. S. Kivitz (eds.), The history of mental retardation: Collected papers, pp. 151–167. Vol. 1. University Park Press, Baltimore, 1976.

Skeels, H. M., and Dye, H. B. 1939. A study of the effects of differential stimulation on mentally retarded children. Proceedings and Addresses of the American Association on Mental Deficiency, pp. 114–136. Vol. 44.

Throne, J. M. 1975. Normalization through the normalization principle. Ment. Retard. 13:23–25.

Wallin, J. E. W. 1956. Mental Deficiency: In Relation to Problems of Genesis,

Social and Occupational Consequences, Utilization, Control, and Prevention. J. Clin. Psychol. Brandon, Vermont.

White, W. D., and Wolfensberger, W. 1969. The evolution of dehumanization in our institutions. Ment. Retard. 7:5–9.

Wilbur, H. B. 1852. First annual report of the New York Asylum for Idiots, pp. 15–16. New York State Document No. 30, 1852.

Wolfensberger, W. 1969. The origin and nature of our institutional models. *In* R. B. Kugel and W. Wolfensberger (eds.), Changing Patterns in Residential Services for the Mentally Retarded, ch. 5. President's Committee on Mental Retardation, Washington, D. C.

Chapter 2

Evaluation

Changing Concepts and Strategies

It is central to the thesis of this book that evaluation concepts and habilitation strategies are closely linked. The manner in which one treats a handicapped individual depends in part upon the way in which all members of that class are regarded. In each generation it is possible to trace the close association between basic concepts of mental retardation and the nature of habilitation treatment available to the mentally retarded.

Some idea of the changing concept of retardation can be gleaned from the evaluative terms that have been used to describe mentally retarded persons. A teacher who labels a child as "trainable retarded" must somehow react differently than one who labels the same child an "imbecile." "Idiot," "feeble-minded," "mentally deficient," "les enfants du bon Dieu," "idiots savantes," "moron," "educable," and "handicapped" are just a few of the terms that have been used, each term with its unique connotations. Each label was intimately related to strategies of identification and measurement and to policies of treatment. This chapter traces the changing nature of the evaluation process as a function of changes in the understanding of mental retardation and discusses some new directions in which evaluation (and treatment) are currently embarking.

MENTAL RETARDATION AS A DIFFERENTIATED CONCEPT

Prior to the efforts of Dorothea Lynde Dix in this country, it seemed to make little difference whether an individual was diagnosed as mentally retarded or mentally ill. In both cases the individual was likely to be confined in cells within prisons, alms houses, or asylums for the poor. In no case was habilitation of the individual seriously considered.

The period of reform ushered in by Dix, Seguin, and Howe accomplished the diagnosis and identification of the mentally retarded as a distinct clinical entity and the establishment of special schools. Notions prevalent at this time regarding the etiology of mental retardation had decided repercussions for both evaluation and treatment. Howe saw the causes of idiocy as being sin, ignorance, and disregard of hereditary "taints" by the parents. Evaluation of the progeny of such waywardness relied heavily on the case history method, which was used to establish familial degeneracy. Observation of the parents and grandparents was an essential part of the assessment procedure, and when these persons were found to be intemperate, licentious, "scrofulous," unhealthy, and given to sensual indulgence, diagnosis was confirmed.

Seguin described idiocy as if it were a unitary phenomenon. Guggenbühl regarded mental deficiency and cretinism as synonomous. Evaluation was largely descriptive, documenting the lowly state of the individual with little concern for individual differences. Perhaps some of the disillusionment that arose in the latter part of the nineteenth century stemmed not so much from the over-optimistic claims of the early workers as from their failure to distinguish what types of mentally retarded people were capable of improvement and what conditions were less likely to improve.

With increasing experience in teaching the mentally retarded, finer distinctions among types of retardation began to be drawn. Howe distinguished among three classes of idiots—"pure idiots," "fools," and "simpletons," or "imbeciles." His criteria were based upon the degree to which the brain and nervous system had command over voluntary muscles and their manifestation of affective and intellectual faculties.

By the end of the American Civil War, idiocy ceased being regarded as a homogeneous condition. The British physician Down first described what he labeled the "Mongolian type of idiocy," basing the diagnosis upon physiognomic characteristics. The era of medical research with the mentally retarded had begun and resulted in identification and descriptions of such conditions as Tay-Sachs disease and tuberosclerosis. This trend continued, and in 1877 an authoritative textbook by William W. Ireland, medical superintendent of the Home and School for Imbeciles in Scotland, described twelve subclassifications of mental deficiency. Ireland (1882) believed that only mongolism and microcephaly were congenital, with other types of mental deficiency stemming from nervous diseases early in life. His concerns about differentiating the "idiotic" child from the deaf or backward child are still relevant today. Ireland made broad distinctions between idiots and imbeciles. He seemed committed to the teaching and occupational training of imbeciles in order to improve their intellectual "power" by exercise and to make them happier. However, a similar commitment to the teaching of idiots seemed to be lacking:

> There are a large number of cases in which the mental fatuity is so complete that training will never be of any use; there are those where it can go no further than habit training, forming habits of cleanliness—a thing, no doubt, of considerable importance, both for the comfort of the idiot and those who have the care of him, and which, is a quite different thing from simply keeping him clean. In reading over the works of the late Dr. Seguin, one is struck by the hopeful way in which he approached cases which seemed to promise little or no improvement. A good deal may sometimes be done in the very worst cases; but this requires an amount of effort and attention and the devotion of time which can only be commanded by those parents who are in affluent circumstances (p. 260).

IMPACT OF MENTAL TESTING

There can be no disputing the impact of the mental testing movement upon evaluation and habilitation of the mentally retarded. While the fledgling science of psychology was firmly enmeshed in Wundt's "structuralism," in which the intent was to discover the general laws governing thought and perception, James McKeen Cattell broke with tradition in a doctoral dissertation dealing with individual differences. Until then such differences in scientific experiments were regarded as error, and Cattell's work met with disfavor in the psychology establishment. In 1890 Cattell first introduced the term "mental test" and described ten assessment procedures for studying individual differences.

The first Binet-Simon scale, published in 1906 in France, was developed to differentiate normal children from feeble-minded children (Binet and Simon, 1916). The project stemmed directly from educational concerns, since the procedure was to be used to weed out mental defectives from the public school system. Binet attacked current methods of diagnosis of the mentally retarded as unscientific, referring specifically to the attribution of mental deficiency to a weakness of the "will." He insisted that scientific diagnosis must be objective and quantitative and offered his procedures as a standard yardstick for this purpose. The criticism that was later leveled at intelligence testing as a sole criterion for determining mental retardation does not vitiate the significance of Binet's contribution to the study of mental retardation.

Goddard's 1910 translation of the scale into English and his application of the procedure in evaluating the mentally retarded residents at the

Vineland Training School had a marked impact on the perceived capabilities of the mentally retarded to respond to special education. From results obtained in testing children at Vineland with the new scale, Goddard provided an educational classification of "idiots," "imbeciles," and "morons." Since none of the children scored above a mental age of twelve years on this scale, Goddard suggested that the twelve-year level be considered a cut-off for the diagnosis of feeble-mindedness. In 1913 Goddard concluded from annual testing of the Vineland children that "the vast majority of feeble-minded children are not changing and are not improving in their intellectual level" (p. 370). He continued:

> From the conclusions that we have so far drawn, it is evident that our educational treatment must be largely modified. When once we have discovered that a child is stopped in his development it is, of course, useless to attempt to teach him to do anything which requires an intelligence above that which he possesses. The notion that by setting him a task somewhat ahead of his ability will somehow draw him up to that capacity, is forever exploded. It is pretty certain that intelligence develops, as we may say, of itself, and yet we only utilize and exercise what is there, and do not create anything new by any of our training methods. Here we may conclude that as a rule, feeble-minded children are trainable but not improvable in intellectual capacity (p. 372).

Intelligence testing was accepted by the medical profession as a scientific advance, and Goddard's conclusions were also accepted, disappointing as they must have been. There is no way of evaluating to what extent this discouragement filtered down to the level of classroom teachers of the mentally retarded, but it is difficult to imagine that it was entirely without effect. The myth of the infallibility of the IQ estimate and its relationship to intellectual capacity, beyond which no further intellectual change was possible, remained unchallenged for several decades.

BROADENED CRITERIA OF CLASSIFICATION

The period of pessimism did not end overnight. It is not possible to pinpoint the beginning of its demise nor the reasons for change. Signs of incipient change could be seen in the dissatisfaction expressed with the prevailing methods of diagnosis and evaluation of the mentally retarded, even with the quantitative accuracy now available in IQ testing. As early as 1924, Edgar Doll, Goddard's second successor as director of research at Vineland, was calling for greater objectivity in the diagnosis of mental retardation by the use of developmental and family history information as well as by direct mental and physical examination. Doll's attack on the use of the IQ as the sole criterion for diagnosis and classification led him toward the development of more standardized measures of social competence and social adjustment (Doll, 1948). The Vineland Social Maturity Scale (Doll, 1965), first published in 1946, avoids the measurement of specific aptitudes or disabilities, focusing instead on social competence in the mastery of maturational tasks at successive age levels. In this procedure Doll succeeded in drawing attention to the child's progression from dependency to self-sufficiency and independence, and away from predetermined conceptions of capacity based on tested mental abilities.

The importance of Doll's contribution is apparent in the current stress placed on social functioning as a criterion of mental retardation. The 1973 *Manual on Terminology and Classification in Mental Retardation* of the American Association on Mental Deficiency thus specifies that the diagnosis of mental retardation must rest on the demonstration of deficiencies along two general dimensions: measured intelligence and adaptive behavior. Adaptive behavior is defined as the success of the individual in adapting to the natural and social demands of his environment. The level of adaptation is assessed in terms of the degree to which the individual is able to function and maintain himself independently and the degree to which he satisfactorily meets the culturally imposed demands of personal and social responsibility. The Adaptive Behavior Scale (Nihira et al., 1969) has gained some acceptance as a measure of these behaviors. That evaluation of the retarded should not be limited to such an assessment of coping behaviors is a thesis that is expounded later in this chapter.

In addition to broadening the criteria of diagnosis of mental retardation to include social adjustment, educators were also calling for more useful systems of classification that would relate to instructional goals. Lightner Witmer (1909), founder of the first American psychological clinic at The University of Pennsylvania, distinguished between psychophysiological and pedagogical retardation. The former was defined as a failure of the child to reach the normal level of development for his age, while the latter refers to the number of years that a child was behind in grade level for his years.

J. E. Wallace Wallin (1924), director of a psychoeducational clinic for the St. Louis public schools, called for a minimum of two distinct special education classes for the mentally retarded, one for children of very limited "mental power" and the other for children of higher mental and educational ability. He attacked the practice of applying the terms "feebleminded," "mentally defective," "imbecilic," and "moronic" to children in special classes as being too vague for purposes of education.

The conception of the IQ as something to be regarded as constant and invariable began to be challenged by studies at the Wayne County Training

School in Northville, Michigan, and at the Child Welfare Research Station and at the Institution for Feeble-minded Children in Glenwood, Iowa. Reports of the variability of intelligence quotients (Hoakley, 1932) were appearing with some regularity. Distinctions between the endogenous, or familial, type of mental retardation and exogenous, or brain-injured, type of retardation began to prove fruitful in predicting response to educational programs (Kephart, 1939; Lehtinen and Strauss, 1944; Strauss and Werner, 1941). The more favorable prognosis for the endogenous group was explained in terms of the intact nervous system of that group and compensation for their deficits by special education programs. The studies of the effects of early education for the mentally retarded youngster, also originating at the Wayne County Training School (Kirk, 1958; Melcher, 1939, 1940), further aided in diminishing faith in the IQ as an inviolate measure of capacity.

Another telling blow that did much to dispel the IQ myth and to change the nature of the evaluation process was dealt by the Iowa Studies. The favorable results of transferring retarded children from an orphanage nursery to a school for the feeble-minded, where they were to receive stimulation and mothering by older, brighter retarded girls, are now well known. However, the idea that IQ could be modified by environmental changes was considered so contradictory to accepted dogma that the results were not fully accepted until thirty years later (Skeels and Dye, 1939).

Once the impact of these studies was felt, the pessimism of Goddard regarding the unimprovability of retarded persons could no longer be justified. Evaluation of the mentally retarded had to be more sophisticated than a one-hour IQ test.

In addition to changing conceptions of the IQ, another research finding had important repercussions for habilitation of the mentally retarded. The results of follow-up evaluations of the adjustment of persons leaving institutions for the mentally retarded, as well as those identified in special education classes in the public schools, were almost unanimously favorable. These studies are considered in detail in Chapter 9. The fact that substantial numbers of mentally retarded persons, even during the years of the depression, were able to be self-supporting and to maintain at least adequate social adjustments in the community was bound to influence the philosophy of evaluation, education, and training of such persons still enrolled within the public school or institution.

During the early 1960s the claims for successful vocational and social adjustments of the mentally retarded were so strong that even as progressive a thinker as Edgar Doll (1964), shortly before his death, urged caution and greater attention to adequate diagnosis and evaluation in studying the effectiveness of habilitation programs:

> We used to know who was feeble-minded (well, we *almost* used to, but now who knows who is mentally retarded?)...We talk about the mentally retarded so glibly without reference to degree, etiology or clinical type. Today nearly all research is suspect without clear validation of the subjects of our research.... False cures, false programs, false hopes are the fruits of such irresponsible, pseudo-professional, pseudo-scientific pronouncements. This is a moral problem which we cannot ignore for long without unhappy reverberations. These efforts are currently most prevalent in the over-optimistic claims of vocational rehabilitation where the validation of mental retardation as feeble-mindedness is rarely set forth (pp. 205–206).

VOCATIONAL EVALUATION

Doll's call for more accurate diagnostic evaluation methods did not go unheeded. Changes in federal legislation in the 1950s and 1960s made the mentally retarded citizen eligible for habilitation services previously used successfully with physically handicapped persons. The desire to apply vocational habilitation strategies to the mentally retarded necessitated the development of new evaluative procedures for assessing vocational functioning and potential. Vocational evaluation became the order of the day.

Industrial psychologists have for many years attempted to develop psychometric tests of ability and interest that would be predictive of work performance and that could be utilized in the selection of personnel and as an aid in making vocational decisions (see Anastasi, 1968; Super and Crites, 1962). The tests most frequently utilized by the vocational counselor are discussed by Super and Crites (1962).

Standardized aptitude and interest-testing procedures suitable for normal populations present many difficulties when they are used with the mentally retarded. Paper and pencil tests contain so many abstract verbal items that most mentally retarded clients score very poorly, often below the norms of the test. Even with nonverbal, performance tests, individual differences among mentally retarded persons are virtually impossible to identify when all tested clients may lie within the first percentile for the general population. The use of national norms with the retarded would result in most retarded persons being classified as unemployable.

The unavailability of meaningful predictors of vocational success for retarded populations was considered serious enough to justify the funding, by federal agencies, of numerous research investigations designed to develop such instruments during the 1950s and 1960s. In such studies various psychometric and behavioral indices are correlated with criteria of vocational and social functioning. Unfortunately these studies have not proven to be productive. In one such study, covered in more detail later in this book, Rosen et al. (1970) reported significant but very modest correlations between perceptual-motor scores and ratings of employment potential and several criteria of community adjustment for clients discharged from the institution. A replication of this study two years later with a comparable population (Rosen, Floor, and Baxter, 1972) failed to cross-validate the original findings.

In 1959 the MacDonald Training Center at Tampa, Florida, undertook the development of a "Vocational Capacity Scale" to assess the abilities, limitations, and potential of mentally retarded young adults (Ferguson, 1959). The scale was validated with a sample of 138 clients divided into three groups: a work activity (day care) group; a sheltered workshop group; and a group working at competitive employment. The scale included five tests—a Disc Assembly, the Pennsylvania Bi-Manual Assembly, the Vineland Social Maturity Scale, the Wide Range Achievement Arithmetic Test, and the Wells Concrete Directions Test. The Vocational Capacity Scale discriminated between the activities program group and the other two groups, but there was considerable overlap between the sheltered workshop and competitive employment groups.

Another approach to evaluating vocational potential involves the use of multidimensional rating scales that will, it is hoped, prove to have predictive validity for criteria of vocational functioning after training. These ratings are usually performed by one or more vocational supervisors at regular intervals during training and include many dimensions of work behavior and attitude.

Vocational evaluation ratings were used at the Edward R. Johnstone Training and Research Center in Bordentown, New Jersey (Parnicky and Kahn, 1963), at Goodwill Industries of Tacoma, Washington (Taylor, 1961), and at the Jewish Vocational Service of Chicago (Gellman, 1960). The latter project resulted in the development of "The Scale of Employability of Handicapped Persons," consisting of three separate scales: a counseling scale, to be completed by the vocational counselor; a workshop scale completed by the foreman in an habilitation workshop program; and a psychology scale completed by the psychologist after his evaluation.

Although vocational evaluation scales generally seem to have some utility in the situation in which they are developed, their reliabilities tend to be low, and their usefulness in other settings and different populations is seldom evaluated. None of the scales described above seems to have been cross-validated. The scales developed by Taylor and by Gellman were also employed in the Elwyn prognostic studies mentioned above, and neither held up as meaningful predictors in cross-validation studies.

Another approach designed to circumvent the problems imposed by standardized aptitude tests with the severely handicapped is the use of work samples (Jewish Employment and Vocational Service, 1968; Rosenberg, 1971). Work samples are simulated job tasks obtained from industry that utilize the same materials, equipment, and tools used on the actual job. Standards of speed and quality are set to conform to standards on the real job. The work sample may be an actual job administered under standard conditions or may be a mock-up of some component of the job. A work sample evaluation may have an advantage over more traditional psychological testing by being more intrinsically interesting to the client. It offers the evaluator the opportunity to observe actual work behavior. The disadvantages lie in the expense involved in time, materials, and standardization of work samples.

The use of vocational evaluations has been severely criticized by Gold (1975), who sees lowered performance levels of the mentally retarded as a function of lowered expectations set for them by society, rather than their own intrinsic deficiencies. Gold advocates a greater emphasis upon training, rather than testing the mentally retarded, and calls for the development of powerful training techniques and greater societal acceptance of broad-based work participation by retarded citizens. Gold's oversimplification about the work capabilities of the retarded and about the injustices perpetuated by underestimations of these capabilities is itself an injustice to the honest efforts to develop meaningful methods of evaluation. Clients can be trained *and* tested. Sophisticated psychological testing can be used to make training more precise and therefore more powerful. Testing need not, as Gold implies, be limited to the screening out of individuals who are difficult to train. Tests may also be used to identify client characteristics and functioning levels as a basis for remediation and strategies of training. Therefore, tests can be conducive, rather than antagonistic, to the development of a training program.

RECENT INNOVATIONS

Gold is neither all wrong nor all right. It is clear that traditional methods of vocational and psychological evaluation have not lived up to expectations and often bear little relation to training efforts or outcomes. Rather than scrap further efforts at evaluation, it seems clear that better methods of evaluation must be developed, using more specific criteria for prediction.

Change in strategies for evaluation is already occurring. Two trends are apparent. The first is the development and use of criterion-referenced rather than norm-referenced tests. The second is the incorporation of behavior modification methods into habilitation programs, along with the use of behavior analysis techniques for assessment.

In education circles the view is increasingly expressed that the variance in performance of students is less important to educational goals than the relation between individual performance and a relevant criterion of functioning. This is usually accepted implicitly in the classroom, where, for example, the teacher of arithmetic is more interested in whether or not a child can reduce fractions to their lowest common denominator than in how well he does in relation to all fifth graders across the country. In this light, norm-referenced tests may be less relevant to habilitation training than more practical assessments of whether or not the retarded individual can handle basic social and vocational behaviors. This point is close to McClelland's (1973) admonition to psychologists to test for competence rather than capacity:

> *The best testing is criterion sampling.* ...If you want to know how well a person can drive a car (the criterion), sample his ability to do so by giving him a driver's test. Do not give him a paper-and-pencil test for following directions, a general intelligence test, etc. ...There is ample evidence that tests which sample job skills will predict proficiency on the job.
>
> Criterion sampling means that testers have got to get out of their offices where they play endless word and paper-and-pencil games and into the field where they actually analyze performance into its components. If you want to test who will be a good policeman, go find out what a policeman does (p. 7).

Perhaps the greatest number of attempts to interface evaluation and treatment goals has come from the application of behavior modification and behavior therapy approaches to the field of habilitation. The early 1960s witnessed a very rapid increase in attempts to develop treatment programs deriving from "modern learning theory," particularly techniques and theory associated with Eysenck (1959), Wolpe (1958), Wolpe and Lazarus (1967), and Skinner (1953).

There is little question that behavior modification techniques often represent radical departures from traditional habilitation efforts, although the same habilitative goals certainly apply. That these techniques can work and can be applied within the more traditional habilitation setting is a matter that is discussed in a later chapter. For the time being it is sufficient to point out that behavior modification tends to do away with traditional approaches to the evaluation of the abilities, traits, assets, and deficits usually assumed to be enduring characteristics somehow resident within the individual. Instead, evaluation focuses on the immediately observable and measurable behaviors that characterize the client's present functioning or malfunctioning.

Evaluation of behavior modification procedures consists of behavior analysis, i.e., the determination of stimulus conditions associated with certain behaviors and the contingencies of "reinforcement" or "reward" that strengthen that behavior. Current behavior modification practices represent the most radical departure from physical, genetic, and moralistic preconceptions that influenced the evaluations of our predecessors.

PERSONAL ADJUSTMENT AND QUALITY OF LIFE

There can be no disputing that the two concepts that have had the strongest influence upon modern habilitation and evaluation programs are the principles of normalization and adaptive behavior. Both concepts are the result of humanitarian concerns about the mentally retarded, and of a desire to evaluate the mentally retarded according to the most relevant criteria and to afford them equal opportunities to basic freedoms available to ordinary citizens.

Yet both concepts have been challenged. Gunzburg (1972) has questioned the indiscriminate use of the normalization principle with persons not equipped for independence. He argues that proponents of normalization tend to overlook real deficits in the mentally retarded where they exist, deficits that will not disappear merely by placing the individual in more normal environmental situations. The criticism of Throne (1975), that the mentally retarded may need more than normal amounts of stimulation, was mentioned earlier. Rosen and Kivitz (1973) have pointed out that normalization is not a psychological principle, and neither normalization nor adaptive behavior can substitute for sound criteria of personal and emotional adjustment. Adequate selection and training of persons for independent living situations must still be the major component of any habilitation program.

The ability to maintain oneself independently and to meet societal demands for social and personal responsibility are indisputedly important criteria of functioning. They are, however, minimal criteria that represent only the lowest levels of functioning. They are not positive in perspective, nor are they consistent with standards of adjustment typically applied to nonretarded populations. Adaptive behaviors represent dimensions of performance, not of personality. The construct does not take into account the many personality, motivational, and emotional variables that may determine a person's adaptive or maladaptive behavior. Acceptance of adaptive behavior as the sole criterion of social adjustment of the mentally retarded could be more detrimental than acceptance of the IQ alone as a criterion. The danger would lie in the abandonment of efforts to provide training conducive to the development of higher order needs than those necessary merely for survival and coping.

Perhaps the most ambitious attempt to learn about adjustment variables for the general population is being conducted by Dr. Angus Campbell, a social psychologist at the Institute for Social Research at the University of Michigan. Campbell (1976) points out that state and federal agencies each year produce a flood of statistics assessing the condition of the population for use in establishing public policy. The bulk of these statistics relate to the material aspects of American life, i.e., to income, expenditures, savings, and the production and sale of goods and services. Such economic indices are popular, Campbell maintains, because they are easy to measure, but they do not adequately represent the quality of national life. Economic indicators, he points out, might be assumed to influence life experience but do not measure that experience directly. Campbell opts for indicators that tap more subjective qualities of experience that are closer to the popular conception of *happiness*. His measures, based upon home interviews with the respondents, who represented all walks of life, sort themselves into three general dimensions, reflecting satisfaction with life, positive or negative affective experience, and perceived stress. He finds that people in different life circumstances (e.g., divorced women, married persons with children, etc.) express different patterns of well-being, patterns that do not correlate strongly with economic indices.

To include criteria of emotional adjustment and quality of life dimensions within the evaluation process for the mentally retarded would be an ambitious undertaking. The variables are subjective and difficult to measure, an obstacle far more devastating with a relatively nonverbal and nonintrospective group than with the populations of normal intelligence that Campbell has studied.

Whether such lofty goals are attainable in evaluating the mentally retarded remains to be seen. Despite the difficulty of measurement, it is our thesis that psychologists can no longer afford to ignore such basic dimensions as self-concept, independence and responsibility for one's own behavior, an accurate perception of reality, ability to feel and express affect appropriately, satisfaction with job, ability to maintain goal-directed behavior, ability to maintain satisfying interpersonal relationships, and the capability for appropriate heterosexual relationships.

Later chapters in this book attempt to develop such personality constructs that will have utility in evaluating mentally retarded persons in light of our better understanding of their capability for community living. Now, as throughout the history of mental retardation, the dimensions we accept as worthy of our evaluation efforts both reflect and determine what we define as habilitation.

LITERATURE CITED

Anastasi, A. 1968. Psychological Testing. 3rd Ed. The MacMillan Company, London.

Binet, A., and Simon, T. 1916. Upon the necessity of establishing a scientific diagnosis of inferior states of intelligence. *In* M. Rosen, G. R. Clark, and M. S. Kivitz (eds.), The History of Mental Retardation: Collected Papers, pp. 329–354. Vol. 1. University Park Press, Baltimore, 1976.

Campbell, A. 1976. Subjective measures of well-being. Amer. Psychol. 31:117–124.

Doll, E. A. 1924. Current problems in mental diagnosis. *In* M. Rosen, G. R. Clark, and M. S. Kivitz (eds.), The History of Mental Retardation: Collected Papers, pp. 23–33. Vol. 2. University Park Press, Baltimore, 1976.

Doll, E. A. 1948. The relation of social competence to social adjustment. *In* M. Rosen, G. R. Clark, and M. S. Kivitz (eds.), The History of Mental Retardation: Collected Papers, pp. 267–275. Vol. 2. University Park Press, Baltimore, 1976.

Doll, E. A. 1964. Yesterday, today and tomorrow. Ment. Retard. 2:203–208.

Doll, E. A. 1965. Vineland Social Maturity Scale. Condensed Manual of Directions. American Guidance Service, Circle Pines, Minnesota.

Eysenck, H. J. 1959. Learning theory and behavior therapy. J. Ment. Sci. 105:61–75.

Ferguson, R. G. 1959. Evaluation of the potential for vocational rehabilitation of mentally retarded youths. MacDonald Training Center, Tampa, Fla.

Gellman, W. 1960. A scale of employability for handicapped persons. Office of Vocational Rehabilitation, Project No. 64–57.

Goddard, H. H. 1910. Four hundred feeble-minded children classified by the Binet method. *In* M. Rosen, G. R. Clark, and M. S. Kivitz (eds.), The History of Mental Retardation: Collected Papers, pp. 355–366. Vol. 1. University Park Press, Baltimore, 1976.

Goddard, H. H. 1913. The improvability of feeble-minded children. *In* M. Rosen, G. R. Clark, and M. S. Kivitz (eds.), The History of Mental Retardation: Collected Papers, pp. 367–376. Vol. 1. University Park Press, Baltimore, 1976.

Gold, M. W. 1975. Vocational training. *In* J. Wortis (ed.), Mental Retardation and Developmental Disabilities. Brunner/Mazel, New York.

Gunzburg, H. C. 1972. (Editorial.) Brit. J. Ment. Subnormal. 28(2):63–65.

Hoakley, Z. P. 1932. The variability of intelligence quotients. Proceedings of the American Association for the Study of the Feebleminded, pp. 119–148. Vol. 37.

Ireland, W. W. 1877. On Idiocy and Imbecility. Churchill Ltd., London.

Ireland, W. W. 1882. On the diagnosis and prognosis of idiocy and imbecility. *In* M. Rosen, G. R. Clark, and M. S. Kivitz (eds.), The History of Mental Retardation: Collected Papers, pp. 247–261. Vol. 1. University Park Press, Baltimore, 1976.

Jewish Employment and Vocational Service. 1968. Work samples. Final report.

Experimental and demonstration project. Contract No. 82-40-67-40. Manpower Administration, U. S. Department of Labor. JEVS, Philadelphia.

Kephart, N. C. 1939. The effect of a highly specialized program upon the I.Q. in high-grade mentally deficient boys. *In* M. Rosen, G. R. Clark, and M. S. Kivitz (eds.), The History of Mental Retardation: Collected Papers, pp. 69–76. Vol. 2. University Park Press, Baltimore, 1976.

Kirk, S. A. 1958. Early Education of the Mentally Retarded: An Experimental Study. University of Illinois Press, Urbana.

Lehtinen, L. E., and Strauss, A. A. 1944. A new approach in educational methods for brain-crippled deficient children. *In* M. Rosen, G. R. Clark, and M. S. Kivitz (eds.), The History of Mental Ratardation: Collected Papers, pp. 89–96. Vol. 2. University Park Press, Baltimore, 1976.

Manual on Terminology and Classification in Mental Retardation. 1973. American Association on Mental Deficiency, Washington, D.C.

McClelland, D. C. 1973. Testing for competence rather than for ''intelligence.'' Amer. Psychol. 28:1–14.

Melcher, R. T. 1939. A program of prolonged pre-academic training for the young mentally handicapped child. Amer. J. Ment. Defic. 44:202–215.

Melcher, R. T. 1940. Developmental progress in young mentally handicapped children who received prolonged pre-academic training. Amer. J. Ment. Defic. 45:265–273.

Nihira, K., Foster, R., Shelhaas, M., and Leland, H. 1969. Adaptive behavior scales. American Association on Mental Deficiency, Washington, D.C.

Parnicky, J. J., and Kahn, H. 1963. Evaluating and developing vocational potential of institutionalized retarded adolescents. Edward R. Johnstone Training Center, Bordentown, N.J.

Rosen, M., Floor, L., and Baxter, D. 1972. Prediction of community adjustment: A failure at cross validation. Amer. J. Ment. Defic. 77:111–112.

Rosen, M., and Kivitz, M. S. 1973. Beyond normalization: Psychological adjustment. Brit. J. Ment. Subnormal. 19(2):64–70.

Rosen, M., Kivitz, M. S., Clark, G. R., and Floor, L. 1970. Prediction of post-institutional adjustment of mentally retarded adults. Amer. J. Ment. Defic. 74:726–734.

Rosenberg, B. 1971. Job evaluation through the ''Tower'' work sample approach. *In* R. N. Pacinelli (ed.), Research Utilization in Rehabilitation Facilities. Proceedings of an International Conference, June 1–18, 1970. Grant No. 22-P-55091/3-01 from the Social and Rehabilitation Service, U. S. Department of Health, Education, and Welfare, Washington, D. C.

Skeels, H. M., and Dye, H. B. 1939. A study of the effects of differential stimulation on mentally retarded children. *In* M. Rosen, G. R. Clark, and M. S. Kivitz (eds.), The History of Mental Retardation: Collected Papers, pp. 241–266. Vol. 2. University Park Press, Baltimore, 1976.

Skinner, B. F. 1953. Science and Human Behavior. The MacMillan Company, New York.

Strauss, A. A., and Werner, H. 1941. The mental organization of the brain-injured mentally defective child. *In* M. Rosen, G. R. Clark, and M. S. Kivitz (eds.), The History of Mental Retardation: Collected Papers, pp. 77–87. Vol. 2. University Park Press, Baltimore, 1976.

Super, D. O., and Crites, J. O. 1962. Appraising Vocational Fitness by Means of Psychological Tests. Harper & Row, New York.

Taylor, J. B. 1961. The prediction of rehabilitation potential among the mentally retarded. Project No. RD 603. Vocational Rehabilitation Administration, Department of Health, Education, and Welfare, Washington, D.C.

Throne, J. M. 1975. Normalization through the normalization principle. Ment. Retard. 13:23–25.

Wallin, J. E. W. 1924. Classification of mentally deficient and retarded children for instruction. *In* M. Rosen, G. R. Clark, and M. S. Kivitz (eds.), The History of Mental Retardation: Collected Papers, pp. 35–50. Vol. 2. University Park Press, Baltimore, 1976.

Witmer, L. 1909. The study and treatment of retardation: A field of applied psychology. *In* M. Rosen, G. R. Clark, and M. S. Kivitz (eds.), The History of Mental Retardation: Collected Papers pp. 5–11. Vol. 2. University Park Press, Baltimore, 1976.

Wolpe, J. 1958. Psychotherapy by Reciprocal Inhibition. Stanford University Press, Stanford.

Wolpe, J., and Lazarus, A. A. 1967. Behavior Therapy Techniques. Pergamon Press Ltd., London.

Chapter 3

Research Utilization

The immediate and long-term effects of habilitation programs upon mentally retarded persons have not been well researched. The opportunity for studying large populations of mentally retarded persons receiving habilitation services therefore offers an exciting possibility for psychological research. There is probably no more fertile area of investigation for a behavioral scientist than the transitional experience of an individual returning to independent community living after spending most of his life within an institution. The motivational changes, cognitive restructuring, and social phenomena that may be associated with this experience are still largely unexplored. The investigator based at a setting offering habilitation programing is in a unique and advantageous position for serving as an observer and a social historian of these processes.

Unfortunately, however, habilitation studies tend to be isolated and without a unified purpose. Workers at each facility are largely insulated from each other and remain preoccupied with their own particular habilitation programs. Despite the recommendation of numerous conferences, a sound model has failed to emerge to guide investigation in a manner that would maximize research utilization. Effective research utilization can become a reality only when research studies are designed to provide answers to meaningful questions.

The most significant issue facing the field of habilitation concerns current trends toward deinstitutionalization and normalization of the mentally retarded. It follows, then, that habilitation research must concern itself with the processes involved in training the mentally retarded to function independently. Yet, despite general acceptance of the attitude that it is necessary to train the mentally retarded in order to decrease their dependence upon family or institution, it is still unknown what can be expected of them in the way of social learning, economic advancement, and integration within community settings. Such data should be available to habilitation personnel in their day-to-day decision-making.

This chapter expresses the bias that behavioral research at habilitation facilities should be directly concerned with the educational or training functions of that facility and should have the specific purpose of affecting important decisions about educational programs and policies. In addition to contributing to the general body of knowledge, the habilitation researcher must take responsibility for the conduct of investigation pertinent to the growth and development of his facility, for dissemination of his findings, and for implementation of results in education, training, or treatment programs.

Two general types of behavioral investigations account for most published research. The first represents basic theory-building efforts in the areas of intelligence, learning, perception, and cognition. This research is conducted primarily at large universities or university-affiliated settings. Rarely are the findings translatable into practical programs. The second type of investigation represents applied research, usually conducted at institutions, habilitation centers, and schools. This research category includes such efforts as test construction and validation as well as evaluation studies of education or habilitation programs. Experimental precision in such studies is often less rigorous than it is in basic research, and practical difficulties in the conduct of such investigation are greater.

This chapter deals with the second type of research, i.e., applied behavioral research performed within habiliation settings. The chapter suggests needed guidelines for such research. Such guidelines should transcend the dictates of governmental funding priorities and should derive, instead, from internal needs of the habilitation facility. The ideas expressed are offered as standards for guiding behavioral research in habilitation settings and for placing limits on research ideas that are not in keeping with the habilitation mission of such facilities.

BASING HABILITATION PROGRAMS ON RESEARCH FINDINGS

Social change occurs slowly; established precedent dies hard. Policy and program changes, when they occur, are often dictated by what has gone before, what is the current ''Zeitgeist,'' and what federal or state funds happen to be available. It is seldom the case that programs and policy derive from meaningful empirical investigations designed to answer specific questions. Today, more than ever, federal granting agencies, by setting research and program priorities for their funds, determine the direction that service-providing agencies must follow. It is the very rare facility that is in the position of charting its own course, let alone doing it on the basis of research results.

Yet the absence of objective empirical guidelines for public policy can sometimes lead to far-reaching and disastrous consequences. As is described in Chapter 1, for over a century the policy toward the mentally retarded was based on outmoded theory and ideas. Programs for the retarded had stagnated or were nonexistent. The growth of institutions, for example, was based on assumptions regarding the genetic determination of mental deficiency, and the detrimental effects the mentally retarded were presumed to have on society. Even when research served to disconfirm these assumptions, institutionalization remained the only alternative available for many mentally retarded persons.

Today we are witnessing an extreme reaction to the policies of previous decades. The outcome of the deinstitutionalization wave of the 1970s is still to be determined. Appropriate research studies are still to be conducted. Yet in many states deinstitutionalization policy decisions of enormous consequence are being made without sufficient evidence concerning the effects of institutional living on the mentally retarded, the effects of drastic environmental change on the retarded persons involved, the relative effectiveness of various community alternatives to institutionalization, the variables affecting adjustment within alternative community settings, the manner in which communities will accept mentally retarded persons discharged from institutions, and the characteristics of the mentally retarded that might be associated with successful or unsuccessful community placement.

It may be argued that few persons have the perspicacity to foresee, even with the advantage of research results, the most advantageous choices in such decision-making situations. Furthermore, it may be argued that few facilities exist that can afford the competent research staff who could conduct research designed to answer relevant questions. We hold that such staff do exist now, that they are already available to habilitation facilities, and that others could be made available if educational institutions would adequately train people in such skills.

This chapter develops a research utilization approach that can be used effectively within habilitation settings. It suggests areas of habilitation for the mentally retarded that require research solutions, and, finally, it describes a research utilization program at one facility that conforms to these guidelines.

RESONANCE, IRREVERENCE, AND RELEVANCE

Since habilitation settings for the mentally retarded lack clearly defined practices for the conduct of research (Tarjan, 1965; Wolfensberger, 1965, 1967), it is incumbent upon the researcher to define his own role. In so doing, he has the opportunity to assume a role as promoter, organizer, clarifier, and ground-breaker for programs and policies of his facility. His research should be *resonant,* in the sense of expounding the philosophy, rationale, and theory underlying facility programs. It should be directed toward innovation in areas previously judged impractical, unsafe, premature, or forbidden when this direction is suggested by valid research conclusions. This latter function may require an attitude of *irreverence* toward traditional policies. Finally, behavioral research should be *relevant* to the primary educational and habilitative goals of the habilitation facility.

A habilitation facility represents much more than the barest components of physical structures, clients, and staff. It may have a long and meaningful history that determines both its course of development and its present programs. It may have a philosophy that is unique or perhaps representative of broader social or cultural phenomena. Unless a researcher operates in a vacuum, he cannot help but be influenced by these factors. To the extent that he is aware of these forces, he can use them in planning his studies and interpreting the findings. The research worker in such facilities can serve as interpreter, monitor, and social historian of agency programs and policies. The research itself can document the effects of programs, evaluate their broader implications, and identify areas of need for future programing. In this sense, the research is "in tune" with the habilitation facility.

If research is conducted within the framework outlined in this chapter, it may well lead in new directions. The conclusions deriving from research findings may not always be consistent with present philosophy or programs. Research serves its most useful function in those cases in which results support conclusions that are in conflict with current policy and unpopular with administration. It is in such cases that dissemination of findings is most crucial and where the necessity for the researcher to fall back upon the objective and unemotional quality of his investigation is greatest. It is often the case in these instances that the most powerful impact of the research will be within the home facility. In such cases the function of research reports as a medium of communication is paramount, and the researcher is obliged more than ever to avoid professional jargon and theorizing.

The scope of behavioral research should be as broad as the number of programs at habilitation facilities. However, identification of relevant research can be facilitated by defining the goals of habilitation. Habilitation is usually considered to be a process by which various professional services are utilized to help a disabled individual to make maximal use of his capacities and to function more effectively. The term can have at least three referents. First is the procedure or treatment that is applied, including the situational milieu, which may vary from facility to facility. Second, because concern is with reversible behaviors, a change in "state" within the individual is implied. In other words, it is presumed that the client is in some way different after receiving services than he was before if habilitation is successful. Finally, habilitation may be defined as an outcome, i.e., a consequence evaluated by some criterion of success or failure. It is clear, then, that even though habilitation is often described as if it were a unitary phenomenon, operationally it encompasses three types of variables. Research relevant to the field of habilitation includes research pertaining to treatment variables, subject variables, and outcome.

TREATMENT VARIABLES

Studies of treatment variables can be further broken down into those dealing with the effects of the physical and social setting in which habilitation programs are administered and those dealing with the design and effects of a specific training, service, or remedial education technique.

Studies of social settings are especially pertinent today. More meaningful than any other goal for the mentally retarded person is the ability to change his role from one of helplessness, dependency, and social inadequacy to one of independence, individuality, and freedom of expression. Ideally, a comprehensive habilitation program should provide the social cues and environmental supports to achieve this goal. The application of the normalization principle has been interpreted as requiring that the mentally retarded individual be treated within the least restrictive alternative in residential and treatment settings. Institutions are under continual attack because of the social constraints, regimentation, and depersonalization that have been associated with such settings.

It is well known that institutions, as they developed at the end of the nineteenth century, were predicated upon an inaccurate theoretical model linking mental deficiency with social depravity. Based on this model, institutions were designed to provide maximum isolation, segregation, and control. However, the modern day institution for the retarded represents a vastly complex social environment, the effects of which are not really understood. Nor has it been established that community settings necessarily provide greater freedom merely by being situated in the community.

Investigations of the situational variables affecting the development of adaptive and coping behaviors within institutions, halfway houses, group homes, and other community living arrangements for the mentally retarded represent an important research utilization problem about which there is almost no information available.

Now more than ever, research-supported guidelines are needed for planning and evaluating specific habilitation strategies that are based on anticipated needs of mentally handicapped persons. Chapter 4 describes the elements of modern vocational and social habilitation programs for the mentally retarded. For the most part, such programs have evolved from practical experience within habilitation settings. Yet habilitation programs are extremely complex. Rarely is it possible to establish which components of a comprehensive program are effective, which require modification, and which ought to be dropped entirely. Since 1965 habilitation centers have tended to focus primarily on vocational evaluation and training. Gunzburg (1968) has suggested that vocational training is less important than training for social competence. The determination of those aspects of an habilitation program that are most vital to community adjustment is an empirical question that can be answered by properly designed, competent research studies. One approach would be a detailed analysis of the living situations of mentally retarded persons in various community situations. Feedback from such studies would be the most relevant source of information for designing or revising training curricula. The habilitation program for an individual being trained for independent living in the community should certainly differ from that designed for a person who will reside in a group home.

At one institution for the mentally retarded, considerable effort was expended in teaching students to complete job application blanks. When interviews with mentally retarded persons indicated that the completion of a job application blank was seldom required, the curriculum was revised. Similarly, the need to know whether the mentally retarded must learn to tell time (when the radio or telephone provide such a service), or to read a newspaper (when TV provides news and entertainment) must be assessed. Appropriate research must be designed to determine the minimal amount of practical information and skills the mentally retarded individual must possess in order to survive in various community settings. Once such information is available, it will be necessary to develop scales measuring various aspects of social achievement. A good beginning has been made with scales of social functioning such as the Vineland Social Maturity Scale (Doll, 1965), the Progress Assessment Chart (Gunzburg, 1968), and the Adaptive Behavior Scales (Nihira et al., 1972). While such scales provide good overall estimates of developmental level, they do not allow a sufficient degree of latitude in measuring specific abilities and skills such as social sight vocabulary, monetary knowledge, measurement, time concepts, use of a post office, use of a newspaper, use of a bank, use of the telephone, and use of public transportation facilities. The Fundamental Achievement Series (Bennett and Doppelt, 1968) has been used for this purpose with culturally disadvantaged populations and may also be useful with the mentally retarded (Rosen and Hoffman, 1975).

Once there is general agreement about which skills should be acquired by mentally retarded persons and measurement techniques have been constructed, the next step will be to determine the effectiveness of intensive remedial instruction in these areas.

Numerous researchable problems derive from vocational training procedures. There seems to be little question that it is possible to teach specific work skills to the mentally retarded or to provide certain critical information. A mentally retarded person can be taught to use a push-broom, to operate a Veritype machine, or to change a light bulb. A specific teaching program for such operations, which are general enough to be applied in a variety of settings, could be developed and evaluated.

A more difficult research question has to do with the motivational determinants of work performance. Variables such as the learning of general work habits and attitudes, the motivation to work and to remain on the job, identification with the American work ethic and striving for achievement, and the development of job satisfaction and specific job preferences represent extremely complicated learning phenomena. Workshops and job training classes within habilitation centers provide excellent laboratories for studying the social and psychological determinants of work-related behaviors. Such settings provide the opportunity to vary and experimentally control work incentive, task difficulty, supervisory conditions, and the social structure of work groups in order to determine the best arrangements for maximizing performance and the benefits of work training. A work laboratory investigating basic processes of work behavior of the mentally retarded would be an important component of any comprehensive habilitation program.

One type of treatment variable that has been almost completely ignored in training the mentally retarded relates to subjective "quality of life" dimensions. Campbell (1976) has criticized studies of the material aspects of American life that ignore more direct measurement of subjective indices of experience and a sense of well-being of the individual. He calls upon psychologists to take up their responsibility in studying what Tolman (1941) labeled "psychological man" and what Maslow (1954) later termed "higher order needs." As mentioned in the preceding chapter, the same criticism can be made in studies of the mentally retarded. The ways in which education and training can be expanded to deal with more subtle and subjective criteria of functioning remain to be explored. Psychologists must learn to develop evaluative constructs for the mentally retarded that encompass the same areas of emotional adjustment generally accepted for nonretarded populations.

INDIVIDUAL VARIABLES

The second referent for the term habilitation is a change in "state" in the individual that is usually implied but seldom demonstrated. The study of individual variables would answer questions concerning what, if anything, happens to the individual client during the time he is exposed to habilitation services. It is necessary to study the mentally retarded individual as a dependent variable in the habilitation process. It is important to identify the essential characteristics that must change if habilitation is to be successful. It is difficult to conceive of the possibility that the intensive stimulation applied to a mentally retarded person in a comprehensive habilitation program would have no effect upon his personality. However, it is not reasonable to accept subject change as a "given" in designing programs.

Numerous studies (Cromwell, 1963; Zisfein and Rosen, 1974*b*) have pointed out the significance of self-concept as a variable affecting performance and adjustment of the mentally retarded. Edgerton (1967) has described the plight of mildly retarded adults discharged from the institution to community living as one of continuously denying their social incompetence. He views the stigma of mental retardation as being so central to self-esteem that, despite their "cloak of competence," the mentally retarded can never really successfully "pass" as normal. One aspect of their living style is to deny their incompetence to themselves and to others.

Perhaps the most useful research awaiting habilitation psychologists concerns the ways in which habilitation programs can enhance self-concept to a degree commensurate with a reasonable likelihood of happiness and self-satisfaction in community settings.

OUTCOME VARIABLES

Finally, the third meaning of habilitation relates to the outcome of training. Outcome studies presume some form of follow-up of persons completing habilitation programs. The purpose may be either predictive, evaluative, or simply descriptive. In predictive studies, the major interest is in determining prognostic indices available before or during the habilitation treatment that relate to some later criterion of success or failure. Presumably, once such indices are available they can be used for selection purposes. Chapter 11 reviews prognostic studies of mentally retarded adults living in the community. As will become clear subsequently, attempts to identify valid predictors of community adjustment of the mentally retarded have been largely unsuccessful. Until a better understanding of the meaning of adequate or poor adjustment has been developed, prediction will be limited by the absence of a meaningful criterion of success. Such criteria can be developed by means of long-term studies of community adjustment of the mentally retarded. The acceptance of standardized measures of functioning used by researchers in different geographic settings will allow the development of normative data so that criteria can be further improved. The greater availability of sound adjustment criteria will improve the chances of identifying predictive indices.

Outcome studies may serve an evaluative purpose if interest is primarily in the adequacy or value of habilitation procedures. Appropriate investigations of the effectiveness of a particular habilitation program require the use of control groups drawn from the same treatment population and matched according to relevant characteristics. Outcome investigations are often limited in precision because of difficulties inherent in selecting appropriate control groups. Furthermore, dimensions chosen for evaluating community adjustment often reflect behaviors that are determined by many circumstances unrelated to the habilitation experience of clients. Variables such as employment stability, income, or reinstitutionalization are extremely difficult to relate to predictor variables. Problems inherent in the conduct of outcome research have considerably limited the number of studies that meet the rigorous demands of scienctific objectivity. Rosen, Floor, and Baxter (1972) have suggested that criteria of success in outcome studies be chosen with sufficient construct validity that potential predictors may be selected from those sharing some conceptual relationship to criteria.

Outcome studies may be classified as descriptive if primary interest lies in obtaining normative data concerning the adjustment of a previously identified group. At the present stage of progress in studying community adjustment of the mentally retarded, it seems likely that most outcome studies will fall in this category. Although in 1958 Tizard called for an end to the purely descriptive follow-up study in favor of predictive investigations, the fact that such predictive studies have not proved productive suggests that we still are in further need of normative information regarding community adjustment of the mentally retarded.

FEEDBACK

Whether interest is in predictive, evaluative, or descriptive studies of habilitation, research efforts serve little value unless the results are appropriately funneled back into training and education programs. The danger of adding a research unit to a habilitation facility is that it may become an isolated, almost exclusive, entity, often divorced from commerce with daily administrative and service problems. To prevent this, an efficient system of information exchange must be established among service personnel. The more that is learned about the process and outcome of habilitating the mentally retarded, the more we can improve training programs. Program development and criterion improvement are parallel and interdependent processes.

AN ILLUSTRATIVE RESEARCH UTILIZATION PROGRAM

An attempt to apply such a research utilization model began at Elwyn Institute in 1964. At this time the Institute was awarded a four-year grant by the Vocational Rehabilitation Administration (now the Social Rehabilitation Service) to evaluate habilitation programs that were then being initiated. This research study evolved into a programmatic research effort with direct input into services at the Institute. The habilitation program that was developed is described in Chapter 5. The results of the follow-up study used to evaluate this program are outlined in Chapter 10. Indeed, various aspects of this research are referred to throughout this volume and provided the major impetus for this book. The remainder of this chapter is intended to describe only the research utilization aspects of the project and to illustrate how applied research can be performed within an habilitation facility.

It seemed evident at the outset that the only manner in which program effectiveness could be demonstrated was by a follow-up of the products of those programs, i.e., the clients themselves, who, completing their training, would be discharged from the institution and returned to the community. A descriptive follow-up study was designed—one that would provide an account of the post-institutional adjustment of all "graduates" of the program as measured by relevant indices of community functioning.

When the project was completed, the final report (Clark, Kivitz, and Rosen, 1968) documented the favorable community adjustment of the majority of persons leaving Elwyn. The recognition afforded the habilitation programs at Elwyn by these results was an important factor in gaining administrative and public support for continuation of programs initiated during the course of the project. One project recommendation pointed out the need for a halfway house in Philadelphia in order to provide a transitional experience between the institution and the community. Several years later this recommendation became a reality.

Relief from the pressure of annual reports and other formal requirements of the funded project brought freedom to continue the research in whatever directions the findings would lead. Follow-up interviews were continued and papers were published describing various aspects of the community living of the identified population. Research reports included studies of work satisfaction (Rosen et al., 1970*b*), sociosexual problems (Floor et al., 1971), marriages (Floor et al., 1975), IQ changes after leaving the institution (Rosen, Floor, and Baxter, 1974) as compared with changes during institutionalization (Rosen et al., 1968), and changes in students' self-perceptions related to their habilitation training (Rosen and Floor, 1970). The employment satisfaction studies had direct relevance to vocational counseling of clients, since our findings indicated that work dissatisfaction often existed because of low wages of "graduates" and the relatively low status they held in their places of employment. Studies of marital adjustments and sexual problems encountered in the community resulted in a greater emphasis at Elwyn on social and sex education programs.

Because little was known about the characteristics of the mentally retarded individual that might be associated with successful or unsuccessful adjustment, the original investigation was also intended to identify what factors might be related to these outcomes. A correlational study was planned that would attempt to relate various psychometric indices, available within the institution, to criteria of social, vocational, economic, and personal functioning in the community. As in similar attempts that had predated our research, this effort was largely unsuccessful. Initially, several measures emerged with significant correlations to criteria (Rosen et al., 1970*a*). Later, when we attempted to cross-validate these findings with a new sample of clients (Rosen, Floor, and Baxter, 1972), the original findings could not be replicated.

The failure to identify meaningful predictive indices of community adjustment led to a reconsideration of the directions we had been exploring. The criteria of adjustment originally used represented extremely complex variables. Dimensions such as income, job stability, and employment satisfaction were determined by many influences not necessarily related to client characteristics. If individual differences did bear upon these criteria, they were apparently not the characteristics being measured.

The investigators returned to the case studies and searched for some commonalities in the experiences and characteristics of the subject population in the community. Many subjects had experienced some type of exploitation after leaving the institution. It was possible that graduates were overly susceptible to such experiences in ways that went beyond their intellectual limitations. Analyses of these histories led to a conceptualization about the personality dimensions that mentally retarded residents of the institution seem to share. These characteristics were labeled "the institutional personality" (Rosen, Floor, and Baxter, 1971). Later these traits were also found to be characteristic of mentally retarded adults living at home with their families. These ideas launched a research program that was to have direct impact upon counseling programs within the institution.

The studies performed included investigations of acquiescence (Rosen, Floor, and Zisfein, 1974*a*, 1974*b*), helplessness (Floor and Rosen, 1975), self-concept (Zisfein and Rosen, 1974a), and inappropriate behavior (Hoffman and Rosen, 1974).

The findings of these studies were translated directly into service programs in the form of in-service training curricula and personal adjustment counseling programs (Zisfein and Rosen, 1973) structured to remediate qualities of acquiescence, helplessness, and low self-esteem in institutional residence. Counseling programs, in turn, stimulated evaluative research to study the effectiveness of the procedures (Zisfein and Rosen, 1974*a*).

The research utilization program described above continues today at Elwyn Institute. Research is planned to answer practical, everyday problems of programing for the mentally retarded. New programs are always planned to include an evaluation component. Service and research thus become two sides of the same coin.

LITERATURE CITED

Bennett, G. K., and Doppelt, J. E. 1968. Fundamental Achievement Series. The Psychological Corporation, New York.

Campbell, A. 1976. Subjective measures of well-being. Amer. Psychol. 31:117–124.

Clark, G. R., Kivitz, M. S., and Rosen, M. 1968. A transitional program for institutionalized adult retarded. Project No. 1275P. Vocational Rehabilitation Administration, Department of Health, Education, and Welfare, Washington, D. C.

Cromwell, R. L. 1963. A social learning approach to mental retardation. *In* N. R. Ellis (ed.), Handbook of Mental Deficiency, pp. 41–91. McGraw-Hill Book Company, New York.

Doll, E. A. 1965. Vineland Social Maturity Scale. Condensed Manual of Directions. American Guidance Service, Circle Pines, Minnesota.

Edgerton, R. B. 1967. The Cloak of Competence. University of California Press, Berkeley.

Floor, L., Baxter, D., Rosen, M., and Zisfein, L. 1975. A survey of marriages among previously institutionalized retardates. Ment. Retard. 13:33–37.

Floor, L., and Rosen, M. 1975. Investigating the phenomenon of helplessness in the mentally subnormal. Amer. J. Ment. Defic. 79:565–572.

Floor, L., Rosen, M., Baxter, D., Horowitz, J., and Weber, C. 1971. Socio-sexual problems in mentally handicapped females. Train. Sch. Bull. (Vinel.) 68:106–112.

Gunzburg, H. C. 1968. Social Competence and Mental Handicap: An Introduction to Social Education. Baillière, Tindall & Cox Ltd., London.

Hoffman, M., and Rosen, M. 1974. An inventory of inappropriate behavior. Train. Sch. Bull. (Vinel.) 71:179–187.

Maslow, A. H. 1954. Motivation and Personality. Harper & Row, New York.

Nihira, K., Foster, R., Shelhaas, M., and Leland, H. 1972. Adaptive behavior scales. American Association on Mental Deficiency, Washington, D. C.

Rosen, M., and Floor, L. 1970. The importance attributed to perceived work competence and scholastic achievement by institutionalized retarded persons. Ment. Retard. 8:33–36.

Rosen, M., Floor, L., and Baxter, D. 1971. The institutional personality. Brit. J. Ment. Subnormal. 17:2–8.

Rosen, M., Floor, L., and Baxter, D. 1972. Prediction of community adjustment: A failure at cross-validation. Amer. J. Ment. Defic. 77:111–112.

Rosen, M., Floor, L., and Baxter, D. 1974. IQ, academic achievement and community adjustment after discharge from the institution. Ment. Retard. 12:51–53.

Rosen, M., Floor, L., and Zisfein, L. 1974*a*. Investigating the phenomenon of acquiescence in the mentally handicapped: I. Theoretical model, test development and normative data. Brit. J. Ment. Subnormal. 20(2):58–68.

Rosen, M., Floor, L., and Zisfein, L. 1974*b*. Investigating the phenomenon of acquiescence in the mentally handicapped: II. Situational determinants. Brit. J. Ment. Subnormal. 20(2):6–9.

Rosen, M., and Hoffman, M. 1975. Use of the Fundamental Achievement Series with a mentally retarded population. J. Spec. Ed. Ment. Retard. 11:87–93.

Rosen, M., Kivitz, M. S., Clark, G. R., and Floor, L. 1970*a*. Prediction of postinstitutional adjustment of mentally retarded adults. Amer. J. Ment. Defic. 74:726–734.

Rosen, M., Nowakiwska, M., Halenda, R., and Floor, L. 1970*b*. Employment satisfaction of previously institutionalized retarded workers. Ment. Retard. 8:35–40.

Rosen, M., Stallings, L., Floor, L., and Nowakiwska, M. 1968. Reliability and stability of Wechsler IQ scores for institutionalized mental subnormals. Amer. J. Ment. Defic. 73:218–225.

Tarjan, G. 1965. Facilitation of research through administration. *In* E. Hart (ed.), Role of the Residential Institution in Mental Retardation Research. National Association for Retarded Children, New York.

Tizard, J. 1958. Longitudinal and follow-up studies. *In* A. Clarke and A. D. B. Clarke (eds.), Mental Deficiency: The Changing Outlook, pp. 422–449. Methuen & Co., Ltd., London.

Tolman, E. C. 1941. Psychological man. J. Soc. Psychol. 13:205–218.

Wolfensberger, W. 1965. Administrative obstacles to behavioral research as perceived by administrators and research psychologists. Ment. Retard. 3:7–12.

Wolfensberger, W. 1967. Research policies and problems in residential institutions. Ment. Retard. 5:12–16.

Zisfein, L., and Rosen, M. 1973. Personal adjustment training: A group counseling program for institutionalized mentally retarded persons. Ment. Retard. 11:16–20.

Zisfein, L., and Rosen, M. 1974*a*. Effects of a personal adjustment training group counseling program. Ment. Retard. 12:50–53.

Zisfein, L., and Rosen, M. 1974*b*. Self-concept and mental retardation: Theory, measurement and clinical utility. Ment. Retard. 12:15–19.

Section II

The Habilitation Process

Chapter 4

Vocational and Social Habilitation

Contemporary textbooks define the rehabilitation concept as a process of "restoring" the handicapped individual to the fullest physical, mental, social, vocational, and economic usefulness of which he is capable (Cull and Hardy, 1972; McGowan and Porter, 1967). The history of the rehabilitation movement in this country has been described in great detail by Cull and Hardy (1972) and Obermann (1965). Evolving from a period of public apathy toward the disabled, attitudes have changed to a recognition of an economic necessity and a social obligation to help the disabled move toward independence and vocational sufficiency.

In the case of the mentally retarded and other developmental disabilities, the rehabilitation concept requires stretching to assume new dimensions. Some writers prefer to use the term "habilitation" when referring to services required to develop capabilities where none previously existed (see Authors' Note, p. ii). Needless to say, such goals are more difficult to achieve than restorative efforts.

The modern period of habilitation efforts began in 1965 when Public Law 333 was passed. This law focused interest on vocational evaluation, sheltered workshops, and vocational habilitation. Vocational habilitation as a service delivery system to the mentally retarded finally came of age.

ELEMENTS OF VOCATIONAL HABILITATION

The process of vocational habilitation has assumed different meanings in different settings. In general, it relates to a sequential use of evaluation and training opportunities necessary to allow a client to function to his maximum capacity in a work setting.

The evaluation phase of a vocational habilitation program is defined by Hardy and Cull (1973) as consisting of both prevocational evaluation and vocational or work evaluation. In their terms, prevocational evaluation means "the evaluation of such factors as activities of daily living, social development and basic educational abilities... characteristics which an individual must have before he can even consider preparing for a vocation or even being evaluated for a vocation" (p. 6). Vocational evaluation is a broad assessment of pertinent medical, psychological, vocational, social, and environmental factors relevant to work adjustment. Work evaluation is a narrower term that refers to the assessment of an individual's vocational strengths and weaknesses using real or simulated work situations. The object of work evaluation is to develop a vocational plan for each client.

The work adjustment phase of vocational habilitation refers to the treatment process designed to improve work behaviors. Work adjustment is the implementation of a vocational plan, the evaluation of success or failure in meeting criteria of vocational competence established by this plan, and the decision to terminate the treatment plan. Vocational and work evaluations include the use of both psychometric testing and situational approaches to assessment. The latter method is used primarily within sheltered workshop operations, using a production line that simulates actual work conditions and activities.

Another evaluation technique is the job tryout or exploratory work situation. This method consists of the use of work stations either within the habilitation center or in business and industry. Within the habilitation facility, the work station may utilize actual service departments in food preparation and handling, laundry, maintenance, and buildings and grounds. It allows the evaluator an opportunity to assess performance, attitude, motivation, and initiative; it affords the client an opportunity to sample various types of jobs in order to form vocational preferences.

Vocational training is intended to develop skills that will allow the handicapped person to be gainfully employed despite his handicap. Such training may be part of the vocational plan and is based upon an assessment of a client's present vocational skills and determination of those areas that might be improved by training. Cull and Hardy (1972) distinguish among four types of training methods:

1. *Personal adjustment training* is designed to develop proper work habits, attitudes, and behaviors to help the client understand and get along in a work situation.
2. *Prevocational training* provides background and supplementary knowledge and skills requisite for an occupation.

3. *Compensatory skill training* provides specific skills needed to enter the labor market but not necessarily directly related to a specific occupation. Speechreading for deaf people is one illustration.
4. *Vocational training* provides specific knowledge and skills necessary for performance within a given occupation. Training methods may involve didactic instruction as well as on-the-job and apprenticeship training.

The choice of vocational training courses for the mentally retarded requires a knowledge of careers suitable for varying levels of ability and skill as well as a knowledge of the current labor market and local employment conditions that would make a specific occupation feasible.

It is generally assumed today that most mildly retarded individuals are capable of benefiting from vocational training and job placement in competitive work settings. More intellectually limited persons may not be able to respond to such programs, and alternative training methods have been developed.

The sheltered workshop is a work-oriented habilitation facility designed to assist the handicapped person in achieving a more normal and productive vocational status. Individual goals for clients are established that allow the client to develop his assets within a remunerative work setting under controlled working conditions. Unskilled packaging and subassembly operations have been used successfully with even very limited mentally retarded workers. The workshop combines a therapeutic and working environment that allows the client to develop a sense of dignity and self-respect as a productive person. While some persons may be prepared to enter a regular labor market, for others the vocational goal may be modified to prepare the person for extended placement in the sheltered workshop or for referral to programs providing further education or supportive services.

A small proportion of the mentally retarded, those with severe mental limitations, are unable to function even within the sheltered setting of a workshop. Such persons lack the attention span needed to perform a regular work task or to do so for any extended period of time.[1] Often, behavioral difficulties present problems of control and supervision that preclude workshop placement. For such persons activities programs provide limited work experience with basic vocational tasks of sorting, matching, and counting, which may lend themselves eventually to workshop performance.

Traditionally, sheltered workshops and pre-workshop programs have been predicated upon the assumption that severely retarded persons are

[1]Some writers have pointed out that even the severely retarded are capable of approximating normal performance levels if society is willing to expend the money, effort, and appropriate technology needed for training (Gold, 1975).

incapable of learning more complex production tasks or of working at levels of productivity of normal intelligence workers. More recently, Gold (1973*a*, 1973*b*, 1975) has challenged these assumptions. Gold maintains that low productivity estimates for the mentally retarded are based upon typical performance levels in sheltered workshops and reflect societal expectations more than they do the true potential of the clients. By distinguishing between acquisition and productivity and by applying task analysis procedures, Gold has demonstrated that productivity levels can be markedly increased and that severely retarded workers' earnings can approximate the piece rate earnings of normal workers. Gold urges a shift away from traditional methods of evaluation, in which test results, he argues, are not predictive of performance after appropriate skill training. Gold's dramatic demonstrations of the effectiveness of task analysis methods are still regarded as controversial. They require and deserve testing in an ongoing workshop facility over an extended time period with appropriate evaluation and follow-up investigation to reveal the overall habilitative value of the training regimes.

Many mentally retarded persons require transitional vocational and community adjustment programs even after they have successfully acquired a sufficient degree of vocational skill to make themselves employable. Transitional on-the-job programs provide the client with more intensified vocational experience on a real job while still maintaining some degree of supervision and control by the habilitation facility. Transitional work experience is particularly helpful for clients who have never worked before and for those leaving institutions for community work. Transitional community work experiences can often best be provided while the client resides at a halfway house or other group living situation in the community. Criteria of success can be established for the transitional experience to serve as operational requirements for final job placement.

Vocational training efforts should result in a vocational placement of the client on a job that is well suited to his interests and abilities. Successful placement requires an accurate matching of job to client and presumes that vocational training has been both realistic in terms of the available job market and sufficient to ensure that the client has attained a degree of proficiency equal to that of nonhandicapped workers competing for the same position. Job placement involves not only a job search for suitable positions, but also job analysis to achieve a proper match with employee qualifications, involvement of the client in the job choice, and preparation of the clients for job interviews and job demands.

Progress of the client through the various phases of the vocational habilitation process usually cannot be accomplished without involving him in an ongoing counseling relationship. Individual and group counseling approaches are essential to successful involvement of the client in the evaluation and training program. Counseling is used to assist the client in understanding his vocational skills, in helping him formulate realistic vocational goals, in instilling appropriate motivation for training, in providing vital information about available jobs and the labor market, in solving specific problems that may arise during the habilitation program, and in helping the client understand and identify with his individual vocational plan. Habilitation counseling is often very concrete and oriented toward practical guidance in vocational and daily coping skills.

The vocational habilitation process does not end with the completion of training and job placement. Most handicapped persons completing vocational habilitation programs require some degree of supportive follow-up service during their initial experiences on the job and often for extended periods of time. This is especially true of the mentally retarded, who may have limited capacities for dealing with emergency situations, loss of job, or responsibilities such as completing income tax forms. Habilitation counselors must make themselves available to successful and unsuccessful graduates of habilitation programs in order to continue counseling relationships, act as advocates, and provide practical assistance or referral service where required.

IMPORTANCE OF SOCIAL EDUCATION

It is the thesis of this book that the most serious deficit of the mentally retarded, from the point of view of providing habilitation services, is not their low intellectual level, nor their educational limitations, nor the problems presented by vocational training. Rather, the most challenging training need and the most important lessons the mentally retarded must learn center on their social inadequacy. Indeed, no other criterion of successful habilitation can be achieved without a modicum of social competence. As is shown below, this fact was fully appreciated by our predecessors, although they seemed to have incorrectly assumed that social competencies could not be taught.

Perhaps the best description of habilitation as a social learning process is provided by Gunzburg (1968):

> ...society—once having made the decision that the mentally handicapped should, so far as possible, live outside the hospital and institution—must provide a type of education and training which will make him competent to survive in the community with relatively little support even if only for comparatively short periods.... (p. 1)

> Although our knowledge of the mentally handicapped person's achievements and development is inadequate and incomplete, the available data provide sufficient support for the thesis that the content of a rehabilitation programme should be *social education* rather than academic education during the junior stage or mere work training during the senior stage (p. 2).

Gunzburg's excellent book provides a discussion of the development of social knowledge and social competence in the mentally retarded, describes an assessment technique for measuring these skills, and suggests a program of social education for correcting deficiencies in social skills. In the present volume the authors hope to carry Gunzburg's thesis one step further by exploring emotional and personality characteristics of the retarded and expanding the concept of social education to include more subtle dimensions of personality that are also relevant to community adjustment.

ANTECEDENTS OF THE SOCIAL HABILITATION CONCEPT

The optimism of E. Seguin, S. G. Howe, and H. B. Wilbur about habilitating the mentally handicapped so that they might take their place in society was all but dead by the close of the Civil War. Dr. Charles T. Wilbur, Superintendent of the Illinois Institution for the Education of Feeble-Minded Children, acknowledged, in an address to the National Conference of Charities and Corrections in 1888, that many persons had graduated from institutions, but he also expressed reservations that "a very large proportion of them could be made independently self-sustaining."

> In the race of life, where an individual who is backward or peculiar attempts to compete with those who are not, the disadvantages are so great that the graduate from the idiot asylum really has no chance to succeed. The capacity of the individual is not at fault; but the world is not full of philanthropic people who are willing to take the individual from the asylum and surround him with the proper guardianship which his case demands. There is a want of the legal authority which the asylum possesses in the matter of discipline and control. The institution cannot so develop the judgement and moral nature that he can always withstand the temptations of life (Wilbur, 1888, p. 299).

Fernald, reporting to the same organization in 1893, makes much the same point when he indicates that 50 percent of "adults of the higher grade" are capable of sufficient work to pay for their support, but, because they lacked "common sense," only 10 to 15 percent of the inmates of the Massachusetts School for the Feeble-minded would be capable of sustaining themselves in the community.

Concern over the social adequacy of the mentally retarded was expressed through the first half of this century. In an article in the *Journal of Psycho-Asthenics* in 1926, Howard Potter, Director of Research of the institution at Letchworth Village, in New York, and Crystal McCollister, parole agent for the institution, describe its programs of parole or extra-institutional living for more capable students. It is clear from their report that parole to the home of the family or an employer involved strict rules of supervision by the institution. Only a small percentage of parolees earned discharge from the institution because of satisfactory adjustment in the community. Reservations about social and emotional traits of the mentally retarded are expressed in the authors' explanation of their finding that males make more satisfactory adjustments than females:

> ...the male parole material had a definite advantage over the female parole material in that it is, almost point for point, made of better stuff. We find that proportionately less than a third of the males as against nearly two-thirds of the females come from anti-social feeble-minded stock....
>
> Furthermore there are certain general considerations which combined with the above differences in clinical make-up tend to explain why our boys are more easily adjusted in an extra-institutional environment. The girl has problems to meet which do not commonly confront the boy. The girl is occupied in-doors at work which affords but little outlet to her emotions. The boy works out-of-doors at labor requiring the use of large muscle groups which provides a safe outlet for fundamental emotional urges. The end of the day finds the girl in a state of nervous tension, not particularly physically tired, and craving some sort of excitement as a relief. The boy is physically tired, experiences no nervous tension, and his chief craving is a comfortable bed.
>
> At times of relaxed supervision the girl is the easy prey of unscrupulous persons and, pursued, falls a ready victim to sex delinquencies. The boy, belonging to the aggressive sex, because of his dull wit, cannot successfully compete with his more normal brethren in the game of procreation (pp. 136–137).

The farm colony, originating around the turn of the century, was an innovative habilitation program. Although Fernald (1903), who is credited with developing the first colony, is often criticized as being primarily motivated by the economics of operation of such colonies, the concept was regarded as part of the industrial principle of training the mentally retarded to be at least semi-autonomous vocationally. In this respect it was not markedly dissimilar to today's concept of the group home except that it was apparently used for the most capable inmates of the institution, who would today be judged candidates for more complete independence in the community.

It is of interest that somewhat less concern over the social inadequacies of the mentally retarded was shown by those who worked within community settings. Perhaps this is because the community residents were more capable socially than those within institutions. It may also reflect the fact that for the professional working within a community setting the retarded were already perceived as realistically functioning within the community without severe social problems. For the professionals within the institution the prospect was not a *fait accompli* but one that aroused their worst expectations. It is important to remember that the institutions were regarded by all concerned as the bastion of defense of society against all the social ills thought to be associated with mental retardation. It seems likely, then, that institutional staff would tend to be somewhat more pessimistic about the capabilities of the retarded than professionals working at community schools or centers would tend to be.

Thus Farrell (1915) reports on the follow-up of 350 persons who left ungraded classes in the New York City schools and finds that 64 percent were ''employable out of their own homes, and for wages'' and only 9 percent of these persons were unemployed at the time of the investigation.

An outstanding example of the more positive thinking about social habilitation is found in the writings of Stanley P. Davies, who was associated with the Department of Mental Hygiene in New York State. Davies (1925) urged the public schools to assume a greater role in the education of mentally retarded children, including the more severely retarded, and emphasized the teaching of social skills:

> *The determination of cases for institutional care should be made on a social rather than an intellectual basis.* This position is taken in the belief that the primary function of the school for both normal and backward children should be to give training for social life, rather than mere intellectual training, or even specific vocational training. If the school cannot be instrumental above all in developing its students to become good members of the social order, it has failed of its mission....
>
> The institution should be left free to provide for those who are too troublesome and too dangerous to remain outside, or those whose home conditions are such as to be unfit for the child, regardless of whether the child's I.Q. is low or high. In such a capacity the institution can be of inestimable service to school and society, and as we are well aware, it will not lack for plenty of work to do, in our generation at least. With its careful discipline, its regularity of regime, its facilities for intensive medical, psychological and psychiatric work, its vocational training courses, its ability to gradually restore patients to the community on trial through the parole and colony systems, the institution is especially equipped to work on the reconstruction of these more difficult types of mental deficiency, and it should be left free to concentrate its energies upon that important work. Let us not clog our expensively constructed and equipped institutions, precious as the bed space in them is, with the dull, harmless type (pp. 232–233).

ELEMENTS OF SOCIAL HABILITATION

Despite the fact that social habilitation represents the most difficult and most challenging habilitation goal, it is also the one in which the least has been accomplished. It is convenient to categorize two types of social habilitation efforts—those provided during formal training programs, including those applied within institutions; and those applied within community settings that represent either long-term community supports for the socially handicapped or transitional experiences toward independence.

Ideally, social habilitation programs must simulate, as closely as possible, the setting in which the client will eventually be living. If total independence in the community is a goal, then the habilitation setting must be prepared to approximate the demands society places upon its normal citizens. This is possible only to a limited extent in most settings; within an institutional setting the problems of simulating a normal environment are compounded by whatever institutional rules and mores that have developed.

Habilitation settings, and particularly institutions, represent artificial environments that, by their very nature, are different from normal society in many important ways. Most habilitation settings represent some degree of shelter or protection for the client. Institutions, for example, were designed explicitly for that reason. While a desire to shelter the mentally retarded represents the best humanitarian motivation, it also may be antagonistic to the goal of placing increasing demands and responsibilities upon the client.

The staff of habilitation settings are not representative of people in general. They consist of professionals, trained to understand and to be tolerant of deviant behavior. This adds to the detrimental sheltered effect of the habilitation facility.

Habilitation facilities, even those located within the community, are free from the requirements of competitive, profit-making goals of business and industry. They are often supported, at least partially, by public funds. Their financial and social structure may be very different from other community organizations. Even where this is more myth than fact, it is the way such facilities may be perceived by clients, staff, and the general public.

Because of these factors, habilitation facilities can simulate the outside world only to a very limited degree. The compromise arrived at is to represent the outside world through facsimile or other indirect methods, such as classroom instruction or counseling. Community trips and excursions are used to familiarize the client with community resources. Transitional experiences at group homes, halfway houses, and foster homes serve to ease the client into more independent living situations.

Adult education classes are used with the retarded to supplement vocational training and provide vital information related to personal, community, and vocational adjustment. Curricula are available for this purpose (Rosen, DiGiovanni, and Peet, 1975; Wilkie, DeWolf, and Younie, 1975). Such curricula include basic information pertaining to employment, insurance, medical emergencies, use of leisure time, banking, restaurants and menus, use of public transportation, use of the telephone, finding a job, and other skills considered critical to coping in the community.

Individual and group counseling approaches have also been devised for the mentally retarded (Zisfein and Rosen, 1973) although evidence concerning the effectiveness of such programs is scanty.

Gunzburg (1968) likens the mentally retarded adult in the community to a stranger traveling in a foreign country. He believes social education of the individual should begin in childhood, which should be geared to prepare him to be a socially efficient person as an adult. He classifies the minimal needs of the adult under four headings: self-help, communication, socialization, and occupation.

In Gunzburg's program, by the time the severely subnormal individual reaches his late teens he is transferred to an adult work environment. Progress is judged by his ability to handle tools and materials reasonably well. Arts and crafts are supplemented by simple repair work. Both men and women learn to prepare simple meals. Industrial training is largely in unskilled labor, where the mentally retarded worker is better able to compete with normal workers. Demands for speed and quality of work are set to be comparable to requirements in normal work settings.

The halfway house for the mentally retarded provides a transition from the institution or home to independent community living. A greater degree of freedom exists, and supervision is considerably less than that within the structured institutional setting. At Chestnut Hall, a community-based halfway house in West Philadelphia, mentally retarded men and women, discharged from private or state institutions, have their own apartments or share them with a roommate. They are free to come and go as they wish, provided they maintain the apartments well, keep reasonable hours, and meet the demands of their community jobs. Residents at the facility are required to pay rent, which is later returned to them when they are ready for discharge from the facility. Chestnut Hall is maintained administratively as part of a comprehensive habilitation program so that students who fail to meet minimal requirements, either vocationally or socially, are reassigned to the institution for further training or counseling.

Such persons are usually given other chances in the program and may eventually succeed after several trials at the halfway house facility. Chestnut Hall is described in more detail in Chapter 5.

When the client appears to require a more long-term program under supervision, a group home is often used. Many persons are independent enough that they no longer require the structure of an institutional setting but will need some minimal supervision. The group home provides community experience to many persons who may never be able to maintain complete independence. In such settings individual or shared apartments are also utilized, but there is a greater degree of planned group activities and supervision. Many mentally retarded persons now live at community-based group homes and walk or commute to community sheltered workshops.

The desire to apply the normalization principle to the mentally retarded is accepted by most as the basis for social habilitation programs despite the fact that critics have questioned whether all mentally retarded persons should be treated according to conditions considered normal for nonretarded populations (Gunzburg, 1972; Rosen and Kivitz, 1973; Throne, 1975). Zipperlin (1975) has pointed out the pitfalls of focusing solely on the modification of deviant behaviors according to societal norms. Instead, she prefers a concept of normalization that includes the teaching of interdependence and socialization and that demands as much a change in society as in the retarded individual. Advocating the sheltered village concept and citing the Camphill (New York) community as an example, Zipperlin wishes to permit the mentally retarded adult to become more social rather than more normal, to provide him the opportunity to give as well as receive, to question the value of competition as a criterion of success, and to recognize that many retarded persons ''march to a different drum.'' The ''spiritual environment'' advocated by proponents of the Camphill movement requires life-long programing. While this model has been applied at a few settings, such as Jean Vanier's L'Arche in the French village of Trosly-Breuil, north of Paris (Clarke, 1974), it is not likely that it will provide widespread solutions to socialization problems of the mentally retarded.

Wolfensberger (1970) has proposed another type of social habilitation system, one that goes far beyond traditional training methods. This proposal, which he calls ''citizen advocacy,'' requires that mature, competent citizens in the community assume responsibility for representing, as if they were their own, the interests of a mentally retarded individual who is impaired in his ability to solve practical everyday problems or to meet his needs for affection. Wolfensberger outlines various types of advocacy, including foster parents, adoptive parents, citizen-guardians, and citizen-friends for the handicapped. Advocacy is seen as an alternative to the types of protective services (primarily institutionalization) that have been previously used by professionals and social agencies. Advocates can function singly or in groups, but the heart of advocacy is one individual serving as an advocate for one other citizen. Difficulties inherent in the advocacy system proposed by Wolfensberger lie in the practical questions of finding a sufficient number of motivated citizen advocates, and in implementing this program and supervising such persons. To offset these problems Wolfensberger advocates the establishment of state and local level advocacy offices to implement, supervise, and follow up such programs.

The change in attitude regarding the capabilities of the mentally retarded for community living has already been described in Chapter 1. This change came about slowly as part of a wave of increased social consciousness and concern over individual liberties that has positive repercussions for all handicapped persons and for minority groups in general. Paradoxically, the impact of this social change has had both positive and negative repercussions for the mentally retarded.

It seems unlikely that mentally retarded persons have changed over the past century any more than they changed between the time of Seguin and the heyday of institutions. The same social deficiencies that alarmed institutional superintendents fifty years ago exist today. Indeed, many workers have been aroused to express reservations about wholesale normalization and deinstitutionalization procedures. Even Gunzburg (1972) has cautioned:

> Do we perhaps tend to forget that the handicapped are also emotionally immature, unstable, insecure, anxious, inadequate, that they are easily disturbed, tend to vegetate, to collapse in face of difficulties and show little confidence in their admittedly meagre abilities?...there is nothing to suggest that sizeable and significant weaknesses in his personality make-up will not still remain after transplanting him to new, more normal, but also more demanding conditions (p. 64).

Such alarm is not unwarranted. Good intentions sometimes wreak havoc and there is no question that recent deinstitutionalization policies have involved risk, especially when mentally retarded persons are placed in community settings without enough supportive services.

The crux of the renewed emphasis on the community's role in mental retardation must involve more than merely a greater tolerance for the amount of risk society is willing to assume for the mentally retarded. Public policies of deinstitutionalization and normalization must incorporate renewed and innovative efforts in order to provide social habilitation training to prepare the retarded for their greater degrees of independence. The community must also be committed to accept, understand, and integrate mentally retarded citizens into community life. If institutions and community training centers do not expand the scope of their training to incorporate more meaningful methods of social education with individual accountability for training outcomes, then we are certain to experience another reaction against the progressive changes of the past decade.

LITERATURE CITED

Clarke, B. S. J. 1974. Enough Room for Joy: Jean Vanier's L'Arche: A Message for Our Time. McClelland & Stewart Ltd., Toronto.

Cull, J. G., and Hardy, R. E. 1972. Vocational Rehabilitation: Profession and Process. Charles C Thomas, Springfield, Ill.

Davies, S. P. 1925. The institution in relation to the school system. *In* M. Rosen, G. R. Clark, and M. S. Kivitz (eds.), The History of Mental Retardation: Collected Papers, pp. 225–239. Vol. 2. University Park Press, Baltimore, 1976.

Farrell, E. E. 1915. A preliminary report on the careers of three hundred fifty children who have left ungraded classes. *In* M. Rosen, G. R. Clark, and M. S. Kivitz (eds.), The History of Mental Retardation: Collected Papers, pp. 13–21. Vol. 2. University Park Press, Baltimore, 1976.

Fernald, W. E. 1893. The history of the treatment of the feeble-minded. *In* M. Rosen, G. R. Clark, and M. S. Kivitz (eds), The History of Mental Retardation: Collected Papers, pp. 321–325. Vol. 1. University Park Press, Baltimore, 1976.

Fernald, W. E. 1903. Farm colony in Massachusetts. *In* M. Rosen, G. R. Clark, and M. S. Kivitz (eds.), The History of Mental Retardation: Collected Papers, pp. 117–126. Vol. 2. University Park Press, Baltimore, 1976.

Gold, M. W. 1973*a*. Factors affecting production by the retarded: Base rate. Ment. Retard. 11:41–44.

Gold, M. W. 1973*b*. Research on the vocational habilitation of the retarded: The present, the future. *In* N. R. Ellis (ed.), International Review of Research in Mental Retardation, pp. 97–147. Vol. 6. Academic Press, New York.

Gold, M. W. 1975. Vocational training. *In* J. Wortis (ed.), Mental Retardation and Developmental Disabilities, pp. 254–264. Vol. VII. Brunner/Mazel, New York.

Gunzburg, H. C. 1968. Social Competence and Mental Handicap: An Introduction to Social Education. Bailliére, Tindall & Cox Ltd., London.

Gunzburg, H. C. 1972. (Editorial). Brit. J. Ment. Subnormal. 28(2):63–65.

Hardy, R. E., and Cull, J. G. 1973. Vocational Evaluation for Rehabilitation Services. Charles C Thomas, Springfield, Ill.

McGowan, J. F., and Porter, T. L. 1967. An introduction to the vocational rehabilitation process, p. 4. Rehabilitation Services Administration, U.S. Department of Health, Education, and Welfare, Washington, D. C.

Obermann, C. E. 1965. A History of Vocational Rehabilitation in America. T. S. Denison & Company, Inc., Minneapolis.

Potter, H. W., and McCollister, C. L. 1926. A resume of parole work at Letchworth Village. *In* M. Rosen, G. R. Clark, and M. S. Kivitz (eds.), The History of Mental Retardation: Collected Papers, pp. 127–143. Vol. 2. University Park Press, Baltimore, 1976.

Rosen, M., DiGiovanni, S., and Peet, D. 1975. Remedial adult education for the physically handicapped: A curriculum outline. Elwyn Institute, Elwyn, Pennsylvania.

Rosen, M., and Kivitz, M. S. 1973. Beyond normalization: Psychological adjustment. Brit. J. Ment. Subnormal. 19(2):64–70.

Throne, J. M. 1975. Normalization through the normalization principle. Ment. Retard. 13:23–25.

Wilbur, C. T. 1888. Institutions for the feeble-minded. *In* M. Rosen, G. R. Clark, and M. S. Kivitz (eds.), The History of Mental Retardation: Collected Papers, pp. 293–301. Vol. 1. University Park Press, Baltimore, 1976.

Wilkie, E. A., DeWolf, L. T., and Younie, W. J. 1975. Guide to the community. Elwyn Institute, Elwyn, Pennsylvania.

Wolfensberger, W. 1970. Toward citizen advocacy for the handicapped. January, 1970. Nebraska Psychiatric Institute, University of Nebraska, Lincoln, Nebraska.

Zipperlin, H. R. 1975. Normalization. *In* J. Wortis (ed.), Mental Retardation and Developmental Disability, ch. 11. Vol. VII. Brunner/Mazel, New York.

Zisfein, L., and Rosen, M. 1973. Personal adjustment training: A group counseling program for institutionalized mentally retarded persons. Ment. Retard. 11:16–20.

Chapter 5

An Institution Transformed

Building a Pattern of Habilitation Services

BEGINNINGS

Eighteen hundred and fifty-two was a year of optimism with regard to the mental defective. Itard's work with the "wild boy" was already history, and Seguin's school in Paris was widely acclaimed. Samuel Gridley Howe had established a school for the retarded in South Boston. James B. Richards, native of Ceylon and a Harvard graduate, had been recommended to Howe by Horace Mann as a teacher best suited to carry out the work of Seguin in this country. For three years he applied Seguin's physiological method as a teacher in Howe's school.

In 1852, Richards came to Philadelphia and opened a private school for mental defectives on School Lane in Germantown. He enlisted the sympathies of Dr. Alfred L. Elwyn, a physician, and together they were able to arouse interest in the movement in Philadelphia. Their efforts led, in 1854, to the incorporation of The Pennsylvania Training School for Feeble-minded Children, later renamed the Elwyn School. An appropriation from the Commonwealth of Pennsylvania of ten thousand dollars and provisions for ten students were obtained. The school and its 17 students were moved to Woodland Avenue in 1855. Edouard Seguin, then a political refugee from France, was appointed educational director the following year. Formerly, Seguin had replaced Richards in Boston but had clashed with Howe. He also left Elwyn, after only a short stay, when conflicts developed over lines of authority.

Before the end of the decade, dissension and financial difficulties threatened to end the new school. Richards retired from the field of special education. Dr. Joseph Parrish was appointed Superintendent and was able to bring about financial stability. An additional appropriation of $20,000 by the Legislature for buildings provided opportunity for expansion, and the search for a permanent location began. Dorothea Dix, who had been so instrumental in paving the way for humanitarian treatment of both the mentally ill and mentally retarded in Massachusetts, assisted in choosing a new site, twenty miles south of Philadelphia at Media. In 1857 the cornerstone of the main building was laid, and the new school was dedicated to the shelter, instruction, and improvement of mentally retarded children.

On September 1, the entire school and its 25 children, attendants, and teachers were loaded into two Conestoga wagons and brought to their new quarters. The formal opening took place on November 2, 1859; John B. Crozer, Chairman of the Board, delivered the opening address at the dedication ceremonies.

The school grew in size despite the financial difficulties that again developed during the Civil War. By 1864 the property, grounds, and buildings held by the institution were valued at $140,000. The student population had increased to 144, many from other states. Eighty of these children were supported by the state. During this year Dr. Parrish retired and was succeeded by Dr. Isaac Kerlin, who served until 1893. Prior to his appointment Dr. Kerlin had served with the Army of the Potomac during the Civil War and had been selected by President Lincoln to direct a program for colonizing newly freed slaves, a plan that was never carried out.

During Kerlin's administration there was further expansion of the institution with the help of additional state appropriations. Kerlin was widely recognized for his scientific interest and study of retardation. The Association of Medical Officers of American Institutions for Idiotic and Feeble-minded Persons was founded and held its first meeting at Elwyn in 1876. Dr. Kerlin, along with Seguin, H. B. Wilbur, C. T. Wilbur of Illinois, Dorin of Ohio, and Knight of Connecticut were the original members of this group, which later changed its name to the American Association on Mental Deficiency. In 1871 Elwyn endorsed the idea of a custodial department. A special act of the Legislature authorized the institution, now called the Pennsylvania Training School, to provide asylum for "idiotic and imbecilic" persons without regard to age. Later, buildings were added for epileptic and paralytic girls. The school, which became an institution after the Civil War, now described its custodial department as the Asylum Village of Elwyn.

Kerlin was a gifted writer. His many papers urged recognition of the "moral imbecile" and the necessity for his life-long guardianship and detention for the protection of society (Kerlin, 1889). Kerlin believed firmly in the growth of institutions and the dependence of the "defective classes" upon the strong arm of a paternal government. His acceptance of a correlation between idiocy, pauperism, and crime led him to assume that the reduction in the number of jails, criminal courts, almshouses, and "grog-shops" awaited only the growth of "villages of the simple."

Leadership at Elwyn was continued by Dr. Martin W. Barr from 1893 to 1930. Dr. Barr is known for his anthropometric research laboratory and for authoring the first American textbook on mental deficiency.[1] He emphasized manual training for students and introduced classes in printing, weaving, and basketry. A strict martinet, Barr followed the tradition of Seguin in relying upon daily exercises for physical training. He organized a student orchestra and chorus. A 34-acre farm was purchased and farming became an important "training area." By 1902 Elwyn's grounds encompassed 137 acres; a staff of 165 employees served a population of 1,041 students, three-fourths of whom were in training programs and one-fourth in custodial care.

Dr. E. Arthur Whitney succeeded Dr. Barr in 1930 and served in that position until 1960. Dr. Whitney continued the tradition of Kerlin and Barr as a recognized leader in the field of mental deficiency. He was a staunch proponent of eugenics and argued repeatedly for the control of feeblemindedness through selective sterilization (Whitney, 1929; Whitney and Shick, 1931). Whitney advocated sterilizations even for the "low-grade imbecile of obscene habits" although they did not reproduce and were permanently segregated: "...(after sterilization) most of them 'brighten up' considerably mentally and the majority seem more easily managed and less temperamental" (Whitney and Shick, 1931; p. 205).

CHANGE

Gerald R. Clark, appointed Superintendent in 1960, was responsible for radical changes in the institution. During the years of his administration, Elwyn has made rapid strides away from the closed custodial model and

---

[1]Seguin wrote the first textbook dealing with mental retardation. However, this book was largely an English translation of his earlier (1843) work *Hygiene et Education des Idiots*.

became a more open school and habilitation center for multiply handicapped children and adults. The emphasis shifted from segregation and shelter toward community-oriented training, with the goal of helping mentally handicapped individuals find a useful role in society. The name Elwyn Training School, which had been used for several decades, was changed to Elwyn School and then to Elwyn Institute to avoid confusion with state and correctional facilities. The use of the term ''children'' for older students, a practice dating back to the establishment of Elwyn, was abandoned.

Physical punishment was discontinued. Instead, students were provided with increasing responsibilities and privileges for appropriate behavior. The staff titles of ''matron'' and ''attendant'' were replaced by ''housemother'' and ''counselor.'' Breaking with tradition, closer relationships with family were encouraged by increasing the frequency of visiting and by family counseling procedures. Vacation periods were introduced at Christmas, Easter, and Thanksgiving. The practice of censoring incoming and outgoing mail was discontinued. All locks were permanently removed from doors of dormitories and dayrooms. Panic bars were installed on all exit doors. For the first time residents were permitted to chew gum, and smoking on the grounds was allowed. Greater provision was made for recreation and entertainment during weekend and evening hours by providing increased employee coverage. Increased opportunity was provided for participation in religious services and receiving religious instruction. By 1968, the staff had been increased from approximately 250 to 600.

Educational programs were expanded with the opening of a new educational center. Rather than having a hundred students in educational programs, services were increased so that all levels of mentally retarded were enrolled in full-day educational programs. The old classifications of moron, imbecile, and idiot were replaced by classifications of mild, moderate, and severe mental retardation.

A director of vocational training and rehabilitation was appointed and given the mandate to develop a vocational training and community preparation program for mildly retarded adults. At this time a large proportion of Elwyn's population consisted of young and middle-aged adults, with IQs between 50 and 80, and with diagnoses of familial retardation and cultural deprivation. Most of these persons had been living at the institution since childhood and were performing useful work within the institution in various service and maintenance departments. Vocational training courses for this population were developed and licensure as a private trade school for the handicapped was obtained from the State Department of Public Instruction. A close working relationship was established with the Pennsylvania Bureau of Vocational Rehabilitation (BVR) and a vocational counselor from the Bureau was located at Elwyn on a full-time basis. BVR provided necessary training funds to supplement vocational training programs. A sheltered workshop program on the institutional grounds was initiated for lower-functioning students. Later, two additional workshops were developed within dormitories for less ambulatory geriatric students.

Almost 100 percent of the 1,100 residential students at Elwyn were enrolled in some form of education or vocational habilitation program. In addition to the residential population, programs were expanded to accommodate day students from the community. Hearing impaired, visually impaired, and multiply handicapped students were also accepted. A volunteer program was initiated to stimulate and direct the interest of service clubs, church groups, and individuals.

An active community preparation program was pursued for the first time at Elwyn to provide students with appropriate experience and training for independent community living.

Changes were made at all levels of the financial and administrative functioning of the institution to provide more efficient business-like procedures and to improve services directly affecting the care, training, and safety of students. By the early 1970s these changes had been consolidated and greater effort was expended in expanding programs into the community by means of community workshops and habilitation centers, a halfway house, and group homes.

IMPLEMENTATION OF AN HABILITATION PROGRAM

Wilkie et al. (1968) describe the transitional period at Elwyn, beginning in 1961, when the habilitation philosophy and orientation were established. The newly identified objectives of the institution were to provide the widest range of services needed to assist every resident to achieve his maximal social, personal, and vocational potential. A survey of the adult residential population revealed three distinct groups of students:

1. The most capable group were functioning at a mildly retarded level. These students had opportunities to return to the community, provided they had adequate family and institutional support for this goal. If such support was lacking they were destined for life-long service in key positions within the institution. When efforts were later made to move these students to more realistic community preparation training areas, work supervisors expressed resistance because they depended so strongly upon them for services.
2. A second group of students were semi-dependent. Intellectually and socially less capable than the first group, they also were destined to

remain within the institution, although their work assignments were often merely busy work.

3. The third group consisted of the most dependent students, who had more severe intellectual and social deficits. Educational goals were poorly defined for these individuals, staff were generally negative in their willingness to work with them, and many were consigned to backward living arrangements.

In order to achieve the goal of training these individuals to function at their highest potential, it was necessary to avoid preconceived conceptions about ability levels. Instead, a graduated series of programs was developed, allowing the student to demonstrate his proficiency within the program and to progress from one activity to another. A coordinated educational-vocational habilitation program was developed, integrated under the direction of one person. Students followed a natural progression from educational classes to vocational training sites of increasing complexity. Programs for all levels of mentally retarded persons and all ages stressed practical knowledge required for work and community living.

Elwyn Industries, the sheltered contract workshop, was established on institutional grounds in 1962. This program was initiated to accommodate large numbers of students who were without an active program and who were judged by many staff as being "not capable of doing anything."

In order to gain institutional support for the program, arrangements were made for key personnel to visit local community workshops. Group meetings were held with the entire staff in order to acquaint them with the function and philosophy of habilitation and to familiarize them with the goals of a sheltered workshop.

A workshop director was employed with experience in supervising a community-based workshop facility. Approximately 2,500 square feet of unused space on the third floor of a building were renovated at comparatively small cost. A hoist was installed so that material and supplies could be moved from the ground to the third floor. Local businesses were contacted by phone or personal visits. These visits were followed with letters describing the services to be rendered by the workshop. Several small contracts were secured and the workshop began operating with 25 men and women selected from the inactive group of adult students.

Brief interviews were held with the students to explain the operation of the workshop at a level they could comprehend. They responded to the work with enthusiasm. Their frequent comments during the first week of operation included remarks such as: "We're not as dumb as they thought."

The workshop was gradually expanded to accommodate greater numbers of students. Satellite workshops were developed in other buildings for geriatric retarded and for physically disabled persons who were unable to travel the distance from their residence to the workshop. In 1968 a large rehabilitation center was constructed to house the workshop and vocational training programs.

For higher-functioning students there was a need to involve the maintenance and service units of the institution in a student training program. Employees in these areas tended to view the service aspect of their jobs as most important. Conversely, training directors tended to view the *training* opportunities provided by the work area as most important. Actually, both are closely interdependent. Successful change in the focus and direction of work area activities had to be accomplished with an awareness of the service needs of the institution and how they could be integrated with the training needs of the student.

A review of existing work areas throughout the institution revealed considerable information regarding problems in providing realistic training opportunities for adult residents. For example, some students were assigned to work areas primarily to meet the needs of the institution. Inservice meetings, daily visits by training department staff, and a sincere attempt to understand and assist work supervisors with their daily problems resulted in a change of focus for these activities from service to the institution to both training and service.

Supervisors were not willing to release their more capable students to other work areas. It was common for students to remain on a work assignment for extended periods of time, regardless of their needs or desires. To change this, supervisors were given a role as instructors. Because of their additional prestige and their involvement in the process, cooperation was obtained and attitudes changed. (Herein lies the success or failure of many vocational programs in residential facilities.)

Several work activities were antiquated relics and served no purpose other than to occupy the student's time. Activities in the broom shop and the mattress shop, for example, had little benefit for the participant. Many other work areas were ill-equipped to provide students with training opportunities because of obsolete tools and equipment. Such equipment and the unrealistic working conditions could not prepare adults for employment.

It was necessary to replace hand ironing with unit presses and automatic shirt units in order to provide realistic training for laundry workers. The bake shop had to be completely renovated, and an up-to-date oven, mixers, and bread slicers replaced obsolete equipment. The print shop was reorganized in order to meet the current demands of industry. With these and other changes, it was felt that the various service areas were able to provide appropriate training, and a multiphase training program was instituted.

THE PROGRAM

The primary concept of the program at Elwyn is a hierarchy of social and work experiences progressing from lesser to greater complexity, with the focus on the remediation of educational and social deficits of mental retardation as well as on institutional or sheltered community experience. Components of the program include a preliminary psychological and vocational evaluation, an activities program, preindustrial experience and exploratory work training, vocational training, adult education, personal adjustment counseling, community work, halfway house experience, and discharge and follow-up services.

A diagnostic evaluation unit assesses all students entering the habilitation program. Standard psychological testing, vocationally oriented tests, and work samples are administered. The evaluation has a decided vocational orientation. It is intended to form a basis for deciding the level at which the student enters the habilitation program. This phase of the program lasts three weeks. The first two weeks are spent in a small, group-testing situation. The third week is spent in a sheltered workshop setting in which work samples can be administered. Because of the low predictive validity of most vocational aptitude tests for an evaluation of the mentally retarded, the assessment relies most heavily upon observations of the individual in a real work situation. Continuous feedback by workshop supervisors to vocational counselors and training associates provides a means for evaluating the progress of each student, during both the evaluation and training phases of the program. This type of information, available through direct on-the-job observations by supervisors, allows for maximum flexibility in structuring vocational training assignments to fit students' needs and capabilities.

Students functioning vocationally below sheltered workshop levels are enrolled in an activities program labeled Adult Adjustment Training. This program, when implemented in the early 1960s, was extremely small because a majority of Elwyn's population at the time was functioning in mildly retarded categories. With increasing deinstitutionalization at Elwyn, and the development of community programs, the adult adjustment classes have grown steadily in size and have become a major component of the habilitation program.

These classes are designed primarily for severely retarded adults. They are intended to provide clients with the basic social and occupational skills required for functioning within sheltered workshops. As in the workshop, activities include basic counting and sorting operations. Because of the higher incidence of behavior management problems in clients, more individualized attention is required, and the curriculum must include help in personal hygiene and appearance, self-help skills, and basic social relationships. Because of the increasing numbers of severely handicapped persons now receiving services, habilitation centers, and particularly institutions, must devote greater attention to the severely retarded adult.

The workshop provides the industrial community with a variety of services, ranging from sub-assembly work to complex packaging. Modern assembly line techniques are utilized, and the equipment includes automatic shrink packaging machines. Students range in age from 16 to 87 years, with IQs ranging from 30 to 75. In addition to mental retardation, many of the workers suffer the disabilities of blindness, deafness, epilepsy, and cerebral palsy. Some workers may advance to more demanding vocational assignments, while others remain as long-time employees of Elwyn Industries.

Students work from nine until three. There is an hour lunch break and a morning coffee break. Each worker punches a time clock upon entering the workshop each morning and punches out when he leaves. Workers are paid on a piece rate basis according to their productivity. Wages are determined according to a formula that reflects the client's degree of disability as compared with a normal worker and his job productivity. Records are audited regularly by the Department of Labor and Industry and must meet minimum wage requirements.

Contracts are obtained by the workshop manager from local businesses and industry. Workers produce a saleable product and perform a useful service for the contracting company. The product must meet the factory standards of the contractor. The workshop is run on a nonprofit basis, with all income used for salaries and operational costs.

The workshop provides a pool of potential workers at higher vocational levels. It furnishes a backup vocational experience for clients who fail to adjust at higher vocational levels. It provides remedial work training for clients with specific problems in adjusting to a work setting. It allows for an on-the-job evaluation of basic work skills and attitudes. For many students it provides a means of achieving self-respect and dignity accruing from gainful employment.

For students who are judged ready to advance beyond a sheltered workshop, a full range of vocational training experiences suitable for the mentally retarded is provided.

Preindustrial training provides exposure to a range of trades suitable for the mentally retarded. The maintenance and service areas of the institution, including the laundry, dietary department, hospital, and custodial departments are organized to provide exploratory work experience for students. In addition, all students are assigned to the sheltered workshop. The length of time students remain in work areas ranges from four to eight weeks, depending on their interests and needs.

After the exploratory work experience, the student is assisted in determining realistic vocational objectives. Training courses are licensed by the Department of Public Instruction of Pennsylvania.

The vocational training areas include: building maintenance (carpentry, painting, plumbing, and electrical work), dietary training, baking, laundry training, custodial work, printing, hospital aide work, stock work, beautician's aide training, business education, and power sewing. These courses include both didactic instruction and on-the-job training. The jobs are taught at an unskilled or semi-skilled level. Trainees reach an apprentice level of functioning rather than becoming journeymen.

One of the basic concepts inherent in this program is the belief that the student must be intimately and actively involved in decisions related to his habilitation process, and he must develop a greater degree of self-responsibility. This requires a realistic appraisal of his assets and liabilities and aid in selecting a realistic vocational objective. Inappropriate attitudes fostered by institutional life have to be counteracted if he is to leave the institution as a responsible citizen. Individual and group counseling sessions are used to aid the student in achieving these goals.

When a student has completed his trade training he is then placed in the community work program. This placement enables him to be employed in the community while still a student at Elwyn. The student resides at the community-based halfway house while enrolled in this program. He commutes to work by public transportation and is responsible for his own budgeting and banking. He continues to receive counseling, guidance, and adult education during his nonworking hours.

An adult education program provides formal practical training in social and academic skills that are essential for independent community living. Recognizing that the entire institutional environment plays an important part in the adjustment of the individual, attempts are made to supplement formal classwork and remedial instruction by creating, within the institutional setting, a milieu conducive to habilitation. This program is intended to alleviate some of the handicaps resulting from prolonged institutional living.

To provide a systematic transition from the institution to employment and to the community, a progression of separate courses was developed. These courses are coordinated with the specific phase of the vocational program in which the individual is engaged. Students receiving personal adjustment training deal with personal hygiene and cleanliness, proper attire, grooming, and self-image. Work adjustment training is designed to instill proper work attitudes and knowledge of basic work procedures, such as time cards, payroll deductions, and income tax. Community adjustment training deals with specific services and responsibilities in the community, such as insurance, banking, budgeting, post office skills, and recreational facilities.

Since 1971 Elwyn has operated a halfway house in West Philadelphia, providing transitional community living and community work experiences for students completing habilitation programs on the main campus. After the program was in operation several years, it led to the establishment of several group homes that serve Elwyn residents as well as adults from the surrounding community and others from Pennsylvania state schools and hospitals. The halfway house program and one of the group homes operate within a 350-unit apartment house. Chestnut Hall houses over 500 inhabitants, most of them college students or instructors at nearby universities. Thirty-five units house mentally retarded persons in either the halfway house or group home program.

The location of the halfway house was chosen because of its proximity to public transportation, medical facilities, laundromats, shopping, and other community resources. Persons accepted into the halfway house program must be over eighteen years of age and employed in full-time community jobs.

The halfway house program at Chestnut Hall encompasses three wings on the second floor of the apartment building. A married couple on each wing and a social worker administrator, operating from an office in the building, and several counselors working 1:00 p.m.–9:00 p.m. schedules comprise the staff. Volunteers from the community also assist in the programs. For students in transition to the community, guidance, rather than strict supervision, is provided. The halfway house serves as a transition for students being trained for independent community living.

For those requiring more long-term living arrangements, group home apartments are available with no time limits. The apartments are either large efficiencies or one-bedroom units. Each accommodates two adults of the same sex and has a private kitchen and bathroom. Residents pay $86.50 a month in rent. Those employed in community jobs have little trouble maintaining their payments. Group home residents are usually employed at one of Elwyn's satellite sheltered workshop programs and supplement their income by public assistance checks.

Both halfway house and group home residents receive their own keys when they move into their apartments. They are free to come and go as they please but must receive permission for being away an entire night or weekend. Each resident is assigned a counselor who initially accompanies him shopping. Counselors advise their clients about bargains but also emphasize independence in shopping and budgeting. Clients continue to receive counseling and adult education classes while enrolled in the transitional program. Evening and weekend recreational programs and community excursions are planned by counselors to help acquaint residents with the city's social and recreational facilities.

Since its inception, most students leaving the institution for more independent living arrangements have spent some time at Chestnut Hall. Many go on to completely independent situations in the community. Others move to Centerpost Village, six apartments scattered throughout a 90-unit garden apartment complex in West Philadelphia, also administered by Elwyn. Most of the neighbors at Chestnut Hall and Centerpost Village are unaware of any "special group" living near them.

After successfully completing the community work program with adequate work adjustment to the community job, the student is eligible for discharge from the institution and permanent placement in the community. In order to be recommended for discharge, he must have been able to adjust socially without any serious behavioral problems during the community work program and have accumulated at least $500 in savings during this time period. Students are aided in obtaining suitable living and employment situations and are discharged to the community. In some cases these individuals remain in the same job they held during the community work programs; in other cases they are assisted in finding similar positions at other companies.

After leaving Elwyn, graduates are encouraged to maintain contact with the staff in order to receive a "continuum of service." Follow-up interviews are scheduled regularly after discharge to provide counseling and assistance if needed and to gather research information about the adjustment of previously institutionalized graduates. Approximately 50 percent of Elwyn graduates sever contact with the institution after discharge. Others develop overly dependent behavior patterns and require help in weaning themselves from the institution. The majority of graduates, however, are able to maintain their independence of the institution, yet visit periodically, attend annual picnics, parties, and special events at the institution, and avail themselves of community support services. One full-time staff member is employed with the primary responsibility of locating jobs, developing community resources, making home visits, helping graduates make the transition to the community, providing continual counseling and assistance when required, and gathering ratings and follow-up information.

The follow-up phases of the program are considered as important a part of the program as any of the training experiences provided before discharge. Although Elwyn maintains no legal responsibility for continuing services after discharge, it is considered a moral obligation to provide help when needed, even when graduates are gone several years from the institution. In several instances habilitation counselors were instrumental in providing emergency services when graduates ran into difficulty and requested such services.

Experience in providing habilitation programs at Elwyn has demonstrated that it is possible to change a traditionally custodial institution into an habilitation facility. As a result of this change, a relatively large percentage of the educable retarded population of the institution can be habilitated and discharged to independent living, even after long years of institutionalization. This habilitation is not restricted to those individuals having parental support. Habilitation workers at Elwyn have demonstrated that many residents can be successfully trained to work and live independently in the community.

With administrative support, the custodial institution can be reorganized so that its maintenance and service departments can be used in providing habilitation training. To successfully make this transition, it is essential that the entire institutional staff be oriented toward and supportive of habilitation philosophy and goals. The vocational rehabilitation counselor and the state vocational rehabilitation agency can play an important role in bringing about institutional change.

Experience with the habilitation programs attests to the value of a progression of training opportunity leading to increasing responsibility and realistic community experiences. Organization of social and vocational training curricula, according to such a model, provides continuing evaluation of students so that selection, assessment, and training are accomplished simultaneously in activities most relevant to community functioning. The high success ratio with discharged persons in the community is attributable, to a large degree, to the utilization of a halfway house, which allows for early detection of community adjustment problems while the individual is still subject to some degree of supervision. Those persons showing severe adjustment problems may be temporarily withdrawn. Recycling for further remediation experience and counseling can thus be provided as often as needed before final discharge. Many students have made successful adjustments on their second or third placement after initial failure in the halfway house program.

Throughout Elwyn's history administrators have expressed protective concerns about returning trained mentally retarded persons to the community. As is seen in Chapter 10, there is little justification in the follow-up data for perpetuation of this attitude. Elwyn's experience lends support to the continued use of community preparation programs, particularly when supplemented by appropriate community-based support services.

LITERATURE CITED

Kerlin, I. N. 1889. Moral imbecility. *In* M. Rosen, G. R. Clark, and M. S. Kivitz (eds.), The History of Mental Retardation: Collected Papers, pp. 303–310. Vol. 1. University Park Press, Baltimore, 1976.

Whitney, E. A. 1929. The control of feeble-mindedness. *In* M. Rosen, G. R. Clark, and M. S. Kivitz (eds.), The History of Mental Retardation: Collected Papers, pp. 197–200. Vol. 2. University Park Press, Baltimore, 1976.

Whitney, E. A., and Shick, M. McD. 1931. Some results of selective sterilization. *In* M. Rosen, G. R. Clark, and M. S. Kivitz (eds.), The History of Mental Retardation: Collected Papers, pp. 201–210. Vol. 2. University Park Press, Baltimore, 1976.

Wilkie, E. A., Kivitz, M. S., Clark, G. R., Byer, M. J., and Cohen, J. S. 1968. Developing a comprehensive rehabilitation program within an institutional setting. Ment. Retard. 6:35–39.

Section III

The Residential Institution and Attempts at Normalization

Chapter 6

Habilitation of the Cerebral Palsied Citizen

PROBLEMS OF THE CEREBRAL PALSIED

Among developmentally disabled persons, those with cerebral palsy frequently represent a combination of physical, mental, social, and vocational disabilities that pose special problems to the habilitation counselor. While a mentally retarded person, functioning with mild intellectual limitations, may demonstrate good potential for community employment, a cerebral palsied individual (CP), functioning at a possibly normal or high intellectual level, may present a much more difficult employment picture. Many occupations available even to the mentally handicapped must be ruled out because of the physical limitations of cerebral palsy. Even if the client can handle the actual job operations, employers are reluctant to make the architectural adjustments or provide the adaptive devices that may be needed for his overall functioning in a work situation. Since his disability is often markedly obvious to others, the cerebral palsied client may be particularly subject to the negative reactions of society toward the handicapped. Even when they can handle the physical requirements of a job, and when society meets them halfway, the cerebral palsied may be emotionally handicapped by their own awareness of their disabilities. For all these reasons, many such persons are restricted to functioning at the sheltered workshop level, although their intellectual capabilities may equip them for potential in more complex and demanding careers.

A summation of the problem can perhaps be best expressed by quoting from a speech made recently to a meeting of habilitation counselors.[1] The speaker is a young woman of normal intelligence with quadriplegic spasticity and a speech impairment; she is nonetheless articulate and eager to express her thoughts. Some of her comments were:

> We (the physically handicapped) play a big part in your community. For every mental retardation patient...there are four of us. Why don't we have a program?...We can't even get housing or jobs. We are qualified, but we need to sit...You look at us as children, as mentally retarded, and a big joke to people. All we want is a chance in our community . . . How can we live from the sheltered workshop when we don't even make our carfare? If some of us didn't have mother or daddy or get social security or welfare...how would we make it?...I'm not asking you for sympathy or pity. All we want is a chance to show *our* skills, *our* brain-power, and *our* know-how...We, the handicapped people and the drug addicts have a whole lot in common...They (the addicts) need a chance to prove themselves *again* . . . and we need a *first* chance to prove ourselves.

In the light of such feelings, the need for counseling and other services for the cerebral palsied is obvious. It is the underlying rationale of the present project that an intensive program of adult education and counseling applied as needed can be a vital supplement to traditional follow-along services, and that persons receiving maximal input of this sort will show significant improvement in various areas of adjustment.

LITERATURE REVIEW

While medical and habilitation journals have offered numerous articles on the diagnosis, evaluation, and treatment of the cerebral palsied, there have been few attempts at follow-up studies of significant numbers of these individuals. One survey of considerable magnitude was performed by Wolfe and Reid (1958), who questioned over 3,000 cerebral palsied children and adults in the state of Texas. A registry of such persons was established through contact with physicians, hospitals, and habilitation centers. Initial questionnaires were sent to adults over 21, and to the parents of the younger group. Present physiological, developmental, and educational status was ascertained. A second survey, given only to those who responded to the first, determined medical and prenatal history, and occupational, social, and economic status. This information was obtained personally at interview centers.

---

[1]Frances Coleman—addressing the West Philadelphia Mental Health/Mental Retardation Consortium, June 12, 1973.

Data from this study were descriptive rather than predictive, since the survey procedure was not a follow-up technique. However, because of the scope of the study, the descriptive information is presented here in some detail as probably typical of cerebral palsied populations throughout the country. The sample was classified according to type of disability, etiology of symptoms, developmental history, social maturity, therapeutic treatment, and employment. Respondents were 56% male, and the median age was 13. Major findings revealed that the sample was 43% spastic and 59% quadriplegic. Ninety percent had been diagnosed at birth as having cerebral palsy. Twenty-three percent were unable to walk even with help; 48% were unable to speak a three-word sentence before age 10. Of the school-age subjects, only 23% were attending school; failure to attend was due to speech problems, inability to walk, mental retardation, convulsions, and lack of toilet training. For older persons the average grade level completed was fifth; it took them approximately 1.5 years longer than normal persons to attain a given grade level.

Seventy-four percent of the subjects needed speech therapy, but only 35% of these were receiving any. Sixteen percent of the sample had had surgery (usually on the legs); a majority had used crutches and/or braces at some point; 16% used wheelchairs.

Only 94 persons in the sample (approximately 3%) were employed; about 20% of these were in semi-professional or managerial jobs; 20% each were in industry (skilled and semi-skilled), agriculture, clerical work, and sales. Twelve percent were in service occupations and 8% in unskilled work. The mean salary (1955) was $2,742. Only 35% of the parents questioned felt their child could ever earn a living.

Although the study just mentioned was descriptive in nature, the research of Klapper and Birch (1966, 1967) may be appropriately termed a follow-up study. A group of 155 children, aged 2–16, had been classified in 1948 according to medical diagnosis and IQ. Eighty-nine of this original sample were given a detailed follow-up interview, conducted in their homes, in 1962. Information was elicited on marital status, social involvement, family organization, schooling, residential stability, extent of physical handicap and degree of self-care, employment, special skills, stated goals, training and training plans, contacts with hospitals, habilitation centers, and private physicians, current treatment programs and needs, and various other factors. The sample comprised 50 males and 39 females between the ages of 15 and 28.

Interviews were analyzed for: 1) level of employment, 2) economic status, 3) self-care status, 4) educational achievement, and 5) social functioning. These variables were related to the initial diagnosis and IQ score as well as to one another. Results showed that over half these young adults were unemployed; less than 20% were in skilled or competitive positions. Over 60% of the group were completely dependent on their families for financial support. There was a marked contrast between economic status and self-care ability, since over 60% of the group were entirely independent in a physical sense, despite the presence of some abnormalities. The subjects were characteristically uninvolved in social functioning (group memberships, community activities, friends) with 25% classified as ''social isolates.''

When the interrelationships among variables were explored, it was found that spastic cases had higher IQs, achieved a higher level of schooling, and were more independent socially, economically, and in self-care than the other CP classifications. Persons with an initial IQ under 50 had minimal education and were totally unemployed; the IQ had less predictive value, however, in the higher ranges. Levels of self-care correlated highly with degree of employability, school achievement, economic status, and degree of social integration. In agreement with other studies of the current status of the cerebral palsied, the authors conclude that ''cerebral palsied adults who are potentially employable and capable of social activity are typically unemployed and socially isolated.''

A study of cerebral palsied college students (Muthard and Hutchison, 1968) used mail questionnaires in a follow-up procedure. Fifty male and thirty female students were interviewed and compared to a sample of nonimpaired students. Some time after graduation both samples returned questionnaires relating to their employment and salary.

The cerebral palsied and control groups were matched for age and home community. However, the CPs tended to have had poorer academic records than the nonimpaired students, and to have parents with lower economic and vocational status. More than three times as many CP as normal students required substantial financial assistance either from parents or state agencies, and frequent help from college counselors in coping with educational, vocational, and personal problems.

A major question of this study was whether the college-going CP should be provided with a general education, or one directed toward vocational goals. The CP students in the sample had fewer exploratory work experiences before or during college than their nonimpaired peers. The authors suggest the desirability of special college programs designed to help handicapped students to secure interim and part-time work.

Follow-up questionnaires revealed that CPs took longer than other graduates in finding employment. However, only 4% of the cerebral palsied college students were unemployed, compared to 70% of adult CPs in general. Thus a college education appears to be a major asset to the physically handicapped, despite the fact that they seldom are able to earn as much as their nonimpaired peers, or to hold jobs on comparable skill levels.

The CP graduates reported considerable dissatisfaction with their post-college jobs. This was interpreted as a result of their inability to secure jobs commensurate with their education. However, those who had done well in college had found jobs more closely related to their educational background than did those with poorer academic records. In addition, it was found that those CPs who had pursued a vocationally oriented education were more often employed than those who had completed nonvocational curricula, liked their work better, earned more, and had fewer adjustment problems. The general implication is that college is a valuable experience for CP students, but could be more valuable if it provided more vocational training and work opportunities.

Two other follow-up studies on which minimal information is available have dealt with both cerebral palsied children and adults. These include an investigation by Ingram (1964) of children in Scotland in 1953. This study was undertaken to determine the prevalence of CP in Edinburgh and to examine its causes and effects on patients and their families. The problems of the subjects in adapting to life as handicapped people in the community were examined ten years later.

A study conducted by *The Exceptional Parent* (1972) re-interviewed three teenagers and their parents after a three-year interval and reported on the general family situation and the degree of progress shown by the children. One girl had entered college and was functioning well both socially and academically, although her physical progress had been minimal. While the other two teenagers continued to present many problems, the parental attitudes had become more realistic and productive over the three-year period.

A significant follow-up study on vocational potential was performed over a five-year period through the Institute for the Crippled and Disabled (Moed and Litwin, 1963). The major aim of this investigation was to assess the employment history of 286 cerebral palsied clients who had been previously evaluated on various vocational and academic skills. They also received vocational counseling during the evaluation process. Of these persons, 64% were estimated to have employment potential, and of that group, 47% eventually found jobs. Jobs held were primarily unskilled (53%) and clerical (28%). Clerical trainees tended to be the best employment risk; they found jobs faster and held them longer than those recommended for other occupational areas.

Factor analysis of evaluation measures revealed that certain skills were particularly related to employability. These included manual dexterity, IQ, handwriting, severity of gait defect, speech intelligibility, and the ability to travel independently.

A related study by the same authors investigated the employability of 243 cerebral palsied persons over a three-year period. Subjects were evaluated on a number of psychological, social, medical, educational, and vocational variables. The sample was divided into two groups: those employable only under sheltered workshop conditions (SWS), and those considered a potentially employable training and placement group (TP). While the groups were very similar according to degree and type of physical disability, significant differences in favor of the TPs were found in speech, gait, and travel ability. TPs were also somewhat better educated, had higher IQs and appeared more stable socially and psychologically than the SWS group. (Significance of those and subsequent differences was not indicated.) Parental attitudes strikingly differentiated the two groups, with the SWS parents revealing a greater degree of emotional disturbance, disinterest, and pessimism than the TP parents, who tended to be supportive and interested. TP parents also exhibited less overprotective behavior than SWS parents.

The recommendations of those studies include emotional guidance or psychotherapy for both clients and their families, as well as greatly expanded workshop facilities for the over 50% of the sample (and of cerebral palsied persons in general) who can function only in a sheltered situation. Intensive prevocational evaluation and counseling are also strongly recommended for all CPs.

A somewhat similar approach has been taken in a study devised by the Jewish Employment and Vocational Service in St. Louis (Lacks and Plax, 1972). Personal interviews were conducted with 75 persons who had previously received services from an habilitation workshop. All subjects had some type of limiting disability: 33% were mentally retarded, 38% had psychological disabilities, and 24% had physical or neurological problems; many of the latter were cerebral palsied. Two thirds were males, and the median age of the sample was 26. Sixty percent were single and most (66%) had not graduated from high school; 75% had never been employed at more than temporary summer jobs.

Intake forms giving pertinent background information were available for all clients; these forms were used as a basis for assessing changes in client status after receiving habilitation services. Follow-up forms were completed during the personal interviews conducted six to nine months after termination of the habilitation program. Follow-up information included types of services subsequently received, and detailed information on employment and income. Clients were also asked to comment on their experiences with the habilitation services and to make suggestions for improving the program.

The most significant data showed client income in terms of initial counselor recommendation. About 60% of the subjects who had been judged employable had found jobs, but only 40% of these were still employed at the time of interview. The average income was at poverty level ($316/month). Completion of the training program did relate to employability, since of those clients who completed the program, 75% got jobs and 50% were still employed, versus 44% and 33% for those who did not complete training.

The major conclusions drawn from this study are: 1) the need for more adequate agency services geared toward helping clients retain jobs or find new employment on their own, and 2) the need for client follow-up as a method for evaluating adequacy of services. The authors state, "Although the directors of many rehabilitation programs recognize the need for client follow-up, many feel that their agencies cannot afford the cost of such outcome studies...The results of this investigation fully substantiated the need for client follow-up, not only to provide information for improvements needed in programs, but also to furnish continuing contacts and additional placement services to clients."

A two-year follow-up study maintained contact with clients in order to determine the validity of the vocational evaluation. In general, it was found that the predictive measures were reliable and that clients were generally able to function at the vocational level which the diagnosis had indicated.

Heal (1972) reports on an ambitious follow-up study that evaluated the program of an habilitation institute in Budapest. Cerebral palsied students had been systematically assessed at admission and discharge, and were recalled later for re-evaluation of level of functioning in a number of areas. (The period since discharge for the total sample ranged from three to eighteen years at the time of retesting.) Of the 866 subjects, 36 had been classified as "totally dependent" at admission, but only 5 were so categorized at retest. While 55 students had been initially classified as "able to work and study outside the home," 536 met this criterion some years after discharge. Similar changes occurred on specific criteria such as eating competence, dressing, writing, speech, and manual dexterity. However, only writing showed a statistically significant improvement between discharge and retest, while eating, dressing, and mobility showed significant regression during that period. Results suggested that there is a decline in self-help skills but a moderate increase in academic skills after discharge from the institute.

A somewhat similar study by Goble and Nichols (1971) followed up 200 patients, ranging in age between 11 and 84 years, admitted to a disabled living research unit. The objective was to assess the effectiveness of a small, high-cost habilitation unit for severely disabled persons. Various subject areas evaluated over a period of time were personality, intellectual functioning, physical impairment, and degree of social and welfare services offered to the patient. The aim was to establish the unit's value to the community.

The United Cerebral Palsy Association study (1969) of the CP individual and his family prefaces a five-year plan of providing services. Follow-up services are included in the projected program design, as well as evaluation and cost analysis.

The need for improved indicators of habilitation success is stressed by Hawryluk (1972) who points out the inadequacy of the "closed-rehabilitated" and "closed-employed" criteria in measuring effects of vocational programs. He quotes a follow-up study by Keer (1971) in which the success measure was a composite of three indicators: 1) major changes in job level subsequent to initial placement, 2) changes in salary since initial placement, and 3) most recent employment status. Harward (1967) also stresses occupational mobility as an indication of the extent to which a client has adapted to a nonhandicapped society. However, as McCoy and Rusk (1953) have pointed out, there are many aspects of self-help capabilities and lessened dependence on others that can result from the habilitation process but cannot be measured in strictly economic or vocational terms. Rather, they postulate an "ability to function" measure, which includes social characteristics, mobility status, daily activity competency, employment status, and an "overall rehabilitation rating" of general progress.

Hawryluk mentions "a study underway" by Rosenberg (1965) in which clients are administered identical instruments upon referral to a habilitation center and one year following referral. Scores will be compared for each person on an item-by-item basis. The client's sense of self-esteem is emphasized, and scores will reflect overall change indicated by the individual. Such a system of measuring habilitation success is seen as encompassing several dimensions of a client's situation and being sensitive to change in status. Because it is capable of registering changes in ''difficult'' as well as normal clients, it is seen as lessening the current bias of present systems toward helping only those clients with easily remediable disabilities.

In designing a prognostic study for the cerebral palsied, the limitations of psychometric techniques for this population must be kept in mind. Such problems have been pointed out by a number of authors. Newland (1971) devotes considerable attention to the psychological assessment of exceptional children and youth, and particularly notes the problems of testing the cerebral palsied. As he points out (p. 140), ''The greatest liberties in endeavoring to adapt individual examinations have been taken with respect to the cerebral-palsied.'' Depending on the individual's particular physical problems, a ''cafeteria'' approach to testing has often been used. Items are selected from various scales on the assumption that all such items taken together would give a general idea of the mental level of functioning. As Newland indicates, however, such a procedure is of little value unless it is done by a highly trained person who can select items with a view toward ''the sampling of consciously presumed or known types of psychological functioning... .'' The need to develop tests that do not rely on either speech or accurate pointing behavior is emphasized.

Others who have discussed the methods of psychologically evaluating the cerebral palsied include Deaver (1967), Rosenberg (1968), and Allen and Jefferson (1962). These authors emphasize the difficulties of adapting standard intelligence tests to the myriad of physical problems that the cerebral palsied represent. As Deaver says, ''There is no suitable test to differentiate between the (individual's) knowledge and his ability to convey this information to another person.''

Allen and Jefferson differentiate between Type 1 tests, which assume the subject understands oral instructions and that no motor manipulation is required, and Type 2 tests, which can be used with subjects whose response is limited by severe impairment. The former category includes the Peabody Picture Vocabulary Test, the Columbia Mental Maturity Scale, Raven Progressive Matrices, and the Leiter Scale. All these can use pointing, pantomime, eye movement, or head-shaking to indicate a correct response. Type 2 tests require the report of an observer, and include the Vineland Social Maturity Scale, the Adaptive Behavior Scale, and the Gesell Behavior Inventory.

Additional tests investigated for use with the cerebral palsied include the Stanford-Binet, WAIS, MMPI, and Bender Gestalt. Methods of adapting sections of these tests to accommodate persons with specific handicaps are discussed.

Vocational testing of the cerebral palsied includes tests of physical functioning as well as intellectual ability. Rosenberg writes at length about evaluating vocational potential for this population, and cites a project in which 300 clients were assessed in an attempt to establish standardized procedures for such evaluations. Performance on over 100 tasks during a seven-week testing period was used as the criterion for placing clients in various categories of employment potential.

Evaluation and classification of the vocational potential of cerebral palsied clients is the subject of a study by Machek and Collins (1961). Here, 29 clients were evaluated on a series of skills tests and psychometric measurements. The data revealed that vocational potential is poor for severely involved CPs, and that IQ is not related to job performance. Rather, a factor that the authors call "adequacy of the individual," and which includes psycho-social considerations such as emotional stability and motivation, is considered more important for utilization of vocational potential. Other findings revealed a significant relationship between years completed in school and work potential. In fact, education was a more crucial factor for employment than reading ability, manual dexterity, or IQ level. The conclusion drawn is that those CPs who stayed in school longer developed more acceptable personalities and better interpersonal relationships, and that these attributes made them more effective employees.

The various studies comprising this literature survey have provided a considerable amount of information on the characteristics, activities, and problems of cerebral palsied persons. In general, these studies have revealed the multiplicity of physical handicaps with which these persons are afflicted, their degree of financial dependence on others, and their difficulties in attaining educational achievement, social adjustment, and vocational satisfaction. The problems of assessing the psychological, intellectual, and vocational capacities of handicapped individuals have been noted. The need for counseling and habilitation services of various sorts has been emphasized, and attempts have been made in a few studies to evaluate the effectiveness of such services for the physically, mentally, and emotionally handicapped.

A COMPARATIVE FOLLOW-UP STUDY

Floor and Rosen (1976) conducted a study designed to evaluate the effectiveness of three service models provided to cerebral palsied adults, most of whom had previously received some form of habilitation training. A group of 140 clients identified as having received services from the Bureau of Vocational Rehabilitation or other agency were divided into three groups. The first group was provided with intensive follow-along counseling, community-oriented didactic instruction, and a variety of further vocational and social habilitation services. This was defined as a maximal treatment condition. A second group of clients received follow-along home counseling and referral services only. This was defined as a moderate treatment condition. The third group received almost no counseling or habilitation service in accordance with criteria for the minimal treatment condition. All subjects received a comprehensive psychological and vocational evaluation before the onset of treatment. Each group also was administered a home interview designed to assess overall vocational, community, and social adjustment on two different occasions, before the onset of treatment and one year after treatment.

In addition, at the beginning of the study clients were administered a series of intelligence, perceptual-motor, and academic achievement tests, and were rated by the interviewer on scales of degree of physical handicap (Katz, 1956) and employment potential (Gellman, 1960).

Clients were then assigned to the three treatment groups, designated as maximum, moderate, and minimum. While the original study design presupposed that these groups would be of equal number and would be matched on such variables as age, sex, IQ, and degree of disability, the practicalities of the situation made it difficult to control these variables experimentally. Factors such as apparent need, geographic location, mobility, and willingness to accept treatment ultimately affected clients' placement in a given treatment group.

Persons in the maximum treatment group received a wide range of services, many of which were tailored to meet individual needs. Major services included adult education (Rosen, DiGiovanni, and Peet, 1975), in which the curriculum provided information on a variety of subject areas, including home and money management, personal hygiene, use of public transportation, and job-hunting procedures. In general, the program stressed the availability of material and service resources and adaptive aids; role-playing and other techniques were utilized in an attempt to focus on individual needs and to give clients a realistic basis for self-assessment. A second major service area was Personal Adjustment Training (Rosen and Peet, 1975), in which group counseling techniques were employed to help clients gain in self-concept and assertiveness; clients' emotional needs were emphasized, and role-playing and social interaction utilized to help the client attain awareness of his own abilities. Home counseling was the third major service provided (Rosen, Phillips, Floor, Peet, and DiGiovanni, 1975). Here, the client as a family member was the focus, with the concern being on developing better family relationships, including for clients a greater degree of independence from overprotective relatives.

Other services provided to persons in the maximum group included workshop training, individual counseling and tutoring, occupational therapy, job placement efforts, and referrals to other resources.

The moderate treatment group received follow-along counseling in their homes and referrals to other agencies. The minimum group received no services between the time of the initial and testing sessions and the final interview.

Data Analysis

Four types of statistical analyses were performed:

1. A population description according to demographic and psychometric variables as well as initial criteria of adjustment.
2. Between-group comparisons of the three treatment groups as well as the "refuser" group of 27 persons who dropped out before the completion of the study.
3. A prognostic study, in which "predictor" variables such as age, IQ, degree of disability and educational level were correlated with "criterion" variables such as income, job history, self-sufficiency, social activity, and other indicators of adjustment.
4. Pre-post treatment comparisons, in which the differential services provided were evaluated by comparing the three groups on selected criteria before and after receiving services, when initial between group differences were statistically controlled by analysis of covariance techniques.

Additional sources of information were gathered by project habilitation staff in the form of a narrative "case history" on each client. These narratives included descriptions of the client's initial status, degree and type of services provided, events in the course of the year's treatment, and final outcome. While these case histories were subjective in nature, they were nonetheless most valuable in helping alter traditional concepts of "good adjustment."

Results

Population Description The population of this project consisted of adults (average age, 28) who had been diagnosed as cerebral palsied in childhood. Subjects were equally divided as to sex, and three quarters of them lived in the city of Philadelphia. Most lived with their parents in private homes, and many were extremely dependent on their parents and/or felt themselves to be "overprotected" at home.

These persons represented a wide range of physical and intellectual abilities. The majority were diagnosed as spastic, and their disabilities included hemiplegia (34%), quadriplegia (25%), and paraplegia (21%). About a third of the clients had some degree of speech impairment.

The average IQ (WAIS Full Scale) was 77, but the group ranged in intellectual functioning from "severe mental retardation" to "bright normal" ability. The mean educational level attained was tenth grade.

About 70% of the clients were totally dependent financially on parents and/or public assistance. While over 50% of these persons were considered to be "employed," over half of these were confined to sheltered workshops. The average earned income from workshop employment was less than $400 annually; those engaged in competitive employment averaged about $2,500.

Although the majority of clients were able to use public transportation, they tended to lead extremely sheltered lives and to have few friends or social involvements.

Group Differences Although the three treatment groups were intended to be matched on basic demographic characteristics, such matching was a practical impossibility. The maximum treatment group in general represented lower socioeconomic, intellectual, and vocational levels. They were also significantly younger, and included higher proportions of both Blacks and females. The subjects in the maximum treatment group were more likely to be dependent financially on others, to be employed in sheltered workshops rather than competitively, and to have the lowest incomes. They scored significantly lower than the other groups on the majority of the psychometric tests, including IQ and rating of employability. In addition, they needed more help in daily living tasks, and were the least likely to feel they had enough friends. The minimum treatment group, on the other hand, were more likely to hold competitive jobs and to have relatively higher incomes. They were comparatively independent in daily living skills and in financial reliance on others. The moderate treatment group tended to fall between the other two on most initial variables. Interestingly, the three groups did not differ significantly in degree or type of physical disability.

Persons who dropped out before the completion of the study were characterized as a "refuser" group, and were compared with the three treatment categories on characteristics revealed by the initial interview. In general, the refusers showed a comparatively high level of adjustment. They were more likely than other clients to live in the suburbs rather than the city, to be financially independent, to hold competitive jobs on a steady

Table 1. Group comparisons on selected variables

Category	Treatment Group											
	Maximum ($N=54$)			Moderate ($N=25$)			Minimum ($N=34$)			Refusers ($N=27$)		
	Mean	SD	%	Mean	SD	%	Mean	SD	%	Mean	SD	%
Sex												
Male			35			64			62			44
Female			65			36			38			56
Age	25.5	7.4		29.5	10.9		30.5	9.7		28.0	7.9	
Race												
White			56			72			82			93
Black			44			28			18			7
Full Scale IQ[a]	70.1	17.1		81.3	11.9		80.3	15.8		83.6	14.9	
Arithmetic Grade Level[b]	3.7	2.7		5.6	3.4		5.6	4.0		6.4	3.8	
Age Equivalent[c]	6.5	3.3		7.8	2.8		8.5	2.6		3.9	2.0	
Employability Rating[d]	76.1	22.3		88.0	18.6		85.9	17.0		87.5	20.3	
Physical Disability Rating[e]	15.1	2.1		14.5	2.7		14.5	2.4		15.8	1.8	
Financial Dependency												
Wholly on others			82			85			58			39
Partially or not at all			18			15			42			61
Type of Employment												
Unemployed			45			56			32			33
Sheltered Workshop			47			16			27			11
Competitive			8			28			41			56

Annual Income	$352	$770		$757	$1,841		$1,574	$2,389		$1,740	$2,284	
Social Adjustment Rating												
Few, or no friends or activities			53			55			47			44
Some, or many friends or activities			47			46			53			56
Daily Living Rating												
Needs help			89			60			70			56
Independent			11			40			30			44

[a]Wechsler Adult Intelligence Scale.

[b]Wide Range Achievement Test.

[c]Bender Visual-Motor Gestalt Test.

[d]Gellman Scale of Employability.

[e]Katz Scale of Physical Handicap (Total Score).

[f]Including unemployed persons with 0 income.

basis, and to earn the highest incomes. They were independent in handling daily living tasks, got along well with others, and were least likely to have friends who were handicapped. The refusers scored highest on the employability scale, on IQ, and on arithmetic achievement; they were the least likely clients to have a speech defect. This comparatively normal status accounted in large measure for the refusal of these persons to receive either services or contacts with the project staff, and for the reluctance of the staff to "pursue" them in attempting to provide services or maintain contact.

A few of the key areas of comparison among the three treatment groups and the refusers are shown in Table 1. (This table represents only 13 of the 111 variables on which treatment groups and refusers were compared.)

Prognostic Relationships Thirty-two predictor and 24 criterion variables were selected for intercorrelation. All predictor variables were drawn from data acquired at the time of the initial interview; criterion variables reflected clients' status at the time of the final interview. Variables selected were considered representative of important demographic, ability, and adjustment factors.

A number of intelligence and achievement test scores (The Wechsler Adult Intelligence Scale (WAIS) Verbal and Full Scale IQ; the Wide Range Achievement Tests of Reading and Arithmetic; and the Fundamental Achievement Series, Verbal & Numerical) related positively to criteria such as job level (unemployed, sheltered, competitive, professional) and vocational skill level as defined by the *Dictionary of Occupational Titles* (1966).

Significant relationships occurred between the Scale of Employability and criteria such as financial dependency, job level, amount of income, and daily living skills. Since this scale covers topics such as language skills, dependency needs, vocational competence and marketability, attitudes and motivations, and physical appearance, it is not surprising that it is an effective predictor of several aspects of client adjustment.

Ratings of physical disability did not relate significantly to criterion variables. Demographic factors such as age, sex, race, and educational level also failed to relate to criteria.

All significant relationships are reported in Table 2.

Pre-post Treatment Comparisons Because effect of differential treatment over a year's time was the most important concern of this project, a study of post-test differences among treatment groups was the crux of the data analysis. Analyses of variance were performed on selected criteria to assess the interaction effect of degree of treatment with passage of time.

Table 2. Significant relationships[a]—predictor versus criterion variables

Predictor Variable	Criterion Relationship	*r*
Gellman Scale of Employability	Financial Dependency	.51
	Level of Employment	.59
	Daily Living Skills Rating	.57
	Earned Income	.55
Wechsler Adult Intelligence Scale		
Verbal IQ:	Level of Employment	.56
	Skill Level (DOT No.)[b]	−.51
Performance IQ:	None	
Full Scale IQ:	Level of Employment	.58
	Skill Level (DOT No.)[b]	−.56
Wide Range Achievement Test		
Reading Grade Level	Type of Employment	.54
Arithmetic Grade Level	Type of Employment	.64
	Skill Level (DOT No.)[b]	−.54**
Fundamental Achievement Series		
Verbal Score	Type of Employment	.55
Numerical Score	Type of Employment	.65
	Skill Level (DOT No.)[b]	−.54
Self Care Skills Rating (Pre-Test)	Use of Public Transportation	.57
	Daily Living Skills Rating (Post-Test)	.50
Daily Living Skills Rating (Pre-Test)	Level of Employment	.50
	Self Care Skills Rating (Post-Test)	.50

[a]Only relationships meeting dual criteria of $r > .50$ and $p < .01$ were considered of practical significance in this study.

[b]A higher skill level is indicated by a lower DOT No., so this relationship is in the expected direction.

Very few such differences were revealed. In comparison with minimum and moderate treatment groups, the maximum group had increased significantly in its use of public assistance, in the amount of time employed, and in job satisfaction. No other apparent effects of the variety and intensity of services offered this group were demonstrated by changes in criterion variables.

However, as has already been noted, the maximum treatment group started out on a lower intellectual, social, and economic level than the comparison group. Such group differences could serve to obscure whatever effects intensive services had for this group compared to the effects it had for those receiving moderate or minimal services. This was extremely likely, since several of the variables on which the groups differed had already been shown to relate to criterion variables.

Accordingly, analyses of covariance were performed to investigate differential effects of the three treatments when initial group differences were controlled. With appropriate statistical controls, differential effects of treatment across the three groups could not be demonstrated.

DISCUSSION

The apparent failure of pre-post treatment comparisons to support the efficacy of counseling, adult education, and other habilitative services raises questions concerning the value of these procedures for the cerebral palsied individual. It also challenges traditional criteria of success for this population.

Effects of traditional habilitation services were relatively inconsequential when compared to the importance of factors such as measured intelligence, scholastic achievement, and rated vocational potential in affecting an individual's ability to benefit from counseling and other services. It is evident that these differences among subjects are more meaningful than type and conditions of treatment in determining traditional vocational and social outcomes. Such differences are not subtle or abstract, but represent client characteristics that are readily measurable. Thus, from a cost benefit standpoint, it would appear a) that time and effort expended in appropriate client evaluation is time effectively utilized, and b) that for a cerebral palsied population traditional services may not be economically justified in terms of traditional criteria of adjustment.

An extremely important outcome of this study concerns the overall potential of the cerebral palsied for vocational and social habilitation. It is impossible to avoid the conclusion that the cerebral palsied represent an extremely difficult population for vocational adjustment, at least in terms of traditional criteria of job placements. Nevertheless, degree of physical handicap per se is not a significant predictor of outcome. This suggests that habilitation successes or failures are related to factors other than those determined by neurological impairment. It holds out the hope that while physical disability is irreversible, vocational and social disabilities may not be.

Another finding of the study concerned the value of workshop placement for many clients of relatively high intelligence. While approximately 75% of clients with normal intelligence had been placed in workshops, such persons often became quickly dissatisfied with the monotony of the work and with the intellectual deficiencies of many of their co-workers.

Consequently, they left workshop employment after only a short time, and attempted, often unsuccessfully, to find jobs more suitable to their mental abilities. Persons at the lower end of the IQ distribution, however, were content with workshop placement and tended to remain so employed for a longer period.

This reasoning substantiates the findings of Olshansky and Beach (1975) who also noted that their more competent clients were less likely to take low-skill competitive jobs than were their less competent peers. The findings from both studies suggest the need to provide separate, higher level workshops that can offer stimulating and rewarding work for intellectually capable clients who, because of their physical disabilities, may be unable to find suitable competitive employment.

As was pointed out by Olshansky and Beach, many of the unemployed physically disabled persons in their survey "seemed to have moved from resentment to resignation. Not infrequently this feeling of resignation was shared and supported by relatives... The question unanswered...is how to combat the feeling of resignation, as disabling in many instances as the disability itself." A significant effort must be initiated to combat such "feelings of resignation" over lack of employment, by offering alternatives to the Protestant work ethic, and providing those unable to work with viable substitutes for self-development and satisfaction.

In contrast to the paucity of statistical data, however, subjective reports suggested that some positive changes had indeed taken place as a result of the habilitation services offered by project staff.

These reports emerged from the case histories written by counselors for each client, from comments by clients to staff members, and from clients' families, many of whom attended a series of parent meetings at the Rehabilitation Center.

In general, it was found that subtle changes in "quality of life" for many persons had taken place, but that these changes were not included in the traditional criteria on which this study was originally based. Examples of such changes include:

1. Increased use of public assistance. While this finding was supported by research data, it may, to the traditionalist, appear to be a step backward rather than forward. However, if one considers that the legitimate use of public funds, of which he may have been previously unaware, gives the client a new independence and enhances his scope of potential activities, then this can be seen as a positive result.
2. Improved family relationships. A combination of family counseling and assertiveness training for clients resulted in many subtle shifts in

intrafamily attitudes and behaviors. A new awareness, on the part of both client and family, of the client's potential for comparative independence was an important concomitant of improvement in the life situation.

3. More effective use of leisure time. Increased knowledge of current events and of the potential for political power for the handicapped, development of a hobby, and exposure to possibilities for volunteer work or educational experiences all gave clients a more positive attitude toward the relatively confined lives to which many of them were committed.
4. Improved self-concept. While this is a most difficult variable to measure, it is crucial to the client's acceptance of himself as a "person with a handicap" rather than as a "handicapped person." Both caseworkers and families noted such changes in the client's approach to social and work situations.

The types of changes listed above can be considered the direct result of counseling and educational services provided. For example, many clients were unaware of their eligibility for public assistance until informed by their counselor or helped in applying for benefits. Assertiveness training in group counseling sessions and follow-along counseling in the home helped the client achieve an enhanced self-concept and improved family relationships. Adult education on topics such as social image, crisis intervention, mobility training, use of adaptive aids, employment orientation, and human sexuality helped clients learn more about the world around them and their own potential role as more active participants in it. Finally, referral services provided clients with new contacts and awareness of available resources.

That few of these changes were directly measurable through statistical analysis of interview data is interpreted to mean 1) that the measuring instrument (the interview questions and rating scales) was not designed to be sufficiently sensitive to such subtle personality changes, and 2) that the criteria utilized in assessing "improved adjustment" were traditionally oriented toward objective vocational and socioeconomic goals rather than toward inner personal satisfactions and overall "life style" of cerebral palsied persons.

CONCLUSIONS AND RECOMMENDATIONS

Three main findings of this study are:

1. The recognition that not all habilitation services are equally effective according to previously accepted criteria of vocational and social ad-

justment. While such services are undeniably important, in many situations they may be relatively ineffective in relation to initial characteristics such as tested intelligence and rated employment potential.

2. The recognition that for many cerebral palsied persons for whom vocational placement is not feasible criteria of successful habilitation should be changed to include improvements in "quality of life." Such criteria might be, among others, realistic acceptance of one's assets and limitations, improved self concept, ability to use leisure time effectively, good interpersonal relationships, and increased independence from parents.
3. The recognition that while the cerebral palsied population represent an extremely difficult client group to habilitate according to traditional goals of vocational placement, degree of physical handicap may not be an important determinant of overall adjustment.

Some specific recommendations that grew out of the findings of this study include:

1. The need for a reassessment of workshop placement as an habilitation goal, since in many cases it represents a compromise measure arousing resentment and dissatisfaction. This is particularly true for clients of higher intellectual functioning, who should be provided with separate workshop facilities in which more stimulating tasks are available.
2. The need for the establishment of group homes for physically handicapped persons, especially where personal growth requires the learning of greater degrees of independence from parents. Such group homes should be located close to feasible work situations to reduce transportation difficulties for such persons.
3. The need for intensive inservice training for habilitation workers who will deal with the complex needs and problems of the cerebral palsied. Such training should include an awareness of the need for new criteria of successful adjustment.
4. The importance of an accurate diagnostic evaluation of client characteristics that may be crucial in predicting ultimate habilitation potential.

In summary, the conclusions and recommendations of this project suggest the need for new models of adjustment for the developmentally disabled. In contrast to the traditional vocational model, new criteria could be based on a model similar to that accepted for retired persons. Here, "work" is no longer the criterion of adjustment; the use of leisure time, range of interests, good health, social and family interrelationships—all are measures of adjustment accepted by our society for senior citizens. This report proposes the adoption of similar criteria for the developmentally disabled for whom competitive employment is a physical or mental impossibility, and for whom workshop placement may be inappropriate. Although it is recongized that adoption of these criteria represents a departure from traditional habilitation philosophy, it is our strong belief that such radical rethinking is necessary for the realistic and effective provision of services to developmentally disabled clients.

LITERATURE CITED

Allen, R., and Jefferson, F. 1962. Psychological Evaluation of the Cerebral Palsied Person. Charles C Thomas, Springfield, Ill.

Deaver, G. G. 1967. Cerebral palsy, methods of evaluation and treatment. Rehabilitation Monograph IX. Institute of Rehabilitation Medicine, N.Y.U. Medical Center.

Dictionary of Occupational Titles, U.S. Department of Labor, Washington, D.C., 1966.

Exceptional Parent, The. Parent to parent: Conclusion, 1972, 1, 4, 3–5.

Floor, L., and Rosen, M. 1976. New Criteria of Adjustment for the Cerebral Palsied, Rehabilitation Literature, Vol. 37, No. 9. pp. 268–274.

Gellman, W. A scale of employability for handicapped persons. Office of Vocational Rehabilitation, Project #64-57, 1960.

Goble, R. E. A., and Nichols, P. S. R. 1971. Rehabilitation of the Severely Disabled. Vol. 1—Evaluation of a Disabled Living Unit. Appleton-Century Crofts, New York.

Harward, N. 1967. Progress report on development of methodology to study ethnic and religious differences in attitudes affecting success of vocational rehabilitation in Central Arizona. Unpublished project report (Project No. RD-1646-P, Appendix C).

Hawryluk, A. 1972. Rehabilitation gain: A better indicator needed. J. Rehab. 38(5):22–25.

Heal, L. W. 1972. Evaluating an integrated approach to the management of cerebral palsy, Vol. IV. Wisconsin University, Eau Claire. (Ed 070-238).

Ingram, T. T. S. 1964. Pediatric Aspects of Cerebral Palsy. The Williams & Wilkins Co., Baltimore.

Katz, E. 1956. Survey of degree of physical handicap. Cerebral Palsy Program, Department of Pediatrics, University of California School of Medicine.

Keer, E. B. 1971. The Relationship Among Disability, Education and Vocational Achievement. Final Project Report, Fred C. Board, Project Director. Just One Break, Inc. Research Grant RD-2656-G.

Klapper, Z.S., and Birch, H. G. 1966. The relation of childhood characteristics to outcome in young adults with cerebral palsy. Developmental Medicine and Child Neurology, 8(6):645–656.

Klapper, Z. S., and Birch, H. G. 1967. A 14-year follow-up study of cerebral palsy—intellectual change and stability. Amer. J. Orthopsychiatr. 37(3):504–547.

Lacks, P. B., and Plax, K. 1972. The need for an honest look. J. Rehab. 41:19–22.

Mácheck, O., and Collins, H. A. 1961. Second year review of evaluating and classifying the vocational potentials of the cerebral palsied. Arch. Phys. Med. 42(2):106–108.

McCoy, G. F., and Rusk, H. A. 1953. An evaluation of rehabilitation. Rehabilitation Monograph #1. The Institute of Physical Medicine and Rehabilitation, New York University, Bellevue Medical Center.

Moed, M., and Litwin, D. 1963. The employability of the cerebral palsied. Rehab. Lit. 24(9):265–296.

Muthard, J. E., and Hutchison, J. 1968. Cerebral palsied college students—their education and employment. University of Florida, Gainesville.

Newland, T. E. 1971. Psychological assessment of children and youth. *In* W. M., Cruickshank (ed.), Psychology of Exceptional Children and Youth, pp. 115–172. Prentice-Hall, Inc., Englewood Cliffs, N.J.

Olshansky, S., and Beach, D. 1975. A five-year follow-up of physically disabled clients. Rehab. Lit. 36(8):251–252, 258.

Rosen, M., DiGiovanni, S., and Peet, D. 1975. Remedial adult education for the physically handicapped: A curriculum outline. Elwyn Institute, Elwyn, Pa.

Rosen, M., and Peet, D. 1975. Treating emotional problems of the physically handicapped: A manual of group counseling procedures for persons with cerebral palsy or other physical disability. Elwyn Institute, Elwyn, Pa.

Rosen, M., Phillips, D., Floor, L., Peet, D., and DiGiovanni, S. 1975. Follow-along, home counseling techniques for physically handicapped clients. Elwyn Institute, Elwyn, Pa.

Rosenberg, B. 1968. Procedures for evaluating the vocational potential of the cerebral palsied. *In* G. N. Wright and A. B. Trotter (eds.), Rehabilitation Research. University of Wisconsin, Madison.

Rosenberg, M. 1965. Society and the Adolescent Self-image. Princeton University Press, Princeton, N.J.

United Cerebral Palsy Association. 1969. The IHF plan: the individual with cerebral palsy and his family. UCPA, Inc., New York. (Ed 031-838).

Wolfe, W. G., and Reid, L. L. 1968. A Survey of Cerebral Palsy in Texas, UCP of Texas, Austin, Texas 78701.

Chapter 7

Institutions and Their Effects

Never before have institutions for the mentally retarded been subjected to such critical attack (Blatt and Kaplan, 1967; White and Wolfensberger, 1969). Proponents of normalization have pointed to the dehumanizing conditions that have existed in many facilities for over a hundred years and called for an end to such facilities (Wolfensberger, 1971a, 1971b). In response to such criticism as well as to pressure by parental groups, to advances in behavioral and educational research that point toward new training models (Bricker, 1970; Bensberg et al., 1965; Giradeau and Spradlin, 1964), and to state and federal legislation and public recognition of the rights of the mentally retarded, many institutions have already responded with programs and policies reflecting marked shifts in philosophy. Medical models have been supplanted by vocational and social habilitation approaches, and "humanitarian" concerns for protection of the retarded (and society) have succumbed to more utilitarian concerns about individual rights and freedoms.

Although changes have already occurred, demands for deinstitutionalization continue. Due process legislation has employed the principle of the "least restrictive alternative" for determining choice of residential settings for the mentally retarded. Institutions, it is argued, are unnatural environments, and many feel that little can be done to overcome a century of neglect and disinterest within such settings. In a President's Committee on Mental Retardation Message in 1968, Mrs. Hubert Humphrey pleaded for small, attractive, homelike residential units for the mentally retarded and, rather than renovating present institutional facilities for such a purpose, suggested it might be cheaper to "bulldoze some of the old institutions away."

Demands for deinstitutionalization have already had vast impact, and many institutional residents have been transferred to small group homes, foster homes, nursing homes, and other sites in the community. While this trend is undoubtedly motivated by the most sincere attitudes towards past injustices, empirical studies of the detrimental effects of institutions have been far from unanimous in documenting detrimental effects of institutions. Nor is it clear what elements of the institution are associated with what effects, even when there is general agreement that the overall effect has been negative. Furthermore, studies of community facilities indicate that many group and foster homes may be no better than the institutions they are meant to replace (Murphy, Rennee, and Luchins, 1972). Because institutions represent extremely complex social situations, it is difficult to determine what specific aspects of institutionalization may be detrimental. The issue of institutional influence is part of a larger research question dealing with the role of environmental factors in affecting personality, behavior, and adjustment of the mentally retarded individual.

Despite the complexity of the issue, decisions concerning the future of our large institutions must be made. Certainly the role of our large institutional structures represents one of the most pressing problems with which planners for the mentally retarded must deal.

INSTITUTIONS: 1890–1950

The philosophy of institutions beginning with the disillusionment in the post–Civil War era encompassed several major principles that continued through the turn of the century and were still largely characteristic of many institutions as late as 1950. These include:

1) Emphasis on manual training and industrial occupations.
2) Distinction between students in educational departments and custodial departments.
3) Concern about life-long segregation of the retarded for their own protection or the protection of society.
4) Concerns about economy of operation and use of inmates of institutions to run the institution.
5) Concerns about orderliness, habit training, discipline, and a well-ordered institutional regime.
6) Concerns about moral deficiencies of certain classes of retarded and about their proper moral training.

Decision-makers advocating institutional change have tended to view the contemporary situation in institutions as absolutes. The snakepits of retardation have been well described and there can be little doubt that shameful conditions existed for the many retarded living within institutions.

Nevertheless, it is wrong to ignore the fact that in many institutions high quality educational programs were also applied. Early lesson plans and photographs at Elwyn Institute depict educational approaches that represented the best of Forebel, Pestalozzi, and Montessori. Rhythmic approaches to teaching physical education, language training, gymnastics, and military drill seem to have been taught with a degree of precision, enthusiasm, and teacher dedication that may have surpassed contemporary programs. Despite these programs, however, it was clear that administrators at institutions had little faith that, even with vocational training, the mentally retarded adult was suited for life outside institutional walls.

In 1893, Walter E. Fernald, Superintendent of the Massachusetts School for the Feeble-minded, wrote:

> With all our training we cannot give our pupils that indispensable something known as good, plain 'common sense.' The amount and value of their labor depends upon the amount of oversight and supervision practicable....
>
> Outside of an institution it would be impossible to secure the experienced and patient supervision and direction necessary to obtain practical, remunerative results from the comparatively unskilled labor of these feeble-minded people (p. 325).

THE SITUATION IN 1965

By 1965 public attitudes and national policy had changed radically from the philosophy depicted above. The conditions of the large state and private institutions had not yet caught up with this change. Such institutions probably represented much the same situation as they had in the half century previously, except for greater overcrowding and fewer attempts at programing. Butterfield's (1969) summary of basic facts about residential institutions compiles the statistical information available at this time:

More than 200,000 persons were residing in approximately 150 public institutions and 20,000 persons were living in 500 private residential facilities for the mentally retarded. More than half of these persons were children. Institutions were filled to over 98 percent capacity, and waiting periods of many years before admission were common in most large states. Many of the institutions were housing as much as 50 percent above the capacity they were constructed to accommodate. In 1962 the President's

Committee on Mental Retardation estimated that over 50,000 additional beds would have to be provided to relieve overcrowding.

Approximately 5 percent of the mentally retarded were residing within institutions, but more money was being spent upon their care than was spent for the remaining 95 percent.

In 1965 about $500,000,000 were being spent annually to maintain public institutions for the mentally retarded. About three-quarters of this expenditure went for staff salaries. Ninety thousand persons were employed within institutions, more than half of these as attendants. Published figures of one attendant to every four residents are deceptive because round the clock coverage must be provided, and attendants work normal eight-hour shifts. Multiplying this figure by three suggests a 1:12 ratio as a more accurate estimate, but it is likely that this figure is higher than the actual coverage during evening and weekend hours. Butterfield reports that the ratio of physicians to residents was 1:270, and for psychologists the ratio was 1:430.

In the past, attendants have had few educational qualifications imposed upon them. One study reports that the majority have less than a twelfth-grade education (Parker, 1951). Butterfield (1967a) provides a comprehensive review of the selection, characteristics, and training of attendant staff within institutions, although he tends to lump together data relating to psychiatric hospitals with that for institutions for the retarded. Although attendants have more contact with residents than any other employee group (Fleming, 1962), studies by Thormahlen (1965) and Oudenne (1963) indicate that very little attendant time in programs for the severely retarded is actually spent on direct patient care. Oudenne found that an average of 132 minutes per day was spent in direct patient services over a four-day period. The turnover rate among attendants is high and occurs mainly in the first few months after employment (McIntire, 1954). Attendants earn among the lowest salaries within the institution, and at least half (Parker, 1951) tend to be dissatisfied with their salaries.

Data summarized by Butterfield (1969) for 192,493 persons within residential institutions indicate that 27 percent of these were profoundly retarded, 33 percent severely retarded, 22 percent moderately retarded, 13 percent mildly retarded, and 5 percent of borderline retardation. Three percent of these were below the age of five, 44 percent between the ages of five and nineteen, 27 percent between the ages of twenty and thirty and 26 percent above thirty.

In 1967 there was great variability of daily maintenance expenditures per resident, with Alaska spending $22.38 and Mississippi spending $2.30. The daily average for the fifty states was $14.64 per resident.

Butterfield noted that nearly half of the states had only one institution for the mentally retarded, which generally was a large multipurpose facility. One-half of the public institutions housed more than 1,000 residents. However, Butterfield also pointed out a growing trend for smaller institutions intended for 500 or fewer residents.

The mid-sixties may have represented a particularly low point in conditions within many institutions although it seems likely that such conditions had not developed overnight. A photographic expose published in 1967 by Burton Blatt was intended to make Americans aware of the deplorable situation in many such facilities. These photographs, obtained with a hidden camera, did much to arouse public indignation. Blatt (1969) described his feelings during this experience:

> In each of the dormitories for severely retarded residents there is what is called, euphemistically, the dayroom or recreation room. The odor in each of these rooms is overpowering, to the degree that after a visit to a dayroom I had to send my clothes to the drycleaners in order to have the stench removed (and, probably because of psychological reactions, whose odor I continued to smell months later whenever I wore certain clothes). The physical facilities often contributed to the visual horror as well as the odor. Floors are sometimes made of wood, and, as a result, excretions are rubbed into the cracks, thus providing a permanent aroma. Most dayrooms have a series of bleacher-like benches on which sit denuded residents, jammed together, without purposeful activity or communication or any type of interaction. In each dayroom is an attendant or two, whose main function seems to be to 'stand around' and, on occasion, hose down the floor, 'driving' excretions into a sewer conveniently located in the center of the room....
>
> The living quarters for older men and women were, for the most part, gloomy and sterile. There were rows and rows of benches on which sat countless human beings, in silent rooms, waiting for dinner call or bedtime. I saw resident after resident in 'institutional garb.' Sometimes the women wore shrouds—inside out. I heard a good deal of laughter but saw little cheer.

There were few things to be cheerful about....

> The children's dormitories depressed me the most. Here, cribs were placed, as in the other dormitories, side by side and head to head. Very young children, one and two years of age, were lying in cribs without any contact with adults, without playthings, without apparent stimulation. In one dormitory that had over 100 infants and was connected to nine other dormitories that totaled 1,000 infants I experienced my deepest sadness. . . .
>
> In some of the children's dormitories I observed 'nursery programs.' What surprised me most was their scarcity and, unfortunately, the primitiveness of those in operation. . . . The special education that I observed at the state schools bore no resemblance to what I would consider to be 'education.' But, it was special. It was a collection of the most depressing 'learning' environments I have ever had the misfortune to witness.

The authors of *Christmas in Purgatory* were subjected to a severe degree of criticism for their study. Many professionals and administrators in the field of mental retardation were concerned that the pictures, while authentic, did not do justice to the many fine programs that existed at the same institutions that housed the wards that Blatt and Kaplan had photographed. Yet Nirje (1969), commenting on the Blatt and Kaplan report on the basis of his own experiences visiting American institutions for the retarded, has written:

> Such conditions are shocking denials of human dignity. They force the retarded to function far below their levels of developmental possibilities. The large institutions where such conditions occur are no schools for proper training, nor are they hospitals for care and betterment, as they really increase mental retardation by producing further handicapping conditions of the mentally retarded.... I have been told that not all the institutions are as bad as some I have seen, or that within a given institution, good buildings and programs may be found as well as bad ones. However, I find this type of apologetics difficult to understand. Even the so-called good institutions or units are too far from a decent interpretation of the rights to life, liberty, and pursuit of happiness—and in the back wards these words are almost quenchable. . . .

There seems little need to document the detrimental effect upon personality development that conditions such as those described by Blatt had. Yet the role institutional living plays on influencing personality is by no means well established. As Butterfield points out (1967b), this issue is only part of the larger question concerning the contribution of environmental factors to the development of the mentally retarded.

The use of psychological, educational, and habilitation treatment for the mentally retarded is based upon the assumption that such environmental changes will have positive effects upon development, even to the extent in some cases of remediating mental retardation or its effects. It is of interest that in Sweden, where cultural deprivation and malnutrition are virtually nonexistent and all cases of mental retardation are registered, published incidence rates of approximately 0.8 percent are markedly lower than comparable figures in the United States, which vary between 3 and 4 percent (Grunewald, 1975). If criteria for defining mental retardation are comparable to those accepted elsewhere (and they seem to be), there is reason to believe that sociocultural factors are extremely important in producing mental retardation.

Butterfield (1967b) has summarized the literature pertaining to the influence of institutional living upon intellectual and personality development of the mentally retarded. He finds results generally supportive of the thesis that institutionalized mentally retarded persons are less intelligent than comparable groups of mentally retarded living in the community. This finding is based on the assumption that such group differences represent effects of institutional living rather than differences in the groups at time of entrance. Differences in intelligence between institutionalized and noninstitutionalized retarded generally tend to be in verbal areas of intellectual functioning with institutionalized retarded demonstrating generally lower verbal IQ scores.

A detrimental effect of institutional living is also consistent with studies demonstrating intellectual superiorities in short-term as compared with long-term residents of the institution. Some studies indicate that IQ change within institutions may be related to diagnosis on admission. Strauss and Kephart (1939) found that endogenous and psychopathic groups tended to show more IQ gains within the institution than exogenous (brain damaged) groups, who tended to show IQ losses. Mixed groups (both brain damaged and familial factors) tended to fall between these extremes. Rosen et al. (1968) found IQ increments within the institution associated with indigent status and length of time in the institution. Those from poorer homes showed the greatest gains. Since most of the students who were indigent came from poor family backgrounds, the results were consistent with previous studies showing relationships between IQ changes and the type of home in which the individual is reared. Clarke and Clarke (1953, 1954), for example, found that 72 percent of subjects from homes rated "very bad" showed IQ increments of eight points or more within the institution, while only 4 percent showed IQ decrements. There was no difference in increment or decrement in subjects from homes rated "less bad." The Clarkes explain this result as the fading of "intellectual scars" induced by bad home conditions.

These findings have not been supported by other studies (Zigler and Williams, 1963) and, as Butterfield points out, may reflect the detrimental effect of the home rather than the positive effect of the institution.

However, if these results are valid, they indicate that the effect of institutions is more complex than might appear superficially. These results are suggestive of an interaction between the institutional environment and the child's original home environment. Even the worst institution conceivably might be relatively better than some home conditions. The authors are reminded of an incident concerning two mentally retarded parents who were placing their child in a group home when it became clear that they could not care for the child. When the parents agreed to place the child, the father remarked that he hoped it would occur soon because he was planning to purchase a new stereo radio and didn't want the child around to damage the set.

Ideally, a major goal of any special training or habilitation program is to so improve the skills of the trainees that they can live and work with no more assistance than the community customarily provides for its "ordinary" citizens. In the specific case of the institutionalized mentally retarded individual, protection, supervision, and financial support exceed that available in the workaday world of the larger community. So it is natural to ask whether the experience of the sheltered institutional setting affects the individual's adequacy in the performance of purposive activity, including his motivation to achieve and his evaluation of himself as a purposive agent in the situation in which he must operate. It might be predicted, for example, that by providing sheltered and specially structured environments where demands, expectations, standards of performance and competition are minimized, institutions might actually heighten such expectations of achievement in the mentally retarded. The noninstitutionalized retardate, on the other hand, is more frequently exposed to unrealistic demands, failures, and rejections in the community, and may be more likely to evaluate himself more poorly.

Partial support for this position is found in a series of studies comparing institutionalized and noninstitutionalized retarded and normal children in degree of outer-directedness and perseverence in problem-solving tasks (Turnure and Zigler, 1964; Green and Zigler, 1962; Zigler, Hodgden, and Stevenson, 1958). Noninstitutionalized retardates were found to be more compliant than matched institutionalized groups and more distrustful of their own solutions to problems. The authors interpreted these findings on the basis of the more protected institutional environment being more conducive to the development of self-confidence and self-direction.

A study by Rosen, Diggory, and Werlinsky (1966) was consistent with this hypothesis. Using a level of aspiration procedure, the authors found that institutionalized retarded set higher goals, predicted higher performance for themselves, and actually produced more on the task than their noninstitutionalized peers. However, the differences between groups, though statistically significant, were relatively small. A replication of this study (Rosen et al., 1971) used normal mental age and chronological age controls in addition to the two groups of retarded subjects. In addition to trial-by-trial levels of aspiration, predictions of performance, and actual performance measurements on the nut and bolt assembly task, subjects also responded to a self-evaluation questionnaire. Neither the detrimental effects of institutionalization upon personality nor enhanced motivational effects suggested by the original study were apparent. Institutionalized and noninstitutionalized retarded showed more striking similarities than differences and both groups behaved extremely differently than subjects of normal intelligence of the same chronological age. Actual performance and expectancy of success were more closely related to mental age than to IQ. The laboratory measures used in the study were closely associated with global self-evaluation responses for the institutionalized group.

It is clear that, as with effects upon intelligence, the influence of the institution upon personality development is very difficult to determine. Simple black and white generalizations cannot be drawn. Institutions are complex social environments differing in size, degree of freedom, or regimentation afforded, in quality of supervision and leadership (which itself may vary in degree of authoritarian control, punitiveness, benevolence), in physical structure, population, and characteristics of residents, and in degree of community involvement, medical versus educational or habilitation orientation, and numerous other variables. In some institutions the degree of overcrowding, dehumanizing practices, and filth may be so great as to overshadow any positive effects of sheltering upon self-concept.

Butterfield and Zigler (1965) studied two institutions in the same state with identical admission policies. In the first institution, all but the most severely retarded were regarded by staff as potentially capable of discharge to the community. Emphasis was placed on developing individual responsibility rather than on security, punishment, and control. In the second institution, residents were regarded as incapable of returning to the community, and there was a great deal of reliance upon locks, isolation as punishment, and external control. The authors predicted and found a heightened need for social reinforcement in residents of the second institution. Not only do institutions differ from each other, they may also differ internally from one building or program to the next or from one point in time to another. Staff coverage in off hours, on holidays, and weekends may be substantially below normal levels. Turnover in institutional personnel may be very high, particularly for attendant staff. It would be naive to assume that the institution remains constant in its structure. It is equally naive to suppose that effects of institutions upon their inhabitants are constant. What would be the effect upon children of normal intelligence level living at home if parents and family members changed as rapidly as caretakers in institutional residence buildings often do?

The factors mentioned above are the more obvious environmental variables operating within the residential institution. More subtle quality of life dimensions of experience make institutions, and probably other group settings drastically different from home environments. Perhaps these variables are the most insidious, although the likelihood that appropriate investigations of their effect will be conducted in the near future is small. What they amount to can best be described in negative terms, such as the absence of warm concern and involvement of parental or family figures; the absence of variability and enrichment in daily living; the absence of opportunities for choice and decision-making; and a freedom from constraints that may also be operative in family situations but that assume a flavor and rigidity unique to institutional settings. Habilitation specialists who attempt to structure normalized living environments for the mentally retarded have acknowledged these deficiencies, but it is doubtful that these qualities can ever really be achieved in group living situations outside of the home.

Recently, an observational strategy was developed at Elwyn Institute in an attempt to understand better the day-to-day institutional living situations of mentally retarded residents. The casual visitor to the institution observes classroom, training, or residential programs by cross-section. He observes a group with a teacher or supervisor engaged in some activity. Even the long-term staff member is exposed only to a series of cross-sections located in time or by function, e.g., the psychologist sees individuals for psychological testing, the teacher sees a class from 9:00 to 3:00, etc. It is rare that institutional staff focus upon a single child on a longitudinal basis even for one day. It would be unrealistic to expect a busy staff member to do so.

In order to learn more about how institutions operate, an observational procedure was developed for observing individual students during all their waking hours. The procedure required three raters; the first from 6:00 a.m. until noon, the second from noon until 5:00 p.m., the third from 5:00 until 11:00 p.m. Raters carried a clipboard and rating forms and made continuous observations of the student's activities and interactions with people or objects. Observations were recorded in fifteen-minute intervals all day long. These written records were later transcribed. Several students have been observed in this manner. The procedure allows for judgments about the richness or paucity of stimulation for given individuals and allows comparisons between residence buildings or programs. Comparisons between students in the same building or between observations of the same student on different days provide information about the diversity of stimulation within the building.

It is clear that institutional effects upon intelligence and personality have not been definitely established. It is not the authors' purpose here to attack or defend institutions or to challenge the deinstitutionalization decisions that have been prevalent over the past few years. Rather, it is important to point out that such decisions have not been made upon empirical grounds. In many cases they have been necessitated because of the existence of conditions that no one concerned about human dignity would allow to be perpetuated. In other cases good institutional programs and environments may have been unfairly attacked and replaced by less beneficial situations on the basis of the normalization principle. In still other cases, competent attempts have been made to socially engineer adequate living environments, but one wonders whether such attempts have even scratched the surface in establishing environments conducive to healthy or normal development.

Wolfensberger (1971b) has taken the position that institutions should and will fade away. His argument rests upon evidence for declining incidence and prevalence of severe mental retardation as a result of birthrate reduction and greater health care available to high risk groups, increased availability of residential alternatives to the institution, general environmental betterment, and increased availability of early childhood education.

A more moderate view is suggested by Roos (1966). Rather than an end to institutions, Roos sees institutions assuming a new role characterized by a blurring of the demarcation between institution and community, the adoption of specialized demonstration programs within institutions, improvement of training methodologies, such as the use of operant conditioning, greater in-service training for attendant staff, greater reliance on research, and changing roles of the professional to include training and supervision of treatment. However, many would argue, within ten years of hindsight, that Roos' optimism in 1966 thus far has not proven valid, nor have the alternative residential service models offered by Wolfensberger proven to be a great panacea for the future.

LITERATURE CITED

Bensberg, G. J., Colwell, C. N., and Cassel, R. M. 1965. Teaching the profoundly retarded self-help activities by behavior shaping techniques. Amer. J. Ment. Defic. 69:674–679.

Blatt, B. 1969. Purgatory. *In* R. B. Kugel and W. Wolfensberger (eds.), Changing Patterns in Residential Services for the Mentally Retarded, pp. 36–49. President's Committee on Mental Retardation, Washington, D.C.

Blatt, B., and Kaplan, F. 1967. Christmas in Purgatory: A Photographic Essay on Mental Retardation. Allyn & Bacon, Boston.

Bricker, W. A. 1970. Identifying and modifying behavioral deficits. Amer. J. Ment. Defic. 75:16–21.

Butterfield, E. C. 1967*a*. The characteristics, selection, and training of institutional personnel. *In* A. A. Baumeister (ed.), Mental Retardation: Appraisal, Education, and Rehabilitation, pp. 305–328. Aldine Publishing Company, Chicago.

Butterfield, E. C. 1967*b*. The role of environmental factors in the treatment of institutionalized mental retardates. *In* A. A. Baumeister (ed.), Mental Retardation: Appraisal, Education, and Rehabiliation, pp. 120–137. Aldine Publishing Company, Chicago.

Butterfield, E. C. 1969. Basic facts about residential facilities for the mentally retarded. *In* R. B. Kugel and W. Wolfensberger (eds.), Changing Patterns in Residential Services for the Mentally Retarded, pp. 15–33. President's Committee on Mental Retardation, Washington, D.C.

Butterfield, E. C., and Zigler, E. 1965. The influence of differing institutional social climates on the effectiveness of social reinforcement in the mentally retarded. Amer. J. Ment. Defic. 70:48–56.

Clarke, A. D. B., and Clarke, A. M. 1953. How constant is the IQ? Lancet 2:877–880.

Clarke, A. D. B., and Clarke, A. M. 1954. Cognitive changes in the feeble-minded. Brit. J. Psychol. 45:173–179.

Fernald, W. E. 1893. The history of the treatment of the feeble-minded. *In* M. Rosen, G. R. Clark, and M. S. Kivitz (eds.), The History of Mental Retardation: Collected Papers, pp. 321–325. Vol. 1. University Park Press, Baltimore, 1976.

Fleming, J. W. 1962. The critical incident technique as an aid to in-service training. Amer. J. Ment. Defic. 67:41–52.

Giradeau, F. L., and Spradlin, J. E. 1964. Token rewards in a cottage program. Ment. Retard. 2:345–351.

Green, C., and Zigler, E. 1962. Social deprivation and the performance of retarded and normal children on a satiation type task. Child Dev. 33:499–508.

Grunewald, K. 1975. Sweden: services and developments. *In* J. Wortis (ed.), Mental Retardation and Developmental Disabilities, Vol. VII, pp. 313–342. Brunner/Mazel, New York.

Murphy, Rennee, H. B., and Luchins, D. 1972. Foster homes: The new back wards? Monograph Supplement #71, Canada's Mental Health.

McIntire, J. T. 1954. Causes of turnover in personnel. Amer. J. Ment. Defic. 58:375.

Nirje, B. 1969. The normalization principle and its human management implications. *In* R. B. Kugel and W. Wolfensberger (eds.), Changing Patterns in Residential Services for the Mentally Retarded, pp. 179–195. President's Committee on Mental Retardation, Washington, D.C.

Oudenne, W. 1963. Development of a cottage staffing ratio: A result of a practicum method of training for administrative positions. Ment. Retard. 1:371–374.

Parker, G. O. 1951. Attendant nurses for the mentally deficient—some evidence. Amer. J. Ment. Defic. 55:326–336.

President's Committee on Mental Retardation. 1968. Challenge, accomplishment and need. PCMR Message, March.

Roos, P. 1966. Changing roles of the residential institution. Ment. Retard. 4:4–6.

Rosen, M., Diggory, J. C., Floor, L., and Nowakiwska, M. 1971. Self-evaluation, expectancy and performance in the mentally subnormal. J. Ment. Defic. Res. 15:(2):81–95.

Rosen, M., Diggory, J. C., and Werlinsky, B. E. 1966. Goal-setting and expectancy of success in institutionalized and noninstitutionalized mental subnormals. Amer. J. Ment. Defic. 71:249–255.

Rosen, M., Stallings, L., Floor, L., and Nowakiwska, M. 1968. Reliability and stability of Wechsler IQ scores for institutionalized mental subnormals. Amer. J. Ment. Defic. 72:218–225.

Strauss, A. A., and Kephart, N. C. 1939. Role of mental growth in a constant environment among higher grade moron and borderline children. Proceedings of the American Association on Mental Deficiency 44:137–142.

Thormahlen, P. W. 1965. A study of on-the-ward training of trainable mentally retarded children in a state institution. California Mental Health Research Monograph, No. 4. California Department of Mental Hygiene, Bureau of Research and Statistics.

Turnure, J., and Zigler, E. 1964. Outer-directedness in the problem solving of normal and retarded children. J. Abnorm. Psychol. 69:427–436.

White, W. D., and Wolfensberger, W. 1969. The evolution of dehumanization in our institutions. Ment. Retard. 7:5–9.

Wolfensberger, W. 1971*a*. Will there always be an institution? I: The impact of epidemiological trends. Ment. Retard. 9:14–20.

Wolfensberger, W. 1971*b*. Will there always be an institution? II: The impact of new service models. Ment. Retard. 9:31–38.

Zigler, E., Hodgden, L., and Stevenson, H. 1958. The effect of support on the performance of normal and feebleminded children. J. Personal. 26:106–122.

Zigler, E., and Williams, J. 1963. Institutionalization and the effectiveness of social reinforcement: A three year follow-up study. J. Abnorm. Psychol. 66:197–205.

Chapter 8

Beyond Normalization

The principle of normalization, popularized in this country by Nirje (1969), has been described as the aim "to let the mentally retarded obtain an experience as close to the normal as possible," and as "making available to the mentally retarded the patterns and conditions of everyday life which are as close as possible to the norms and patterns of the mainstream of society." Nirje (1969, 1970) has discussed some of the facets and implications of this philosophy as it would apply to all levels of the mentally retarded in a variety of living situations. These include a normal daily rhythm of sleep, meals, and dressing; a normal routine of daily activities, including school or work and leisure time activities; a normal yearly rhythm of holidays, vacations, personal days; normal developmental experiences structured by a few significant adults who are consistent in their lives, and with opportunities for interactions with peers; opportunities for the development of competence in social skills and independence in daily living skills; opportunities to express their own desires and preferences in structuring their lives and making decisions; opportunities for normal sexual development and participation in a bisexual world; normal financial privileges and compensations and the application of normal economic standards; and, in living facilities, application of normal standards, of size, structure, and location, including the opportunities for integration in normal community life.

These various facets of normal living are regarded by proponents of normalization as minimal requisites for the development of a healthy self-regard and a sense of personal identity.

Gunzburg (1973*a)* has published a convenient checklist for evaluating group homes, hospitals, and institutional residential units. The list includes such things as the physical construction of toilets and bathrooms (e.g., whether sinks have mixing valves or separate hot and cold taps, whether mirrors are available), the amount of privacy available, the decor and furnishings, the use of uniforms by staff, access to kitchen appliances by residents, regimentation in movements, opportunity for personal possessions, use of locks on doors, and the amount of supervision or independence available to residents.

While many have seen normalization as desirable in restructuring the existing facilities that serve the mentally retarded or in building social education programs, other have used the principle to challenge the very existence of programs and facilities that have traditionally been associated with the mentally retarded (Wolfensberger, 1971*a,* 1971*b)* and to find new community models for helping the mentally retarded lead nearly normal lives (Wolfensberger, 1972*a;* Sarason, 1969).

No sooner had the normalization definition been popularized than controversy was generated regarding the appropriateness of this principle. The crux of the matter pertains both to the lengths to which one wishes to extend the principle and to how one defines normal. The term normalization can be interpreted in various ways, and, despite attempts by Wolfensberger (1972*b)* and others to clarify the meaning, confusion still exists. Normalization may be interpreted as meaning to make normal, i.e., to make or conform to a standard generally regarded as appropriate or acceptable for the ordinary citizen. Gunzburg (1972) has criticized this as denying real differences between the mentally retarded and other persons where they exist. Throne (1975) has pointed out that the mentally retarded are diagnosed as such specifically because they do not respond to normal conditions of stimulation and because they require special attention in the form of education, training, and habilitation.

Wolfensberger (1972*b)* broadens the definition to ''utilization of means which are as culturally normative as possible in order to establish or maintain personal behaviors and characteristics which are as culturally normative as possible'' (p. 28). This definition seems not to preclude the use of special procedures designed to teach behaviors that approximate the norm or what is typical. It also allows for differences between cultures or subcultures in defining what is normal. For most writers, the term appears to connote modification of behavior away from that which is considered deviant from the mainstream of society to that which is considered more typical. Gold (1975) offers an interesting commentary on the normalization principle. He distinguishes between the teaching of competence, a positive concept, and the elimination of what is deviant, a negative approach. He speculates that the more an individual is perceived by others as competent, the more they will tolerate his deviance. In any event, he believes that normalization should encompass both concepts.

Rosen and Kivitz (1973) have suggested that the principle of normalization has been linked to the acceptance of adaptive behavior as a criterion of functioning of the mentally retarded. While normalization reflects a desire to treat the mentally retarded as normally as possible, adaptive behavior has been offered as a criterion of how well the mentally retarded individual conforms to society's demands for independence and personal responsibility.

The concept of normalization seems a humanitarian, legal, and moral principle. It reflects the desire to afford the mentally handicapped their full measure of legal and human rights. It encompasses the belief, or at least the hope, that greater normalization of the environmental conditions to which the mentally retarded are exposed will have significant repercussions in terms of their personal growth and development and will make them "more normal." It acknowledges that to focus solely on the mentally retarded as individuals can never succeed without changes in the social context in which they function.

Since normalization must be linked to societal definitions, it is basically a statistical concept. What society considers normal (or deviant) can only be defined in relation to a range of behaviors or conditions around a central tendency. The normal or bell-shaped distribution curve depicts the frequency of behaviors that, being more or less frequent, are regarded as more or less normal. In actuality, all behaviors along the bell-shaped curve are normal. Low intelligence is no less frequent than high intelligence, for example. The incidence of a behavior tells us nothing about the functional value of that behavior. Truly adaptive responses may indeed be quite rare.

If we were to accept "normal" (e.g. usual or frequent) behavior as a criterion of what is acceptable adjustment, or acceptable conditions for adjustment, we would also be forced to define adjustment differently from one culture to another. The dilemma of cultural relativism has plagued students of abnormal psychology for generations. The logical resolution of this dilemma is to anchor our criteria of adjustment firmly within the individual rather than in society. The Alaskan chief who communicates with his ancestors is performing a function highly valued by his tribe. Since his delusions have no personal meaning to his own adjustment, they should not be considered pathological. The delusions of the paranoid schizophrenic, on the other hand, are a mechanism for dealing with unacceptable thoughts or impulses. They are considered pathological in any society because they represent an inadequate and unrealistic resolution of internal conflict. Similarly, unless we accept some personal reference of adjustment for the mentally retarded, we will be forced to accept criteria for evaluation and training that may change with the time and the tide.

Normalization, unfortunately, does not speak to the personal attributes of the mentally retarded that are relevant to whether or not they achieve normal levels or modes of behavior. It does not speak to the strategies of training that will be required to teach normal behaviors. Individual differences among retarded as well as between retarded and non-retarded populations must dictate the manner of applying the normalization principle. Adequate selection and training of persons for community living must remain the major emphasis in applying normalizing procedures. Normalization is not a psychological principle, nor can it substitute for broader criteria of functioning than what is considered normal or typical.

As suggested above, the philosophy of normalization has been partially responsible for the incorporation of criteria of adaptive behavior into habilitation programs. The focus has been the teaching of basic coping skills for competence on the job, in the community, or for better functioning within the institution. There is little question that this approach has been productive in shaking off the apathy and pessimism associated with previous conceptions of mental retardation. It has been consistent with the development and utilization of behavior modification techniques for shaping socially desirable behavior or eliminating undesirable behavior (Bensberg, Colwell, and Cossel, 1965; Blackwood, 1962; Gardner, 1971; Giradeau and Spradlin, 1964; Wolf, Risley, and Mees, 1964). Yet it is also possible to challenge the goals associated with normalization, behavior modification, and adaptive behavior as not going far enough. In our fervor for the development of powerful new training strategies, we may have lost sight of basic constructs of emotional health and personal adjustment commonly accepted for intellectually normal populations.

The ability to maintain oneself independently and meet societal demands for responsibility of action are undoubtedly important criteria of functioning. Yet these are minimal demands that represent only the lowest levels of functioning. In the follow-up of mentally retarded persons discharged from the institution to independent arrangements in the community, the authors have encountered many individuals who work steadily, pay their bills, stay out of trouble, are accepted by their neighbors and co-workers, yet are socially withdrawn, lonely, uncomfortable in social situations, frustrated economically, and generally unhappy.

A focus solely upon normalization of the mentally retarded would fail to take into account the many personality, motivational, and emotional variables that may determine daily functioning. Acceptance of normalization, i.e., performance according to a standard that is considered typical, under conditions considered typical, rules out the possibility of training for more positive adjustment.

More recent expositions of normalization are beginning to give recognition to this very issue. Nirje (1973) expands the definition of normalization first stated by Bank Mikkelsen, as follows:

> The application of the normalization principle will not make the subnormal normal, but will make life conditions of the mentally subnormal normal as far as possible bearing in mind the degree of his handicap, his competence and maturity, as well as the need for training activities and availability of services. Thus aims of care and services as well as goals of training—in striving to develop a better adjustment to society—are also part of the normalization principle (p. 30).

Nirje describes the problem of mental subnormality as the result of not one, but three factors: cognitive deficit, including adaptive behavior and learning difficulties; imposed or acquired subnormality as a result of environmental deficiencies, lack of training and educational experiences; and distortions in the self-concept and self-awareness. Efforts at normalization for the mentally retarded can deal directly with only the second factor.

Gunzburg and Gunzburg (1973) have conceptualized normalization as only one aspect of a three-pronged approach toward social habilitation of the mentally retarded. This philosophy is expressed diagrammatically in the form of a triangle, with the three components "personalization," "socialization," and "normalization" forming the apices:

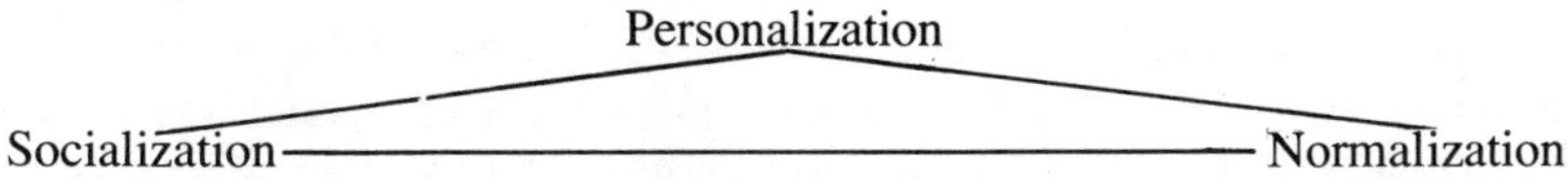

Personalization

Socialization —— Normalization

Socialization is defined as the acquisition of skills that enable the mentally handicapped to participate more fully in life situations. Socialization is the aim of social education in areas such as table habits, cooking, budgeting, and other life management skills. Normalization is required to make the process of socialization more effective by environmental structuring. Personalization refers to the development of the mentally retarded individual as a personality, including the expression of individual tastes, desires, choices, and decisions. The authors point out that the mentally handicapped individual must learn to be himself, in addition to conforming to the requirements of his own community. They see the principle of personalization as a safeguard on normalization by acknowledging that not all aspects of a normal environment are necessarily beneficial to the socialization of the mentally handicapped. While Gunzburg himself has provided invaluable material pertaining to the structuring of social education and socialization programs, and numerous guidelines now exist for creating normalizing environments, particularly in hospital and institutional settings (Gunzburg, 1973*b*), there still exists only scanty information regarding the development of personalization programs. Later chapters of this text attempt to deal with this area while the remainder of this chapter is reserved for a brief mention of the directions such thinking must take.

The search for criteria of adjustment that go ''beyond normalization'' is an area in which little has been done. Theoretical conceptualizations are scarce and empirical research is almost completely nonexistent. It is of interest that criteria for defining adjustment within intellectually normal populations are seldom applied to the mentally retarded. Even those investigations of social and personality variables for the mentally retarded population that are available have generally been attempts to validate theoretical positions rather than to develop useable criteria of functioning in evaluating or planning for mentally retarded persons. Bialer's (1967) suggestion, for example, that the mentally retarded may have trouble shifting from an external to an internal locus of control has interesting clinical implications, yet the locus of control measure has not been used in helping to decide whether or not a mentally retarded person is ready for independent living.

This chapter searches for more positive concepts of personal adjustment, first in the mental hygiene literature for normal populations, then in the research literature dealing with personality and emotional characteristics of the retarded.

Most introductory and abnormal psychology texts (Coleman, 1964; Hilgard, 1971; Krech and Crutchfield, 1970; Morgan, 1971) describe adjustment in roughly similar terms, i.e., as a dynamic process. Adjustment is a reaction to conflict between motives or roles or a reaction to frustration, threat, or stress. Aggressive behavior, anxiety, defense mechanisms, productive problem-solving, neurosis, and psychosis are all cited as possible adjustment or maladjustment reactions. While such processes are probably more difficult to measure and evaluate in the intellectually subnormal, accepted criteria should be flexible enough to encompass the total range of adjustment reactions for this population as well.

Mental hygienists have distinguished between the ''normal'' or modal personality and the healthy personality. Freud defined mental health as consisting of the ability to love and to do productive work, and implied a harmony among the separate conflicting components of personality. Neo-Freudians have defined health as a social feeling (Adler), the attainment of selfhood with a unique purpose or meaning for one's existence (Jung), individuality and creativity (Rank), and accurate, realistic perceptions of other people (Sullivan).

Shaffer and Shoben (1956) describe a maladjusted person as "impulsive, and lacking in foresight and self-control. He cannot persist in tasks and becomes fatigued too readily. He is unable or unwilling to endure personal discomfort in order to meet social expectations. He reacts poorly to stress, and shows decrements of performance when subjected to frustrations and conflicts" (p. 359). According to many authoritative sources, these characteristics would easily pass as a depiction of the mentally retarded personality.

Maslow (1954) used the term self-actualization to define what he considered to be the highest need that man can develop. Once the individual has satisfied physical, safety, love, and esteem needs, he is free to devote his energies to some cause outside the self, such as the quest for beauty, truth, or justice. Among the traits Maslow described in self-actualizing people were such attributes as problem-centeredness, a strong ethical sense, an unhostile sense of humor, and a high degree of self-acceptance.

A comprehensive review of conceptions of the "healthy personality" has been provided by Jourard (1963). A healthy person is one who has adequately coped with his basic needs and is therefore able to set goals and find challenges in problems beyond basic need fulfillment. He is characterized by a relative absence of anxious self-consciousness and by an interest in goals beyond security, love, status, or recognition. He has an efficient contact with reality, undistorted by emotion and need-tensions. He has the freedom to express feeling and the capacity to control emotional expression. He accurately perceives his own bodily structure and capacities and can accept them. He holds a set of beliefs and attitudes that are congruent with his "real self." His defensive structure is not so rigid that it produces compulsive patterns of conduct or distortions in self-perception. His behavior is congruent with social mores, yet he is free of unremitting guilt. He has sufficient interpersonal competence to attain gratification from other people. He is capable of feeling concern for other people and of being interested in the subjective and personal aspects of their lives. He has the ability to identify with a loved one and to accept love from others. He is capable of sexual arousal, has an accepting attitude towards sex, and is able to integrate his sexuality with his overall value system.

Despite their generality, Jourard's criteria of a healthy personality are rarely, if ever, attributed, no less applied, to the mentally retarded. Quite the contrary, descriptive accounts of the personalities of the mentally handicapped have indicated basic conflicts in many of the areas described by Jourard. Cromwell (1963) predicts that retarded persons will have a lower generalized expectancy for success than normals and a higher tendency toward avoidance behavior as a result of having had fewer successes in past situations. This is substantiated by studies demonstrating differential effects, in normal and retarded subjects, of failure in experimental situations (Gardner, 1958; Heber, 1957).

Bialer reports that mentally retarded persons are developmentally delayed in learning to shift the locus of control from external to internal, i.e., to attribute the outcomes of certain goal-directed behaviors to personal success and failure. The mature child can conceive of an unfavorable outcome as being caused by his own shortcomings and is thus able to construe it as failure. Zigler (1966) has predicted and found decrements in performance in the retarded to be a function of reduced social stimulation. Zigler interprets the results of his studies (Green and Zigler, 1962; Turner and Zigler, 1964; Zigler, Hodgden, and Stevenson, 1958) as indicating that retardates are distrustful of their own solutions to problems and are more outer-directed in their problem-solving than are normals of the same mental age. The greater outer-directedness of retardates is viewed as an outgrowth of their higher incidence of failure experiences.

Criteria of personal adjustment have been applied to the mentally retarded by those who have attempted to apply psychotherapeutic methods to the amelioration of their emotional or behavioral problems. Bialer (1967) defines three major goals of workers who direct psychotherapeutic efforts toward the mentally retarded: IQ change, emotional or behavioral adjustment, and milieu (or environmental) modification. He contends that some children diagnosed as defective are capable of making significant improvements in IQ following psychotherapy, but tends to view emotional or behavioral adjustment as the more relevant criterion of psychotherapeutic success.

Attempting to relate psychotherapeutic outcome with predetermined goals, Sternlicht (1966) presents a prognostic-etiological model for the psychological treatment of mental retardation. This model is based on the assumption that psychotherapeutic goals must take into account the etiology of the mental retardation for a particular individual. Thus, if IQ elevation is the goal, psychotherapy is indicated when the etiology is "primary emotional maladjustment," but not when etiology is related to neurological deficit or severe cultural deprivation. If the goal is improved adaptive behavior, on the other hand, psychotherapy is indicated when etiology is emotional disturbance or a secondary emotional reaction to existing intellectual deficits.

Leland and Smith (1965) have developed a play therapy procedure designed to increase self-recognition, to promote an understanding that impulses can be controlled, and to teach children to live within social boundaries. Shadow therapy (Robertson, 1964) was designed to facilitate therapeutic communication and to foster the integration of a severely disturbed child's fantasy life with reality.

While psychotherapeutic models do incorporate personal adjustment variables as outcome criteria, such approaches often fail to acknowledge the special needs and specific situations of stress of a retarded population. Just what should we mean when we describe a mentally retarded adult as well adjusted? That he stays out of jail or an institution? That he lives in the institution but does as he is told? That he has a job? That he marries? That he accepts responsibility for his own actions? That he reacts to frustration in a nonaggressive manner? It seems easier to define poor adjustment. It is, therefore, easily understandable that psychologists have so readily settled for adaptive behavior as an objective criterion of functioning.

Follow-up studies of mentally subnormal persons returned to independent community living have been consistent in reporting favorable community social and vocational adjustments (Clark, Kivitz, and Rosen, 1968; Fernald, 1910; Floor et al., 1975; Hegge, 1944; Windle, 1962; Wolfson, 1956). Studies at Elwyn Institute have likewise been generally positive in reporting successful community adjustment utilizing, however, only minimal criteria. Within the last ten years, approximately 250 persons have left Elwyn to return to independent living situations. To the degree that these persons have managed to maintain themselves in the community, remain employed, stay out of trouble with the law, and remain off welfare rosters, they have adjusted and the normalization effort has been successful. However, like other persons of their socioeconomic level, social adjustment has often been sporadic and marginal. Persons have lost jobs, illegitimacies have occurred. Individuals have been evicted from their living quarters. Persons have been exploited, both sexually and financially (Floor et al., 1971). There has been dissatisfaction with salary levels and low status positions (Rosen et al., 1970).

If we wish to define personal adjustment from the standpoint of the handicapped, it would seem essential to give cognizance to our collective clinical experiences with such individuals. This includes experience with the mentally handicapped living within institutions, with those in sheltered workshops and group living situations in the community, with those in special education classes, and finally, with the results of empirical studies of the personality and behavior of the mentally retarded. If the constructs that arise out of such a framework resemble those that have been developed for nonhandicapped populations, then we need not look further. This is unlikely, however. The acceptance of specific, concrete, and realistic criteria of adjustment would facilitate therapy, education, and training by making goals more explicit.

The available literature reveals seven dimensions of personal adjustment that would need to be considered:

1) Self-concept—Ideally, the adjusted retarded person has a recognition of his learning problems as well as an awareness of the limitations they impose for a specific set of learning-related behaviors. On the other hand, he also recognizes that other areas concerning his self-esteem are not contingent upon his learning deficits. He has the ability to set realistic goals, i.e., to strive for something somewhat above what can be inferred from his past experience, yet not so high that the goal is unattainable. The goals that he sets for himself do not exceed his ability to understand them. More important, however, he does not feel compromised in accepting realistic goals. He is aware of himself as having certain handicaps but does not react to those handicaps so as to afford them an all-encompassing place in his self-image. Once he has accepted goals that are reasonable and feasible for himself, he is able to view himself as possessing the necessary capacities for achieving those goals, either the required skills or the potential for achieving those skills. He has a keen sense of his own individuality and sees himself as responsible for his own behavior and achievement. He believes himself to be a whole person and basically a worthwhile person despite his handicap. Because of his belief in his own value as an individual, he is able to resist attempts at exploitation or coercion. He accepts his handicap as one of many attributes, without overemphasizing its significance.
2) Independence — The adjusted personality has an orientation to life in which he accepts responsibility for his own achievement, gratification, successes, and failures. He is willing to assume the burden of his own destiny and to be ultimately accountable for his successes and failures. He is motivated and able to take action when the circumstances warrant it. Although his actions may not always be maximally effective, he is motivated to keep trying. In Bialer's terms, he has assured an internal locus of control. Even in a dependent position, at home or within an institution, a retarded person has options and may assume an independent orientation to life.
3) Reality Testing — The adjusted personality has developed a perception of reality that is sufficient to make him aware of behavior considered the norm by society. He is likewise able to monitor his own behavior according to the norm. He is sensitive to and can utilize social feedback

as a behavioral guideline. If he demonstrates inappropriate behaviors that he cannot control, he is at least aware that his behavior is deviant.

4) Emotional Development — The adjusted personality is able to express appropriate affect when the situation demands, or to control it when it is inappropriate. He is capable of a full range of emotional expression. His expressions are neither excessive, effusive, nor blunted. He should be capable of expressing positive feeling as well as anger. His reality testing should be sufficient to discern when to express and when to control his feelings.
5) Goal-directed Behavior — The adjusted personality demonstrates a purpose of striving toward some goal such as an occupational choice. He demonstrates a sufficient degree of motivation to move consistently toward that goal, even when rewards are distant. He can visualize his goal and project himself as successful in attaining it. He shows perseverance in pursuing such goals. This pertains to vocational and personal-social goals.
6) Interpersonal Relationships — The adjusted personality has a capacity to assume a role required for successful interpersonal relationships, especially in those casual, day-to-day relationships of work and community living. He has the flexibility to participate in give-and-take cooperative ventures. He can empathize with others and express interest in their personal problems. He can divorce himself from an exclusive focus upon his own problems. He feels a need for frequent and varied social contacts and is able to gratify this need.
7) Sexual Development — The adjusted personality is capable of appropriate heterosexual relationships. He has a sufficient degree of information and coping skills that he can perform adequately in both casual and intense sexual relationships without anxiety or guilt. Although there may be gaps in his sexual information and knowledge, expecially with regard to anatomical and physiological aspects of sex, he has a behavioral repertoire that is sufficient to allow him a full range of sexual responses. He also demonstrates an adequate degree of knowledge of the consequences of sexual behaviors so as to allow him to behave responsibly and with an appropriate degree of planning, foresight, or precaution.

It is likely that these attributes will be amended. It is to be hoped that evaluative techniques for assessing such personality constructs can be developed, and a more enthusiastic attempt will be made to apply positive mental health constructs in evaluating mentally retarded persons in terms of their capabilities for handling normalizing experiences.

LITERATURE CITED

Bensberg, G. J., Colwell, C. N., and Cossel, R. H. 1965. Teaching the profoundly retarded self-help activities by behavior-shaping techniques. Amer. J. Ment. Defic. 69:674–679.

Bialer, I. 1967. Psychotherapy and other adjustment techniques with the mentally retarded. *In* A. A. Baumeister (ed.), Mental Retardation: Appraisal, Education and Rehabilitation. Aldine Publishing Company, Chicago.

Blackwood, R. O. 1962. Operant conditioning as a method of training the mentally retarded. University Microfilms, Ann Arbor, Michigan.

Clark, G. R., Kivitz, M. S., and Rosen, M. 1968. A transitional program for institutionalized adult retarded, VRA Project No. 1275P, U.S. Department of Health, Education, and Welfare, Washington, D. C.

Coleman, J. C. 1964. Abnormal Psychology and Modern Life. Scott, Foresman & Company, Chicago.

Cromwell, R. L. 1963. A social learning approach to mental retardation. *In* N. R. Ellis (ed.), Handbook of Mental Deficiency, pp. 41–91. McGraw-Hill Book Company, New York.

Fernald, W. E. 1919. After-care study of the patients discharged from Waverly for a period of twenty-five years. Ungraded 5:25–31.

Floor, L., Baxter, D., Rosen, M., and Zisfein, L. 1975. A survey of marriages among previously institutionalized retardates. Ment. Retard. 13:33–37.

Floor, L., Rosen, M., Baxter, D., Horowitz, J., and Weber, C. 1971. Socio-sexual problems in mentally subnormal females. Train. Sch. Bull. 68:106–112.

Gardner, W. I. 1958. Reactions of intellectually normal and retarded boys after experimentally induced failure—a social learning interpretation. University Microfilms, Ann Arbor, Michigan.

Gardner, W. I. 1971. Behavior Modification in Mental Retardation: The Education and Rehabilitation of the Mentally Retarded Adolescent and Adult. Aldine Publishing Company, Chicago.

Giradeau, F. L., and Spradlin, J. E. 1964. Token rewards in a cottage program. Ment. Retard. 2:345–351.

Gold, M. W. 1975. Vocational training. *In* J. Wortis (ed.), Mental Retardation and Developmental Disabilities VII, pp. 254–264. Brunner/Mazel, New York.

Green, C., and Zigler, E. 1962. Social deprivation and the performance of retarded and normal children in a satiation type task. Child Dev. 33:499–508.

Gunzburg, H. C. 1972. (Editorial). Brit. J. Ment. Subnormal. 28(2):63–65.

Gunzburg, H. C. 1973*a*. The physical environment of the mentally handicapped VIII. 39 steps leading towards normalized living practices in living units for the mentally handicapped. Brit. J. Ment. Subnormal. 37(XIX, 2):91–99.

Gunzburg, H. C. 1973*b*. The hospital as a normalizing training environment. *In* H. C. Gunzburg (ed.), Advances in the Care of the Mentally Handicapped, pp. 47–60. Bailliére, Tindall & Cox Ltd., London.

Gunzburg, H. C., and Gunzburg, A. L. 1973. Mental Handicap and Physical Environment. Bailliére, Tindall & Cox Ltd., London.

Heber, R. F. 1957. Expectancy and expectancy changes in normal and mentally retarded boys. University Microfilms, Ann Arbor, Michigan.

Hegge, T. G. 1944. The occupational status of higher-grade mental defectives in the present emergency. A study of parolees from the Wayne County Training School at Northville, Michigan. Amer. J. Ment. Defic. 49:86–98.

Hilgard, E. R. 1971. Introduction to Psychology. Harcourt, Brace & Co., New York.

Joint Commission on Accreditation of Hospitals. 1971. Standards for residential facilities for the mentally retarded. JCAH, Chicago.

Jourard, S. M. 1963. Personal Adjustment: An Approach Through the Study of Healthy Personality. 2nd Ed. The Macmillan Company, New York.

Krech, D., and Crutchfield, R. S. 1970. Elements of Psychology. Alfred A. Knopf Inc., New York.

Leland, H., and Smith, D. 1965. Play Therapy with Mentally Subnormal Children. Grune & Stratton Inc., New York.

Maslow, A. H. 1954. Motivation and Personality. Harper & Row, New York.

Morgan, C. T. 1971. Introduction to Psychology. McGraw-Hill Book Company, New York.

Nirje, B. 1969. The normalization principle and its human management implications. *In* R. B. Kugel and W. Wolfensberger (eds.), Changing Patterns in Residential Services for the Mentally Retarded, pp. 179–195. President's Committee on Mental Retardation, Washington, D. C.

Nirje, B. 1970. The normalization principle—implications and comments. J. Ment. Subnormal., XVI, 31:62–70.

Nirje, B. 1973. The normalization principle—implications and comments. *In* H. C. Gunzburg (ed.), Advances in the Care of the Mentally Handicapped, pp. 29–38. Bailliére, Tindall & Cox Ltd., London.

Robertson, M. F. 1964. Shadow therapy. Ment. Retard. 2:219–223.

Rosen, M., Halenda, R., Nowakiwska, M., and Floor, L. 1970. Employment satisfaction of previously institutionalized mentally subnormal workers. Ment. Retard. 8:35–40.

Rosen, M., and Kivitz, M. S. 1973. Beyond normalization: Psychological adjustment. Brit. J. Ment. Subnormal. 19:64–70.

Sarason, S. B. 1969. The creation of settings. *In* R. B. Kugel and W. Wolfensberger (eds.), Changing Patterns in Residential Services for the Mentally Retarded, pp. 341–357. President's Committee on Mental Retardation, Washington, D.C.

Shaffer, L. F., and Shoben, E. J. 1956. The Psychology of Adjustment: A Dynamic and Experimental Approach to Personality and Mental Hygiene. Houghton Mifflin Company, Boston.

Sternlicht, M. 1966. Psychotherapeutic procedures with the retarded. *In* N. R. Ellis (ed.), International Review of Research in Mental Retardation, pp. 279–354. Vol. 2. Academic Press, New York.

Throne, J. M. 1975. Normalization through the normalization principle. Ment. Retard. 13:23–25.

Turner, J., and Zigler, E. 1964. Outer-directedness in the problem solving of normal and retarded children. J. Abnorm. Psychol. 69:427–436.

Windle, C. 1962. Prognosis of mental subnormals. Monograph Supplement to the American Journal of Mental Deficiency 66, No. 5.

Wolf, M., Risley, T., and Mees, H. 1964. Application of operant conditioning procedures to the behavior problems of an autistic child. Behav. Res. Ther. 1:305–312.

Wolfensberger, W. 1971*a*. Will there always be an institution? I: The impact of epidemiological trends. Ment. Retard. 9:14–20.

Wolfensberger, W. 1971*b*. Will there always be an institution? II: The impact of new service models. Ment. Retard. 9:31–38.

Wolfensberger, W. 1972*a*. Citizen advocacy for the handicapped, impaired, and disadvantaged. President's Committee on Mental Retardation, Washington, D.C.

Wolfensberger, W. 1972*b*. Normalization. National Institute on Mental Retardation, 1972, Toronto.

Wolfson, N. 1956. Follow-up study of 92 male and 121 female patients who were discharged from Newark State School in 1946. Amer. J. Ment. Defic. 61:224–238.

Zigler, E. 1966. Motivational determinants in the performance of retarded children. Amer. J. Orthopsychiatry 36:848–856.

Zigler, E., Hodgden, T., and Stevenson, H. 1958. The effect of support on the performance of normal and feebleminded children. J. Pers. 26:106–122.

Section IV

Community Adjustment of the Mentally Retarded

Chapter 9

Follow-up Studies and Their Implications

Follow-up studies of previously diagnosed mental retardates living in the community have been performed by many investigators and have dealt with formerly institutionalized individuals as well as with graduates of special schools or special classes in the public schools. These studies can be divided into those with prognostic intent (discussed in Chapter 11) and those designed to investigate the general adjustment of mentally subnormal persons after a period of time in the community. This type of purely descriptive study is the concern of this chapter. The findings of such studies have been reviewed in several sources (Eagle, 1967; Goldstein, 1964; McCarver and Craig, 1974; Tizard, 1958) and are well known. While a number of follow-up studies are described here, our main purpose is to study the implications of such studies in understanding the adjustment of the mentally retarded living in community situations and in planning future directions for programs and research.

POST-INSTITUTIONAL STUDIES

The earliest recorded follow-up study was performed by Walter E. Fernald in 1919, and is considered a classic in the establishment of procedures that have been used, with some variations, in succeeding studies.

Early in 1916 a letter was sent to friends and families of all patients discharged from Waverly State School in Massachusetts during the twenty-five years between 1890–1914. The letter, which requested information about the present status of these former pupils, stressed the fact that such information would be helpful in programing for present residents of the institution.

Information was gathered by a social worker who visited former patients' families, pastors, local officials and agencies, and the police with the aim of learning "all we can of our former pupils—whether they are now living, where they are now living, how they have occupied themselves, whether they have been useful and helpful at home, or are able to wholly or partially support themselves by work at home, or for wages, whether they have been able to look out for themselves, their problems, trials, experiences, etc." (Fernald, 1919, p. 2).

Of the 1,537 patients discharged from Waverly over the twenty-five year period, the community histories of 646, 470 males and 176 females, could be obtained. Of these, 78 had died and 101 had been readmitted to the school. Of the remainder, the majority had left Waverly either by running away or being discharged under administrative protest. In short, they were not a group about which the institution was optimistic in terms of their potential for leading well adjusted lives in the community.

Fernald was surprised, therefore, to find that many of these persons were leading "useful and blameless lives." A few were living independently and were self-supporting, while many others lived with their relatives under fairly close supervision. Many persons were either earning wages in the community or were doing useful work in their homes. While an appreciable number had been arrested, and some had been sentenced to penal institutions, the majority of both males and females "constituted no serious menace to the community at the time of the investigation." The persons who were successful in terms of employment, as well as in avoiding arrest for antisocial behaviors, were most frequently aided or counseled by friends and relatives. The 26 percent who had records of sexual offenses, alcoholism, or theft were more likely to be living without friends or relatives to supervise them.

Fernald found what was, to him,

> . . . a surprisingly small amount of criminality and sex offense, and especially of illegitimacy. . . . The survey shows that there are bad defectives and good defectives. It also shows that even some apparently bad do 'settle down. . . .' And it shows much justice with the plea of the well-behaved adult defective to be given a 'trial outside,' for apparently a few defectives do not need or deserve lifelong segregation. It is most important that the limited facilities for segregation should be used for the many who can be protected in no other way.

Fernald's study was important both in terms of the methodology it introduced, and also in its administrative implications. It was performed at a time when many mentally retarded were considered to be "moral imbeciles,'' prone to criminal tendencies, and a potential danger to the community. In his review of social and occupational adjustment, Goldstein (1964) points out, ''The results of this study were diametrically opposed to the commonly held expectations of administrators, including Fernald'' (p. 222). Davies (1930) indicates that Fernald hesitated for two years before publishing the results of this study because they seemed so much at variance with the then accepted theories dealing with mental deficiency.

Fernald's results are widely interpreted today as supportive of deinstitutionalization policies. ''If some mentally retarded persons, with serious records of misbehavior who have been discharged from the institution under protest of the administration can make adequate adjustment to their communities despite minimal training, chance placement, and chance supervision, what might be expected of those who receive relevant training, selective placement, and supportive supervision?'' (Goldstein, 1964).

Fernald's study inspired others to pursue similar follow-up investigations. In general, these studies have utilized such criteria of community ''success'' or ''failure'' as employment, avoidance of arrest or antisocial behavior, and ability to remain out of an institution of any sort. Typical of the earlier studies of previously institutionalized retardates are those by Hegge (1944), Coakley (1945), Wardell (1946), Wolfson (1956), and Windle, Stewart, and Brown (1961). These illustrative studies are briefly summarized below in terms of their major findings.

Hegge reported on 177 formerly institutionalized parolees whose average age was 17, and whose average IQ was 71.8 (with a range of 50 to 96). Eighty-eight percent of these persons were employed. Since this study was conducted during the war years, most males were in the service or working in defense plants. Women tended to be working in their own homes, although many had civilian jobs. Hegge concluded that these persons would be employable under normal conditions and not merely in a ''stop-gap'' situation. Many were working above the unskilled level and had been capable of finding their jobs independently.

In a similar study, Coakley investigated the adjustment of 37 formerly institutionalized retarded persons placed in the community because of the manpower shortage in World War II. The sample ranged in age from 20 to 46, with an IQ range of 40 to 75. Most of these persons obtained their jobs independently or through the U.S. Employment Service.

In Wardell's study, groups of male inmates of Sonoma State Home were placed in jobs in a community hospital. They were placed in groups to provide a ''community within a community'' feeling and to facilitate supervision. Eighty percent were reported to have made ''an adequate social and occupational adjustment.''

Wolfson was able to locate 89 males and 119 females discharged from Newark State School during 1946. His data were obtained through correspondence with families and employers and through social agencies that had contact with these subjects. Using a four-point scale that combined both social and vocational adjustment, Wolfson found that 62 percent of the 59 mildly retarded males made "a continuous satisfactory social and economic adjustment in the community." Of the 99 mildly retarded females, 73 percent made a satisfactory adjustment.

Windle et al. studied three groups of patients released from Pacific State Hospital on different types of leave: vocational placement, home placement, and family-care placement. Each person was followed for a four-year period, and reasons for community failure were analyzed. Failure was defined as return to the hospital. The authors found that persons on vocational leave failed most often because of inadequate work performance and inadequate interpersonal relations. Persons on home leave failed mainly for antisocial behavior; those placed in family care failed because of lack of environmental support or because of intolerable behavior. However, while the reasons for failures differed, the percentages of failure were about the same—50 percent—for all three groups.

These represent but a few of the many follow-up studies that have been conducted on previously institutionalized retardates. It is obvious from this review that the interpretation of "success" and "failure" depends not only on the investigator's choice of criteria, but also on his individual value or moral judgments about what to accept as a high or low success ratio. Eagle (1967) summarizes 36 publications since 1941 for a total of 7,436 releases from state institutions. These include vocational placements, family care, independent living, and a combination of these placements. By adding the total number of successful and unsuccessful outcomes of these reports, he found, "an agonizingly high failure record of 39.6 percent for these releases." He continues,

> If we confine ourselves solely to those papers published from 1960 to present—on the assumption that the placement process has benefitted within recent years from new developments in the various disciplines involved—we find that the overall placement failure rate from the 1,830 releases reported in 11 publications during this period proves to be 52 percent. This is considerably higher than the failure rate (36.9 percent) for the total literature sample for the past twenty-five years (pp. 239–240).

It should be emphasized, however, that in making these remarks Eagle based his conclusions on a very broad spectrum of criteria, including antisocial actions, undesirable personal conduct, personality problems, unsatisfactory work, health problems, voluntary return to the institution, adverse environmental factors, and transfer to other facilities. Other investigators, using narrower criteria to define "adjustment" would doubtless come out with a much lower failure rate.

Thus, the absence of uniform and consistent criteria from study to study, differences in the samples being followed, in the type of community placement, the length of time in the community, and the economic conditions during the years studied make comparison of the various follow-up investigations quite difficult. The conclusion of Goldstein (1964) that "...the majority of higher grade mentally retarded inmates of public institutions will make a relatively successful adjustment in the communities when training, selection, placement, and supervision are all at an optimum" probably represents the collective attitude of most workers with the retarded. However, none of the studies has adequately dealt with the question of how to evaluate success or failure rates. While Eagle finds 39.6 percent failure "agonizingly high," we have already noted that Fernald found 24–35 percent failure so low that he hesitated to report his results for two years. Furthermore, the effect of deinstitutionalization, particularly of the higher-functioning mentally retarded, may have so changed the composition of institutions that Goldstein's conclusion may be no longer valid. The higher grade mentally retarded within institutions today may not be the same type of individual within the 1964 institutions. None of the studies reviewed has dealt specifically with the impact of the community as it affects the mentally retarded graduate of the institution.

The monumental study of Edgerton (1967) addresses this problem. Edgerton intensively studied 53 persons who had graduated from the training and habilitation programs of Pacific State Hospital. All were diagnosed as mildly retarded and were considered to have social competence and emotional stability. Their ages ranged from 20 to 75 with a mean of 34; mean IQ of the group was 65. The average stay in the institution was 20 years. Data were collected by personal interviews as well as interviews with friends, relatives, and employers of the ex-patients. A total of 17 hours was spent per each respondent in seeking detailed information on factors such as housing, employment, interpersonal relations, sex, marriage and parenthood, spare time activities, self-perceptions, and practical problems of maintaining oneself in the community. The aim was to present detailed portraits of these individuals with particular emphasis being placed on reactions to the stigma associated with retardation. In general, Edgerton found that subjects were coping with the community but spent their lives trying to conceal the stigma of retardation and incompetence, which never can truly be hidden.

Edgerton found that the central concerns of his population were making a living, management of sex, marriage, and reproduction, and utilization of leisure time activity. He described various mechanisms of "passing" and "denial" by which subjects attempted to appear normal. Subjects spent their lives, Edgerton maintained, attempting to avoid revealing their past to others and to avoid confirmation of their incompetence to themselves. Often they acquired normally intelligent "benefactors" in the community who knew about their past and entered into a "benevolent conspiracy" to help them conceal their secret and assist them in coping with the community. Edgerton's description of the thin and transparent "cloak of competence" of the mentally retarded has been influential in shaping professional attitudes toward the potential of the mentally retarded for independent community living.

Recently, Edgerton published a follow-up study of 30 of the original subjects who were reinterviewed twelve years later (Edgerton and Bercovici, 1976). When compared with the original criteria of social competence and independence, some of the subjects proved to have improved their level of adjustment, some had stayed the same, and some had gotten worse. The authors found they could not predict from their original data who would improve and who would deteriorate. He found that the lives of the subjects underwent major fluctuations from year to year and often from month to month. In contrast to his earlier findings, Edgerton concludes that after longer time periods in the community, his subjects were less stigmatized by their retardation. They appeared less concerned about deceiving themselves or others. Despite the fact that they were older and less employable, they showed less reliance upon benefactors. While the incidence of unemployment was higher, quality of life was heightened. The subjects appeared more occupied with things other than work. Recreation, hobbies, friends, and family rendered their lives more varied and pleasurable. Their increased gratification with life was not a function of employment; subjects regarded themselves as normal despite their vocational failures.

The authors draw several important conclusions from these findings. The variability in adjustment that subjects demonstrated over time is interpreted as being related to the absence of reliable resources in periods of emergency or stress. While normally intelligent populations can fall back upon savings, insurance, or family ties to stabilize them, the retarded citizen is less well able to deal with the loss of a job, spouse, or benefactor, and such occurrences make larger changes in their lives. Edgerton's willingness to change drastically his thesis from the generality of incompetence to a greater appreciation of quality of life dimensions is significant. He points out that adjustment criteria are complex and multidimensional. He is willing to admit a discrepancy between how professionals define adjustment and how the mentally retarded define it. He indicates that competence is less important than individual confidence and that independence as a criterion of success may pale alongside a subjective sense of well being. Whether these changes are a result of increased time spent within independent living arrangements in the community or whether they reflect more general changes in society and the demands of all workers for improved quality of life is difficult to determine because the authors' findings are largely subjective judgments derived from their interviews. It is of interest that Edgerton's suggestion for greater concern of professionals in mental retardation with the more subjective side of life is precisely what the present volume is attempting to explore.

STUDIES OF NONINSTITUTIONALIZED RETARDATES

The previous reflections have been based on a series of follow-up studies on formerly institutionalized persons. Other studies have been performed dealing with subjects who have been identified as retarded by community agencies or the public schools but who have not been institutionalized.

While a number of studies of this population have been conducted, a few stand out because of the rigor and sophistication of their research designs. These include studies by Fairbanks (1933), Baller (1936), Muench (1944), Kennedy (1948, 1966), Charles (1953), Dinger (1961), Miller (1965), and Baller, Charles, and Miller (1967) that have been reviewed in various sources. Again, our concern here is with the later studies, or those that were recently repeated with the original populations.

The study by Dinger assessed the adjustment made by 333 former pupils of classes for the educable retarded in Altoona, Pennsylvania. In reporting his study, Dinger states that the "atmosphere of negativism and hopelessness" surrounding the retarded in the minds of the public has inhibited educational progress. He asserts that his study "has been planned to determine which *positive adjustments can* and *are* being made by former pupils of classes for the educable retarded and thus set forth some modern goals for educators of retarded children" (p. 353). Approximately 13 percent of the persons studied were unemployed, 59 percent employed, and 22 percent were full-time housewives. IQs ranged from 50 to 85. Clients were interviewed in their homes so that the family living conditions could be observed and biographical information obtained. Employers were also visited and asked to perform a job analysis of positions held by employed clients.

Sixty-five percent of the eligible males had served in the armed forces, where, as a group, they had achieved promotions, been assigned responsible duties, and had experiences in foreign service and combat. In general, their contributions and experiences were similar to that of most "normal" personnel.

Those persons who were working at the time of the study had jobs that were primarily unskilled. Wages ranged from $365 to $7,800 annually, with a mean of $3,327 (1958).

Fifty-five percent of the group were married, and divorces had occurred in only 3 percent of the sample. Most clients had married persons who were better educated than themselves. The mean IQ of the spouses was 95. A total of 79 children had been born to these couples at the time of the study. Of the school-age children the majority had IQs higher than their parents.

None of the group was on public welfare, and 82 percent were entirely self-supporting. Fifty-one percent had savings accounts, 73 percent had charge accounts, 84 percent had life insurance, 73 percent carried medical insurance, and 24 percent had checking accounts.

Thirty-four percent had voted in the last election, and 86 percent belonged to a church. However, only 25 percent belonged to any social group or formal activity such as a club, team, or lodge. Most used their leisure time for family-type activities or visiting with friends.

Dinger concludes that adult retardates are capable of successful adjustment in unskilled jobs and, as determined by previous investigators, that intelligence is not a major criterion of job success. He adds that the results of this study justify the effectiveness of the training curriculum that had been offered in the school district to educable retarded pupils, and that periodic modifications of the program would be made based on needs revealed by similar follow-up analyses. Since no effort was made to relate the training curriculum to community outcomes, the latter conclusion appears unjustified.

The investigations of Baller and Kennedy differ from the others in that the retarded groups were compared with normal controls. All subjects originally identified by Baller have been followed in later years by Charles and Miller, and again by Baller in the early 1960s. At the time of Baller's latest study (1967) many subjects were well into mid-life, with their average age being in the 50s.

Because the same population was involved, this interesting series of studies is considered as a unit in this review. These studies have been referred to by Tizard (1958) as "outstanding in thoroughness."

The original sample consisted of 206 persons from special classes in the Lincoln, Nebraska public schools. Each subject had been classified as mentally deficient on the basis of an IQ of 70 or below and failure to do acceptable work in regular school classes. The retarded sample was matched with a control group on the basis of sex, age, race, and ethnic origin. IQs of the controls ranged from 100 to 120.

Social variables investigated in the studies of Charles, Miller, and Baller et al. included: location, mortality, institutionalization, marital status, family characteristics, occupation, employment, economic status, legal status, citizenship, and social activities. Whenever possible, intelligence tests were administered. In the most recent study subjects were interviewed about peer relations, health, recreational activities, and educational history.

According to the report of Baller et al. (1967), 75 percent of the original retarded group were relocated at midlife; 5 percent of these were in nonpenal institutions. As Charles had earlier noted, this population had an unusually high death rate—30 percent—compared to the expected 6 percent. About half the subjects were married; more than 20 percent had been divorced, but half of these had remarried. Almost 80 percent of the group were "usually employed" and 65 percent were entirely self-supporting. Over half the employed group had held the same job throughout the period studied (1951–1962). A third of the females and half the males were in unskilled occupations; the majority of the remainder were in semi-skilled work.

As reported by Miller, law violations were relatively rare. Two-thirds of the group had no violations, 3 percent had civil offenses, 27 percent had traffic violations, and 3 percent had both. However, one person accounted for eight of the twelve civil offenses reported.

Nearly half the subjects reported voting regularly, although this voting was apparently uninformed. Only two persons reported active participation in community clubs or organizations. More than half were church members, but few reported regular attendance or participation in church-related activities.

When the retarded and control groups were compared, it was found that the retarded group had a higher death rate, were consistently less successful in getting and keeping mates, and were more likely to be living alone. The retarded group was also less mobile, tending to have remained in the home community. The retarded group was also more likely to depend on public assistance for support and was generally less likely to be self-supporting than the control group. However, the retarded subjects did show a steady improvement over the time between Baller's initial investigation, 1935, when 27 percent were self-supporting, and 1962, when 62 percent met this criterion.

A serious criticism of these studies is the lack of similarity between the retarded and control groups on dimensions other than IQ. Goldstein has pointed out the problems in comparing groups of unequal socioeconomic levels. He suggests that researchers should compare the retarded with a nonretarded sample "drawn from a common and contemporary sociophysical milieu."

An attempt to correct this deficiency is provided by two studies conducted by Kennedy (1948, 1966) on the social adjustment of a mildly retarded group in a Connecticut city. Here, 256 mentally deficient persons were matched with 129 normal controls according to social and economic backgrounds and status. This procedure, in the original study and in the 1960 reevaluation, was intended to make the groups so comparable in all socioeconomic aspects that the chief difference between them would be their intelligence levels.

The retarded persons studied were all drawn from a single community, and none had been institutionalized. The purpose of the study was to examine adjustment according to five broad criteria: employment record, economic status, marital and family patterns, academic progress of offspring, and social functioning as reflected in antisocial behaviors and community participation. These indices were evaluated for both normal and control subjects in both the earlier and later studies with the added objectives of replicating earlier findings and studying changes that had recurred over the twelve-year intervening period. Approximately 70 percent of the original sample was located for the 1960 study.

At the outset of this study, IQ tests revealed that the retarded group had scores ranging from 50 to 75, while the controls all had IQs of 70 and above. These differences held up in the later study, despite subject attrition, as did the comparability of the retarded with the controls on sex, age, religion, and nationality. As had been found by Baller, the retarded subjects were less mobile than the controls. Slightly more than twice as many controls as subjects had moved from the home community and were thus unavailable for interviews.

In general, Kennedy's findings showed both similarities and differences between the two groups. A large majority of both subjects and controls had married. The average number of children was the same for both groups (2.1). However, while subjects and controls had similar proportions of normal IQ children, the subjects' children were four times as likely to be of subnormal intelligence, while the controls' children were more likely to have superior IQs.

About three-fourths of both groups were totally self-supporting. Five times as many controls were employed in high-level occupations, while three times as many subjects were in unskilled work. Both groups had attained a high degree of job stability, and both showed upward mobility during the two years of the study. Average earnings in 1960 were $78.80 per week for the subjects and $88.30 for the controls.

Of the married persons in both groups, an equal number (92 percent) were living independently as opposed to living with relatives. More than half these people in both groups owned their own homes. Of those paying rent, the amount paid was similar for both groups.

Ninety-three percent of the controls and 84 percent of the subjects owned a car. A similar percentage of both groups (61 percent) used installment buying. Ninety percent of both groups held some form of insurance, and the majority of both groups said they were saving money.

When employers were interviewed about work performance, the two groups compared favorably on absenteeism and promptness. On all other criteria (including learning rate, carelessness, judgment, decision-making, etc.) the subjects fell far short of the controls.

There were no significant differences between the two groups in terms of court records, number of arrests, or disposition of arrests. Ninety percent of both groups had never been arrested.

Favorite recreational activities for both groups were TV and radio, sports participation, and card-playing. While newspapers, magazines, and books were preferred in that order by both groups, more than twice as many controls as subjects reported reading books. Ninety-eight percent of the controls and 86 percent of the subjects reported that they voted regularly.

In defining personal, social, and economic adjustment in terms of the criteria of her study, Kennedy is quite optimistic in her conclusions:

> ...adjustment in each area of behavior may and does range from a minimal to an extremely high level with, however, the 'norm of expectancy' still being attained because two important criteria have been: to care adequately (even though minimally) for themselves and those dependent upon them; and to be law-abiding....the overwhelming majority of both subjects and controls have made acceptable and remarkably similar adjustment to all three areas: per-

> sonal, social and economic. The main differences are in degree rather than in kind... (p. 51).

The results of Kennedy's study have been reported in detail because her investigations covered a broad range of criteria, many of which have been used in subsequent follow-up studies. However, while Kennedy's study is notable for its completeness, the question can be raised about the similarities of adjustment between the subjects and the controls. In attempting to equalize the two groups on all variables but IQ, Kennedy selected subjects and controls from similarly low socioeconomic levels. In addition, some of her controls had IQs as low as 70. Consequently one may wonder whether the similarities reported are due to the achievement of the retardates, or merely to the initial socioeconomic and intelligence deficits of the controls. The use of control groups in follow-up studies allows for more precise comparisons between retarded and nonretarded populations. However, it does not answer all questions that require answering. Nor does it provide information regarding factors that determine successful or unsuccessful adjustment.

In his review of the follow-up literature on noninstitutional subjects up to 1951, Charles makes this summary statement: "The studies of the social adjustment of persons judged to be mentally deficient present a fairly bright picture, suggesting that many, if not most such persons, can find happy and useful lives in the community if given understanding and guidance."

CRITERIA OF ADJUSTMENT

While many earlier researchers considered "success" or "failure" to be determined by whether or not a person was reinstitutionalized, later investigators have considered many other criteria of adjustment. In their comprehensive review of follow-up studies and procedures, McCarver and Craig (1975) have listed the following criteria:

1) Living environment (type of residence, amount of rent or mortgage payments, residential stability, satisfaction with living quarters)
2) Type of employment (place of work, skill level, job requirements)
3) Job changes (general stability, mobility up or down)
4) Savings and money management (debts, bank accounts, budgeting, installment buying)
5) Sexual problems (venereal disease, promiscuity, prostitution, homosexuality, illegitimacies, marital adjustment, exploitation)
6) Antisocial behavior (legal problems, arrests, delinquency, acts of violence)

7) Marriage and children (sexual adjustment, contraception, parental responsibility, health of children)
8) Use of leisure time (social contacts, recreational activities, hobbies, reading, travel)

McCarver and Craig also suggest the need for consistency in defining such criteria. While some researchers consider a person to be a success as long as he remains in the community and a failure in the event that he requires institutionalization, others advocate the development of behavioral norms in a variety of areas (Rosen, 1967*a;* Windle, 1962). As Windle has pointed out, regardless of a retardate's assets, his behavior has to meet some minimal standard in a number of areas in order for him to be tolerated in the community. Clark, Kivitz, and Rosen (1968) suggest that the level of functioning and personal cost to the individual, as well as the costs to society, must be determined in assessing the value of releasing retardates from an institution to independent living. It is possible, they point out, that for certain individuals marginal and unhappy community existence may be comparable to what Freeman and Simmons (1963), studying the post-hospital adjustment of ex–mental patients, termed a "chronic ward of one."

As Rosen, Floor, and Baxter (1971) have suggested, personality variables should also be considered in determining criteria of adjustment, because these strongly influence interpersonal relations, job stability, satisfaction with one's existence, and other measures of adjustment that are commonly used as criteria.

NEED FOR FURTHER RESEARCH

Because the majority of follow-up studies have resulted in fairly optimistic thinking, it might be said that no further time need be spent in pursuing such studies. This point was made by Tizard, who suggested that the purely descriptive follow-up study has little further interest and should be replaced by predictive investigations. To reason this way, however, is to ignore the gaps that still exist in our understanding of those retarded persons who are capable of community adjustment. Further investigations might fill some of the following research needs:

Need for Longitudinal Follow-up Data

Numerous researchers have stated that comparing the results of different studies may not be valid if the subjects of the various investigations have been in the community for different lengths of time. In addition, there is a conspicuous absence of longitudinal studies in obtaining a sequence of behavior over a time interval. Only by observing the individual over a period of time can we derive insights about his progress in making the necessary adjustments to community living. As Edgerton has pointed out, with the passage of time "successes" may become "failures" and vice versa. Repeated assessments are needed to determine accurately the manner in which a retarded person copes with marriage, child-rearing, job changes, unemployment, and other factors that represent change in his environment.

Need for Understanding the Attitudes and Feelings of Retarded Persons Undergoing the Transition to Independent Community Living

Statistical summaries of the frequency of unemployment, arrests, economic difficulties, and marital problems seldom make provision for understanding the personal reactions of individuals to these critical events. The feelings of previously institutionalized retardates toward their institutional background, their future expectations, and their identification as retarded are still largely unstudied. Cromwell (1963), Rosen et al. (1971), Zigler (1966), and others have stressed the negative effects that the lowered levels of aspiration and expectancies of success held by the retarded have upon levels of learning and performance. Detection of any changes in these cognitions that might occur following discharge from an institution or upon leaving any sheltered environment would provide important information about level of functioning and would also have important implications in planning habilitation programs.

Need for a More Precise Definition of the Retarded Population Capable of Independent Functioning

Criticism can probably be leveled with some justification at most follow-up studies in which IQ has been used as the sole criterion for defining the subject groups. Whether the subjects were previously in special public school classes or were institutionalized, they were usually identified from past records without benefit of comprehensive diagnostic procedures. In some cases, an implicit assumption was made that enrollment in a special class or confinement to an institution constituted an operational definition of retardation. In other cases, IQ estimates may have been lacking in stability between the time of initial identification of the sample and subsequent follow-up. Ranges of IQs of retarded subjects have differed widely from study to study, with few attempts to differentiate borderline or near normal subjects from those with more severe deficits.

Need for Studying the Relation Between Previous Training and Later Success

It is important to ask what types of training, either in special classes or in institutions, are most justifiable in terms of community adjustment. A follow-up would have merit even if its only purposes were to describe which community activities reflect former education or training, which activities could have been handled without previous training, and what the subject still needs to know so that he can learn under more effective training procedures. A better understanding of what the retarded person is required to do in order to remain out of an institution will lead to the development of better habilitative techniques. As Tizard (1958) points out,

> What are most needed today are properly controlled experimental studies and surveys designed to answer particular questions about the social costs of various types of administrative arrangements for dealing with mentally subnormal individuals. On the psychological side, we need to discover the most efficient methods of teaching or training those who are grossly subnormal in intelligence or handicapped in other ways.... How to teach social skills to dull, badly educated people has hardly been studied at all as yet, nor has the treatment of emotional maladjustment or psychopathic instability.

Need to Assess Interaction of the Retardate with the Community

Goldstein notes that "two areas of study are consistently absent from follow-up studies.... These are (1) the relationship of community tolerance to success or failure in community adjustment and (2) the changes, if any, effected by a non-institutional environment on (individuals)." Goldstein explains that while the study of community tolerance is difficult, it is only through this type of study that institutions or schools can make "their training programs more meaningful, their screening techniques more effective, and their placement procedures more efficient" (p. 229).

Edgerton's study of feelings of stigma resulting from reactions of the community to the retarded individual is a significant contribution in this area. He suggests the need for institutions to counteract such feelings by helping the retarded person "to explain his relative incompetence without suggesting that his affliction is one of basic and ineradicable stupidity" (p. 213).

With respect to the effect of the community on the intellectual level of the retardate, a study by Marchand (1956) revealed a significant gain in IQ over an eleven-year period of living in the community for previously institutionalized adults. Charles (1953) had found substantial gains over a thirty-year period. On the other hand, Rosen, Floor, and Baxter (1974) found no significant IQ or achievement test score gains after a three-year period. They conclude that, "For this population intellectual and scholastic ability seem largely unrelated to community functioning and unresponsive to the experience of independent living." Such contradictory results suggest the need for further exploration in this area.

RESEARCH PROBLEMS

While the preceding considerations appear to justify future follow-up studies, it is at the same time necessary to recognize the difficulties that the researcher may encounter in the course of such investigations.

First, there is the problem of obtaining a sufficiently large sample of persons who will agree to participate in the study. When the subjects are residents of an institution or members of special public school classes, they are readily available for the obtaining of initial data. However, when subjects are already in the community they must be contacted by letter and/or telephone or via community agencies.

The methods of obtaining information utilized by researchers have included: 1) requesting information by letter from persons supervising the individual in either a work or home situation; 2) visiting the subject and observing him in the conduct of his daily life; 3) interviewing relatives or others familiar with the subject; 4) contacting agencies, such as welfare departments, police, or habilitation centers, that may have had contact with the subject; and 5) interviewing the subject himself.

Most authors of follow-up studies have utilized one or a combination of the above techniques. For example, Kaplun (1935) noted that information obtained solely by letter was often found to be discrepant with facts actually observed later. Hartzler (1951) reported that second-party data might be unreliable in that information on successful clients might be more readily given than on unsuccessful ones. Wolfson concluded that information typically obtained does not provide a good picture of the subject's emotional or psychological adjustment.

As McCarver and Craig point out,

> It can probably be assumed that most researchers have obtained only rather superficial information. Notable exceptions are the studies of Edgerton, whose staff spent an average of 17 hours with each subject, and the Elwyn Institute studies (e.g., Clark et al., 1968; Rosen, 1967*a*, 1967*b*) in which detailed interviews were obtained at six-month intervals the first year and annually thereafter.

Probably the most effective method of conducting a follow-up study is a direct, comprehensive personal interview with the subject combined with additional objective information obtained from a variety of other sources.

A second major problem facing those conducting follow-up studies is the attrition of the sample over a period of time. For example, Muench (1944) was able to obtain follow-up data on only eight of his original 40 subjects, and Edgerton (1967), 48 out of 191. The reasons for subject loss include geographical limitations, change of address, refusal to cooperate, and death. Many persons also wish to hide their background of institutionalization or attendance at special schools or classes. The stigma of being labeled ''retarded'' may be so devastating that a major portion of the person's efforts are directed toward attempting to pass as normal (Edgerton, 1967). In such cases, potential subjects may refuse to participate in a study that labels them retarded. When Floor, Baxter, and Rosen (1972) explored the effects of subject loss on the validity of conclusions drawn from follow-up studies, they found that subjects married to ''normal'' spouses were unlikely to agree to participate in a series of interviews.

While attrition is an obvious problem, McCarver and Craig assert that ''virtually all subjects can be located if enough time and effort are expended.'' They cite the example of Hoffman (1969) who found 98 percent of a sample of 511 subjects who had been discharged from an institution four to ten years earlier. As the authors suggest in advocating the use of good sampling techniques, ''It would seem much more reasonable to randomly select 50 subjects out of a cohort of 500 and make an intensive effort to locate all of them than to begin with a cohort of 500 and end up with 50.''

It has already been noted that the length of time a subject has been in the community is an important variable to be considered in conducting follow-up studies. After reviewing 36 studies, Eagle found that the mean length of time in the community before follow-up was 5.3 years. However, many subjects of various studies had been in the community for less than six months, and many studies simply fail to report the time interval involved. In any case, the time lapse should be consistent for all subjects in a given study and should probably not be less than one year.

SUMMARY

The studies reported in this chapter, as well as the need for further investigation and the research problems to be considered, may be summarized by the following points:

1) Follow-up studies on both formerly institutionalized retardates and ''graduates'' of special public school classes indicate generally that such persons are capable of independent functioning in the community.

2) Criteria of "success" and "failure" need to be standardized for clarification of results and accurate comparisons of different populations.
3) Specific criteria can include: living environment, type of employment, job stability, money management, sexual adjustment, social behavior, marriage and parenthood, and use of leisure time.
4) Personality variables and the psychological and emotional adjustment of the subject, including his mechanisms for coping with the stigma of mental retardation, should be studied.
5) Areas for further investigation include: longitudinal studies, understanding of an individual's feelings during transition to the community, a more precise definition of retardation, and an awareness of relation between previous training and community adjustment.
6) Research problems include: adequate sampling, population attrition, and time intervals for follow-up.

DISCUSSION

The follow-up study has been with us for a long time and has played its role in shaping changing attitudes toward the mentally retarded. A number of such studies have been reviewed here and their findings, the criteria utilized, and the gaps that suggest the need for further research have been summarized. But what, exactly, is the potential value of follow-up? We take the view that continued attempts at such studies should be made, but with more sophisticated research goals than were used in previous investigations.

Fernald's original study, according to his own words, was undertaken to help future generations of mentally retarded persons passing through his institution. There is good reason to believe that on the basis of his results he was able to modify his earlier endorsement of ideas concerning the menace of retardation, and, we may assume, he was able to modify administrative policies at Waverly State School and within the American Association on Mental Deficiency, where he served as president.

Later investigations appeared to share Fernald's findings and conclusions yet they were not followed by radical changes in attitude toward the retarded. As methodology for follow-up became more rigorous, with the attempt to use comparable control populations, the focus apparently subtly shifted from the adjustment process and implications for policy toward comparative studies with normals. We have already discussed the difficulties in choosing comparable controls. In Kennedy's study, for example, since both controls and subjects were chosen from a low socioeconomic population, it is little wonder that few differences between the groups were uncovered. The study does not answer why the retarded subjects were of low socioeconomic level to begin with. To date, follow-up studies have not explored the factors that determine socioeconomic status in mentally retarded populations.

The researcher must be willing to ask himself about the value of his studies to the planners and policy makers in the field of mental retardation. He must be aware of the important questions that remain to be answered concerning the capacity of mentally retarded citizens, at all levels of ability and social competence, to adjust to and function in the community. The fact that a large majority of mildly retarded individuals should be capable of independent community living and competitive unskilled employment seems to be well established. The actual percentages found capable of this goal in previous studies may not be useful to the habilitation counselor or administrator contemplating the community release of one mentally retarded resident of an institution. On the other hand, the collective experiences of comparable mentally retarded persons previously discharged, the problems they encountered, the factors related to successful or unsuccessful adjustment, and the reactions of the community in which they lived might prove extremely beneficial.

This argument merely restates the need for the application of the research utilization model described in Chapter 3. Applied specifically to follow-up, this involves the development of criteria of adjustment that are more specific, more relevant to training goals, and potentially more closely related to measurable characteristics of the individual or his training program. Global criteria such as reinstitutionalization, employment record, arrests, and other social factors traditionally utilized in such studies are too far removed from the kinds of personality variables that we can measure in mentally retarded persons.

We suggest as an alternative that future studies make more sophisticated criterion analysis of the behaviors exhibited by mentally retarded persons in the community, of their encounters with significant others in their lives (landlords, work supervisors, advocates), of their approaches to the social structures and organizations (clubs, businesses, services), and of their style of life in numerous daily personal situations (e.g., medical problems, saving, credit, recreation).

The accomplishment of these goals must entail intensive studies of smaller numbers of persons, rather than more superficial nose-counting with larger populations. Despite the emphasis on normalization of experiences and opportunities for the retarded, such an approach may be productive in revealing a characteristic life style of the mentally retarded in communities that is different from more "normal" living. Follow-up data suggest that such a style does exist and that it may prove to have general implications for program development.

LITERATURE CITED

Baller, W. R. 1936. A study of the present social status of a group of adults who, when they were in elementary schools, were classified as mentally deficient. Genet. Psychol. Monogr. 18:165–244.

Baller, W. R., Charles, D. C., and Miller, E. L. 1967. Mid-life attainment of the mentally retarded: A longitudinal study. Gent. Psychol. Monogr. 75:235–329.

Charles, D. C. 1953. Ability and accomplishment of persons earlier judged mentally deficient. Genet. Psychol. Monogr. 47:3–71.

Clark, G. R., Kivitz, M. S., and Rosen, M. 1968. A transitional program for institutionalized adult retarded. Project No. RD 1275-P. Vocational Rehabilitation Administration, Division of Research and Demonstration, U.S. Department of Health, Education, and Welfare, Washington, D. C.

Coakley, F. 1945. Study of feebleminded wards employed in war industries. Amer. J. Ment. Defic. 50:301–306.

Cromwell, R. L. 1963. A social learning approach to mental retardation. *In* N. R. Ellis (ed.), Handbook of Mental Deficiency, pp. 41–91. McGraw Hill Book Company, New York.

Davies, S. P. 1930. Social Control of the Mentally Deficient. Thomas Y. Crowell Company, New York.

Dinger, J. C. 1961. Post-school adjustment of former educable retarded pupils. Except. Child. 27:353–360.

Eagle, E. 1967. Prognosis and outcome of community placement of institutionalized retardates. Amer. J. Ment. Defic. 72:232–243.

Edgerton, R. B. 1967. The Cloak of Competence: Stigma in the Lives of the Mentally Retarded. University of California Press, Berkeley.

Edgerton, R. B., and Bercovici, S. M. 1976. The cloak of competence: Years later. Amer. J. Ment. Defic. 80:485–497.

Fairbanks, R. 1933. The subnormal child: Seventeen years after. Ment. Hyg. 17:177–208.

Fernald, W. E. 1919. After-care study of the patients discharged from Waverly for a period of twenty-five years. Ungraded 5:25–31.

Floor, L., Baxter, D., and Rosen, M. 1972. Subject loss in a follow-up study. Ment. Retard. 10:3–5.

Freeman, H. E., and Simmons, O. G. 1963. The Mental Patient Comes Home. John Wiley & Sons Inc., New York.

Goldstein, J. 1964. Social and occupational adjustment. *In* H. A. Stevens and R. Heber (eds.), Mental Retardation. University of Chicago Press, Chicago.

Hartzler, E. A. 1951. A follow-up study of girls discharged from the Laurelton State Village. Amer. J. Ment. Defic. 55:612–618.

Hegge, T. G. 1944. The occupational status of higher-grade mental defectives in the present emergency. A study of parolees from the Wayne County Training School at Northville, Michigan. Amer. J. Ment. Defic. 49:86–98.

Hoffman, J. L. 1969. The location of missing subjects. Ment. Retard. 7:18–21.

Kaplun, D. 1935. The high grade moron—A study of institutional admissions over

a ten year period. Proceedings of the American Association for Mental Deficiency 40:69–91.
Kennedy, R. J. R. 1948. The social adjustment of morons in a Connecticut city. Millport, Connecticut. Commission to Survey Resources in Connecticut, Hartford.
Kennedy, R. J. R. 1966. A Connecticut community revisited: A study of the social adjustment of a group of mentally deficient adults in 1948 and 1960. Project No. 655. Office of Vocational Rehabilitation. U. S. Department of Health, Education, and Welfare, Washington, D. C.
Marchand J. G., Jr. 1956. Changes of psychometric test results in mental defective employment care patients. Amer. J. Ment. Defic. 60:852–859.
McCarver, R. B., and Craig, E. M. 1974. Placement of the retarded in the community: Prognosis and outcome. *In* N. R. Ellis (ed.), International Review of Research in Mental Retardation, pp. 145–207. Vol. 7. Academic Press, New York.
Miller, E. L. 1965. Ability and social adjustment at mid-life of persons earlier judged mentally deficient. Genet. Psychol. Monogr. 72:139–198.
Muench, G. A. 1944. A follow-up of mental defectives after 18 years. J. Abnorm. Social Psychol. 39:407–418.
Rosen, M. 1967*a*. Rehabilitation, research and follow-up within the institutional setting. Ment. Retard. 5:7–11.
Rosen, M. 1967*b*. The retardate in the community: A post-institutional follow-up study. Paper presented at the annual convention of the American Association for Mental Deficiency, Denver, May, 1967.
Rosen, M., Diggory, J. C., Floor, L., and Nowakiwska, M. 1971. Self-evaluation, expectancy and performance in the mentally subnormal. J. Ment. Defic. Res. 15:81–95.
Rosen, M., Floor, L., and Baxter, D. 1971. The institutional personality. Brit. J. Ment. Subnormal. 17:2–8.
Rosen, M., Floor, L., and Baxter, D. 1974. IQ, academic achievement and community adjustment after discharge from the institution. Ment. Retard. 12:51–53.
Tizard, J. 1958. Longitudinal and follow-up studies. *In* A. Clarke and A. D. B. Clarke (eds.), Mental Deficiency: The Changing Outlook, pp. 422–429. Methuen & Co. Ltd., London.
Wardell, W. R. 1946. Adjustment of moron males in a group placement. Amer. J. Ment. Defic. 50:425–433.
Windle, C. 1962. Prognosis of mental subnormals. Amer. J. Ment. Defic. Monograph Supplement 66:No. 5.
Windle, C. P., Stewart, E., and Brown, S. J. 1961. Reasons for community failure of released patients. Amer. J. Ment. Defic. 66:213–217.
Wolfson, I. N. 1956. Follow-up study of 92 male and 131 female patients who were discharged from Newark State School in 1946. Amer. J. Ment. Defic. 61:224–238.
Zigler, E. 1966. Motivational determinants in the performance of retarded children. Amer. J. Orthopsychiatry 36:848–856.

Chapter 10

Coping with the Community

A Post-Institutional Follow-up Study

The preceding chapter has included brief summaries of a number of follow-up studies. It is the purpose here to describe a specific study in detail, with attention both to the methodology of conducting such a project and to its results and implications. A description of the population of this study will provide insight into the manner in which mildly retarded adults make the transition from institutional to community living.

A follow-up study of considerable magnitude was begun at Elwyn Institute in 1964 (Clark et al., 1968).[1] It combined both descriptive and prognostic elements and was designed to assess the level of community adjustment of previously institutionalized adults, and to determine the relationship of specific criteria of community success to a number of predictor variables. The habilitation program at Elwyn is described in Chapter 5. The prognostic aspect of the study is described in Chapter 11. In an attempt to evaluate the success of this program, it was decided to follow up persons who had been living independently for at least six months. The assumption was that the cost-benefit savings would be considerable if those persons who had formerly been state-supported could now be self-supporting con-

[1]Although the original follow-up investigation was conducted between 1964 and 1968, Elwyn has maintained this research project over the past twelve years. The results of later studies of intellectual functioning, also included in this chapter, were not part of the original research procedure.

tributors to society. An ultimate goal of the project was the development of improved institutional services to provide such persons with a graduated transitional program as an effective means of preparation for future adjustment in the community.

Persons involved in the study were previously institutionalized retarded adults between 20 and 55 years of age with IQs between 50 and 80. Only those persons without suitable families to accept them into their homes were included. Thus, the sample was limited to individuals who were orphaned or abandoned. All subjects had been through the habilitation program, including adult education and community work experience. Before discharge, these individuals had worked for at least six months at an "outside" job and had saved at least $500 from their paychecks. The client has been assisted in obtaining a suitable room or apartment. Thus, criteria for discharge also included previous training, present employment, savings, and a place to live.

By the time the study was concluded there were 130 "graduates" who met all of the above criteria. They had been living independently from six months to two years. Letters were sent to these persons requesting an appointment for an interview in their homes. A return postcard was enclosed on which the interview date and time could be confirmed. Sixty-five persons agreed to be interviewed. The remainder either refused to cooperate or had changed their addresses and could not be located.

Interviews were performed by a "community evaluator," who had previously known most of the subjects during their participation in the habilitation programs. The interview usually lasted about two hours and consisted of structured questionnaire items, including forced choices on linear rating scales and open-ended questions. Graphic aids were used for the scales to convey the idea of a dimension. There was little difficulty encountered in communicating the idea of a scale to the subject population. Documentation was requested for items such as salary, rent, and savings. Subjects were contacted by mail or phone before the interview and asked to have materials such as W-2 forms, rent receipts, and bankbooks available.

The interview procedure dealt with three major categories of functioning in the community—vocational adjustment, economic adjustment, and personal-social adjustment. Ratings generally conformed to what would popularly be accepted as better or poorer adjustments in each area, i.e., higher salary better than lower salary, fewer complaints or dissatisfaction better than greater dissatisfaction. Each of the criteria was analyzed separately as a dimension of adjustment.

The indices of vocational adjustment included: job tenure and mobility, unemployment, absenteeism, promotions, salary changes, and accident reports at work. (Employers were not contacted in order to avoid drawing attention to the subjects on their jobs, and to respect their personal privacy.) In addition to the more objective indices, the Minnesota Employment Satisfaction Scale (Carlson et al., 1962, and Scott et al., 1960) was used to provide published norms for eight comparison groups, including handicapped (nonretarded) and nonhandicapped, skilled and unskilled, blue- and white-collar workers.

Economic characteristics included items such as gross annual income, bank accounts, debts, installment buying, charge accounts, and the use of credit cards. Evaluations of the type of housing arrangements the subjects had effected were also rated, as well as the adequacy of their furnishings and the extent of their possessions. The purchase of automobiles and of life and medical insurance was examined.

The assessment of social adjustment covered a broad range of topics that included: the frequency of arrests, marriages, child-bearing, religious affiliation and church attendance, voting, leisure time activities, social relationships, and memberships in clubs and organizations. An attempt was also made to measure the attitudes and self-perceptions of the subjects, including sources of dissatisfaction.

A later study also evaluated the effect of community living experience on intellectual functioning and academic achievement scores.

These subjects were predominantly male (82 percent) and Caucasian (94 percent). The great majority (97 percent) had originally been referred to the institution by public agencies and were state-supported during their institutionalization. Their average age at admission had been 13.3 years and their average admission IQ was 64.3. At the time of discharge the subjects averaged 28.8 years in age and 75.6 in IQ. All had severe educational deficits; the majority were functioning below a fourth-grade reading level.

VOCATIONAL ADJUSTMENT

Approximately 90 percent of the subjects were employed at the time of interview and had worked at least half-time since discharge. Jobs were primarily in unskilled or semi-skilled occupations in personal, food, or building services, or as laborers or stock and factory workers. The most common occupations were those of kitchen workers, custodial or maintenance workers, and orderlies. In terms of job stability, 54 percent of the subjects had maintained the same job they had at the time of discharge. As might be expected, there was an increased tendency for more job changes as a function of time spent in the community.

Gross annual incomes were derived from W-2 forms. Where this figure represented less than a full year of employment, and the individual had been employed steadily since discharge, a projection was made for the full year's salary. (Persons who were employed at live-in situations where they worked were not included in the subsequent data analyses because it was not possible to obtain reliable information about the actual monetary value of room and board.)

Incomes ranged from $247 (for a married housewife working part-time) to $9,000 (for a licensed barber). The average income for single males and females (not including live-ins) was $2,918 (in 1963–67). This figure compared to a $3,391 average for the U.S. population as a whole in 1964. Earnings ranged from $1,770 to $5,075 and corresponded to those of the lowest third of the population according to published census information.

Employment satisfaction was evaluated along several dimensions, including supervision, co-workers, salary, job status, and chances for advancement (Rosen et al., 1970*a*). Results with the mentally retarded workers were not significantly different from norms available for other groups of nonretarded, handicapped, unskilled, and blue-collar workers. The greatest degree of expressed dissatisfaction occurred with regard to receiving what the retarded workers considered inadequate compensation and with being relegated to lower status positions in the company. In addition to responding to the Minnesota Scales of Employment Satisfaction, subjects were also asked: "What are the five most important things about a job that make it attractive to you?" Each subject made his choices from a list of 17 job characteristics that had frequently been reported in studies of normal workers. Compensation was overwhelmingly chosen as the most important job characteristic, with 81 percent of the sample listing it as a choice. Job security and adequate supervision were chosen in second position, with 53 percent of the sample listing each of these factors.

In general, the subjects in the study were able to retain jobs in unskilled and semi-skilled occupations. However, they tended to be somewhat dissatisfied with their relatively low wages and the poor social status of their jobs. The areas of greatest dissatisfaction among retarded workers (Compensation and Sensitivity Scales) were also chosen by the Minnesota groups as areas of least satisfaction. Nevertheless, they may be realistic concerns of retarded workers about their salary levels and status positions in community work settings. While the Minnesota studies weigh each of the satisfaction scales equally, it may be that the retarded worker's dissatisfaction with his salary is a more serious source of discontent and poor work adjustment than is his dissatisfaction with other work characteristics. We have found that retardates are somewhat less satisfied with their pay than other handicapped workers, and considerably less satisfied than nonhandicapped unskilled employees. These findings may reflect the relatively low pay received by retarded workers, and also suggest their intense desire for financial improvement.

These facts are supported by the high rank that retarded workers attribute to compensation as the most important job incentive. This is an apparent contradiction with reported job incentives of normal workers. Attitude surveys report that the need for security is widespread and far outweighs income as a preferred job characteristic. This has been observed in factory employees (National Industrial Conference Board, 1947), high school students (Dipboye and Anderson, 1959), applicants for employment (Jurgensen, 1947, 1948), department store employees (Hardin, Reif, and Heneman, 1951), building trade workers (Davis, 1942), and union members (Rose, 1952). The rankings are also in contrast to observations (Cohen and Rusalem, 1964) of nonretarded and institutionalized and noninstitutionalized retarded adolescents. In this study, subjects assigned low ranks to "independence," "prestige," and "salary" and placed a high value on "chance for advancement," regardless of their intellectual ability or institutional status.

There are several possible implications of the differences in rated job incentives between the institutional sample and nonretarded workers. The lesser concern of the present subjects with "security" than with compensation may mean that retarded workers are less likely to plan effectively for their futures and to postpone gratification. However, since retarded workers earn lower salaries and may have less opportunity for gaining security in their positions than their nonretarded peers, monetary considerations might naturally play a more important role in their motivational structure. The relatively low rank given "salary" by a younger sample of retarded in the Cohen and Rusalem study suggests that practical considerations play a diminished role in determining incentives during the time when shelter and care are provided by others.

The Elwyn subjects were apparently sensitive to the fact that they occupied the lowest status positions in their respective work organizations. The Minnesota study describes the Sensitivity Scale as reflecting "a negative, suspicious, thin-skinned attitude toward various aspects of the work environment...." The sensitivity cluster appeared for all Minnesota groups except skilled white-collar workers. It was chosen as a low satisfaction area, second to compensation, by all blue-collar groups. The Elwyn results indicate that retarded workers were also well aware that they occupied low-prestige jobs and that they were more negative toward their positions in the work hierarchy than are other types of handicapped workers. On the other hand, the retardates were less sensitive to low status than the nonhandicapped unskilled workers. This suggests that, despite his comparatively high sensitivity, the retarded worker may be more willing to accept socially perceived low-level jobs than is the nonhandicapped unskilled employee.

Another area in which the sample reflected dissatisfaction when compared to the nonhandicapped group was in that of attitudes toward supervision. This may indicate an inability on the part of handicapped workers to communicate with supervisory personnel or to receive adequate indications of concern for their problems. It may also reflect a bias on the part of supervisors toward known retardates.

The dearth of long-term follow-up studies of the work adjustment of retarded individuals makes vocational planning a hazardous endeavor. Although the relationship between job satisfaction and other work variables such as job competence is unknown, it may represent an important consideration in an individual's community adjustment. The realistic basis for job dissatisfaction, where it exists, may lie in actual work deficits or handicaps of the retarded, and it may also reflect situational variables such as employer bias. It is possible too that dissatisfaction finds its roots in unrealistic levels of aspiration and in poor work attitudes fostered by years of sheltered institutional living. This study points out a need for providing the mentally retarded with a more realistic expectation of the roles they will play in industry after leaving the institution or sheltered workshop setting. This can be accomplished by practical counseling about salary and prestige levels in community jobs suitable for retarded workers, by training in relationship to supervision, and by more realistic work experiences and pay structures for retarded workers during their vocational training period.

ECONOMIC ADJUSTMENT

The majority of people were living in either rented rooms or apartments. A few had rented homes, always in conjunction with several other inhabitants. A typical rooming situation included a one-room living unit, furnished with chairs, bed, bureau, night-table, and mirror. Bathroom facilities were shared with the landlord or other tenants. A typical apartment consisted of one to three rooms with a bathroom and kitchen. In most cases, the furnishings were more elaborate than those in rented rooms and were owned by the inhabitants. There were often colorful and decorative items such as pictures, bright curtains, and throw rugs in the apartments. The homes offered the most spacious living and were usually on pleasant residential streets. The mean monthly rental for all types of accommodations was $54.00, with a range of $19.00 to $92.00. Over 80 percent of all subjects had a TV in their living-room quarters, either as their own possession or as part of their furnishings in a rented unit. Over 50 percent subscribed to their own telephone; most others had a phone available in their residences.

As has already been noted, upon discharge each person had an established bank account. These accounts were begun when the "graduates" entered the Community Work Program and represented a certain portion of their weekly pay that was set aside for savings. The average savings account at discharge was $500. At the time of the interview most persons had retained their savings accounts, although the average amount had dropped to slightly under $500, and the range was from $1.00 to $5,000. The general trend was a decrease in savings with extended time in the community as more persons made major purchases. Debts appeared to increase with time in the community and included loans from finance companies, unpaid medical bills, and the like. Approximately 20 percent of the subjects were making regular installment payments on purchases. Fourteen persons had purchased automobiles, and sixteen had driver's licenses. Over 60 percent of the subjects had purchased some form of life insurance. This often was in the form of term insurance as a part of employment benefits. Percentages of persons having life insurance tended to increase with time in the community. While over 60 percent had health insurance, there appeared to be a decreasing trend to keep up with hospitalization insurance payments once the individual was discharged from the institution. This probably reflects a tendency for subjects to change jobs to situations that provide fewer benefits once they have returned to the community.

Only two of the subjects received welfare payments. The first received a total of $60.00 during three weeks of unemployment. The second received payments of $45.00 every two weeks during two and a half months of unemployment following hospitalization for surgery.

SOCIAL ADJUSTMENT

Twenty of the 65 subjects involved in the study were married at the time of the interview. Of these persons, 11 (55 percent) married other Elwyn residents. An additional two persons married ex-residents of a neighboring state institution for the retarded, and one married a person who had been a day student in a work-study program at Elwyn. Six persons married individuals who had not been identified as retarded. There were a total of ten children born to eight couples and one born out of wedlock. The children all appeared to be receiving appropriate medical care, and none were reported to be mentally retarded.

The results suggested that mildly retarded persons can sustain a marital relationship for several years with reasonable competence. However, the types of difficulties encountered by many couples emphasize the importance of preparing institutional residents to assume the responsibilities of marriage and parenthood. More recent data concerning marriages is presented in Chapter 16.

Other areas affecting social adjustment included antisocial or aberrant behavior. Involvement with the law was a rare occurrence. One male was arrested for speeding; his driver's license was suspended. Another subject was accused of rape by the parents of two sisters, both of whom were pregnant, presumably by the subject. This case came to trial, and the charge was changed to "fathering an illegitimate child." He spent one night in jail until bail was arranged. Upon the advice of his landlady, he obtained help from the Legal Aid Society. The case was subsequently dismissed when evidence was revealed that the relationship with the girls had existed for some time with mutual compliance.

In an attempt to discover other areas of difficulty in social and emotional adjustment, each person was asked: "Which of the following problems have given you some trouble or cause for concern?" and "Which is so serious a cause for concern that you would desire some help with it?" Although several items were chosen by subjects in response to the first question, no one indicated a desire for help with his problems. The areas presenting the greatest frequency of reported difficulty were: budgeting finances, saving money, controlling one's temper, and using profanity. While 14 percent of the respondents reported occasional difficulties, none was considered by the interviewer to be an unreliable or irresponsible individual.

Subjects were also questioned about problems relating to a list of symptoms and social behaviors selected from the Katz Adjustment Scale (Katz, 1963). Very few psychiatric symptoms were reported. Symptoms were usually in the "sometimes" category of response and were not considered severe. Reported symptoms included such items as: "feels lonely," "feels restless," "can't stop moving," "gets sad, blue," "gets nervous or upset," "worries about things," "gets very angry at people," "prefers to be alone," "not getting along with co-workers," "feels people are talking about him," "feels unhappy," and "feels unfriendly toward others." The items chosen suggested that several persons were experiencing restless, uneasy, lonely feelings in the community.

Involvement in formal social groups was apparently minimal among these persons. Only 18 percent belonged to clubs or participated regularly in organized activities. Those that did participate tended to join loosely organized activity groups such as bowling or skating clubs. Approximately 40 percent reported attending church services at least once a month. Informal entertaining and social participation with friends was quite common.

Subjects were asked if they had been able to make new friends since leaving the institution and whether or not their friends were former institutional residents. Over 90 percent reported being able to make new friends, and over 80 percent reported having more noninstitutional than institutional friends. However, most of the subjects still maintained a circle of friends who were former institutional students.

The most frequent leisure time pursuits, in order of precedence, were "watching TV," "listening to the radio," "visiting friends," "going shopping," "taking auto rides," "going to the movies," and "entertaining friends."

Relatively few of the subjects had become involved in registration or voting. Reasons for not voting included the feeling that all politicians are "no good," and a fear that registration would result in being tapped for jury duty. The majority had filed Federal Income Tax returns, and most had required help with this process. Assistance was often supplied by institutional counseling personnel.

Subjects were rated at time of interview on various items relating to housekeeping, personal hygiene, health and medical care, money and financial management, transportation, and everyday decision-making. Many persons reported that they were often at a loss about how to make appropriate social contacts with the opposite sex. However, the majority of the group were doing at least an adequate job in handling all other related areas.

Socially most of them had managed to avoid serious legal difficulties and had been able to cope adequately with everyday living problems. They tended to be reliable in paying bills and taxes. While they had avoided participation in social groups and activities, their success at making new friends suggests a level of social adjustment at least comparable to that of nonretarded persons of similar socioeconomic levels. Some of the group had married, produced children, and in most cases appeared to be adequate parents. Personal complaints about psychiatric symptoms (and symptomatology as observed by the interviewer) were almost completely lacking.

These persons appeared to do better in areas in which they had had the most experience. The closer the approximation of the institutional training to the actual community living and work situation, the easier the transition from institution to community. Thus, they handled their jobs well, were steady workers, and made friends. On the other hand, many reported problems in budgeting and handling finances, areas in which it is relatively more difficult to provide realistic experiences within an institution.

INTELLECTUAL FUNCTIONING AND ACADEMIC ACHIEVEMENT

Many of the subjects were diagnosed as "moron" or "imbecile" at the time of their admission to the institution. The group averaged 15 years of institutionalization, during which time significant increments in IQ were achieved. (Average IQ rose from 64.3 at admission to 75.6 at discharge.) Since most of these people came from extremely deprived backgrounds, it is not too surprising that the care and stimulation provided by the institution were reflected in cognitive as well as physical development.

If such IQ changes can occur within the institution, the question arises whether the challenges of independent living might also produce cognitive increments. The very problems that might cause difficulties in community adjustment (budgeting, shopping, banking, traveling, adjusting to marriage, raising a child) might also provide motivation for intellectual or academic growth.

While intellectual ability and scholastic achievement have been evaluated as possible predictors of later adjustment (McCarver and Craig, 1974; Rosen et al., 1970*b*; Windle, 1962), there have been few reports dealing with the effects of community experience upon intellectual functioning.

An investigation by Rosen, Floor, and Baxter (1974) sought to explore this relationship by retesting 50 persons who had averaged over three years in the community. All these individuals had been given the Wechsler Adult Intelligence Scale (Wechsler, 1955) and the Metropolitan Achievement Test (Harcourt, Brace, and World, 1959) before discharge. The Wechsler Test explores facets of intellectual ability such as general information, reasoning, vocabulary, and perceptual-motor skills. The achievement test emphasized reading and language skills, arithmetic computation, and problem-solving. These tests were readministered to subjects in their own homes.

When the scores obtained in the community were compared with those obtained before discharge, no significant differences were found for the group as a whole on either test. While some individual gains were substantial, others showed decreases of almost the same magnitude.

The IQ and achievement retest scores were also evaluated in relation to four criteria of community adjustment. These criteria, which were derived from interview data and other sources of information, were income, job stability, coping with daily problems, and social adjustment. Each item was scored one or zero depending on the individual's standing in comparison to the group median for income or number of problems encountered in a given area. Thus, a maximum score of four was possible. Statistical analysis revealed no significant relationship between an individual's score on these combined criteria and his scores on the IQ and achievement retests. The lack of relationship between measures of cognitive ability and criteria of community adjustment has been corroborated by other investigators (see Chapter 11).

CASE HISTORIES

While the preceding section has provided a summary of the general characteristics of this population, some illustrative case studies can bring into sharper focus the manner in which some of these persons have made the transition from institutional to community living. The cases presented here have been chosen to illustrate both the difficulties and achievements of a cross-section of the 65 subjects of this study. While most of the data reported were obtained from the original interview, additional information, when available, has been added to make these histories as up-to-date as possible. Monetary data are drawn from the interviews and should be considered in the context of 1967.

J.D.

J. was referred to the institution by the Department of Public Welfare, and was admitted at age 14. He was noted to have a severe stutter and was classified a "middle-grade imbecile."

After completing school, J. worked in the kitchen at the institution, where he was considered a "faithful and valuable worker, the pride and joy of the kitchen, having the ability to be a second cook." However, a psychological evaluation in 1947 concluded that J. "could not adjust successfully in the community or become self-supporting."

J. was employed as a kitchen worker at a nearby trade school while still residing at the institution. He began work at a salary of $41.00 per week. Once a week he returned to the institution for speech therapy. After six months, he received a $5.00 a week raise. Two months later, J. began work at a nearby military academy on a conditional release. He was unhappy with this situation and was placed in a live-in job at a nursing home. This placement proved to be very successful, and J. was discharged. At this time, he had $690 in savings. His final diagnosis was "borderline intelligence," and his IQ was 77. He was 50 years old and had been institutionalized for 36 years.

J. has continued working at the nursing home, where he is considered an outstanding employee. His salary in 1967 was $236 per month, and he has managed to increase his savings to over $900.

Four years after discharge J. married another middle-aged ex-institution resident, and they moved to a small apartment and purchased their own furniture. J.'s wife is also employed. The couple attend baseball and basketball games, visit with friends (mostly ex-institution residents), make frequent shopping trips, and go to the seashore for their vacation. In general, they seem a devoted and mutually supportive couple. J. has succeeded in completely disproving the negative psychological evaluation made over 20 years earlier.

E.T.

E. was one of twins born in a family of nine children. She was referred to the institution at the age of nine by the Department of Public Welfare after spending a year in a foster home and attending special classes. At the time of admission, she was diagnosed as a "low-grade moron." E. did well in the academic program for several years but was considered "...mean, defiant, and stubborn." After ten years she completed the academic program and was placed in the sewing room for training. She was considered a good worker, but her record was filled with incidents that constantly indicated conflict with authority, hostility, and open rebellion. She worked in the sewing room for eight years and received training in the institution's sheltered workshop, as well as training as a hospital aide, housekeeper, and dietary aide.

E. was helped to find employment as an aide in a local nursing home. She was withdrawn after four weeks for insubordination to her employer after an infraction of the rules. After a year, E. was again placed in the community in another nursing home. This time, she remained on the job for two months and was then returned, reportedly for entertaining boys in her room. She remained at the institution a month, working in the laundry, and was then placed in a Civil Service job as a laundry worker. After suitable living quarters were found, she was discharged to live independently. Her IQ at this time was 78, and her age at discharge was 33.

E. did well in this job for two months. She was married to a man who had left the institution ten years earlier. This individual had been married previously and was divorced. He was employed as a painter at a local college and was earning over $5,200 a year when they were married. A year after the marriage, E. suffered a miscarriage. One and a half years later, she gave birth to a daughter. The family lived in a sparsely furnished, but adequate, apartment where the child had a room of her own and appeared to be adequately cared for and normal in intelligence. However, in the following year, E. became pregnant by a visiting salesman, and her husband left her. She gave birth to a second daughter. After this, contact with E. was lost. The most recent information is over two years old. At this time, E. was unemployed, living with her two chidren, and receiving welfare payments and some support from her husband.

J.N.

J. lived with his parents until age sixteen, when his mother died and his father remarried and was unable to provide support and care for him. He was unsuccessfully placed in a foster home, and, because of increasing difficulties in the community, was admitted to the institution. Here, his initial diagnosis ranged from "low-grade moron" to "high-grade imbecile." In a psychological evaluation, administered six weeks after admission, it was noted that J.

"...lacks the ability to respond to trade training," and that he is "...a custodial-type case who barely meets our minimum requirements for admission." Subsequently J. received training as an orderly and as a kitchen worker, where he was considered a "willing, hard worker."

J. was accepted for employment as a dishwasher in a newly opened department store in the local community. His starting salary was $1.25 an hour. There was no difficulty in adjusting to this work. His supervisor considered him very adaptable to any kitchen job. His vocational counselor considered J. to be one of the most conscientious students in the Community Work Program. After six months in the program, J. had saved $694 and was discharged.

J. first lived in a private room in a boarding house. He lived there one year. His initial job placement lasted fourteen months, after which he was fired for allegedly stealing a tie clasp. He was given a work reference, however, and obtained a dishwashing job at a diner through the State Employment Agency. He worked in this job five months and then obtained a job as a maintenance man at a nearby manufacturing plant at $1.40 an hour. One year after discharge, J. married a former institutional resident. At his wife's mother's insistence, J. underwent an operation for sterilization before marriage, and both had accepted this willingly. During this period, he and his wife lived in a two-room apartment that his wife kept spotlessly clean. His wife was hospitalized twice during their first year of marriage, and this caused considerable strain on their budget. After one year of marriage, his wife insisted on their returning to her home town to be near her mother. To do this, J. borrowed $1,000 from a loan company. His savings had been depleted earlier. When the move was made, J. found no employment except for occasional diswashing jobs at $1.00 an hour. He worked at two such jobs simultaneously in order to meet his expenses. In addition, he purchased several items for the holiday season, which further indebted him. He bought a refrigerator, an expensive stereo, a complex tape recorder system, new rugs, and many small electric kitchen appliances. At the time of the last visit, this graduate was very depressed. An effort was made by the institution's Placement Counselor to obtain a position for J. in a nearby state hospital. This was done, and he started work at $1.65 an hour. After working there about two months, he did not report to work for several days and was fired. Three months later, J. was seen working at a service station in the western part of the state and was known to have sought employment at a hospital in the same community. At last report, J. has been separated from his wife and has returned to his third job, that of maintenance man at the manufacturing plant. He is currently living with a married couple, both of whom are former institutional students.

M. and E.H.

M. and E.H. are a married couple with two children. After the birth of the second child, E. was sterilized at her own request.

The family lives in a run-down house that is badly in need of repair. They are purchasing the house on the installment plan, with their $150 per month rental payments going toward eventual ownership. E. is a poor housekeeper and keeps the house in a dirty and disorderly manner. The family is in debt, having purchased such items as an electric organ and a sewing machine on credit. It has been typical of this family to spend money on non-essentials while living in squalid conditions.

The children attend special classes for the learning disabled in the public schools. They appear to be healthy and reasonably well cared for and well behaved.

M. was admitted to the institution at the age of nine. In the school program, he was also found to have a hearing problem. He was considered the "best behaved boy" in all his classes. After completing the school programs, he began trade training as a plasterer's helper and was later assigned to be a loader on the supply truck. During this time, he had two operations to correct his hearing.

E. was born in a state institution while her mother was serving a term for prostitution. Her father is unknown. She was referred to the institution by a social welfare agency after fourteen previous placements, which included two other institutions. After completing the school program, she was placed in the laundry for vocational training. After six years in this area, she was assigned to the kitchen as a cook's helper. In addition, she received further training as a nurse's helper and as a seamstress.

In the Community Work Program, M. was employed as a custodian in a manufacturing plant at $1.50 per hour. After eight months, with no problems of adjustment, M. was discharged to the same job, and suitable living quarters were found for him. At this time, he had $804 in savings. He had been institutionalized for 13 years, and his discharge IQ was 78.

E.'s initial community job was as a dining room worker at a nearby retirement home at a salary of $35 per week. She also did some cooking, and, on one occasion, she cooked two meals for 110 persons when the regular cook was off duty. However, after two months on the job, E. was removed because of problems with supervisors and the need for closer supervision. After a year and a half, she was again placed in a community job at a local department store as a sandwich girl, starting at $1.25 per hour. E. made good progress on this job, saved over $500 and was discharged from the institution after six months to live independently. She had been institutionalized for 21 years; her discharge IQ was 77.

E. had been in the community five months and M. one month when they were married. At this time, E. had an annual income of $2,560 but owed $500 on her charge account at the store where she worked. After the marriage, M. handled both their paychecks and paid off their debts in one year. M. continued to work at the same job and had two raises the first year. After one year of marriage, their joint income was $3,750. In 1967 with only M. working, the gross income was $5,000.

In addition to their constant indebtedness, the family continues to be plagued by M.'s recurrent ear problems. However, despite all their difficulties, they seem to be surviving disaster. E. has started working part-time for a housecleaning service, and her income helps in paying off some of their debts.

The preceding case histories and the general results of the follow-up study corroborate the findings of previous investigations—i.e., that large numbers of institutionalized and abandoned retarded individuals can be habilitated through vocational and social habilitation and discharged to independent community living. Although a number of these persons were found to be having difficulties in economic, vocational, or social adjustment, none were "failures" in terms of a need for reinstitutionalization. Presumably, if institutionalized mentally retarded persons can make satisfactory adjustments in the community, comparable groups of mentally retarded who have remained within the community are also capable of such adjustments. This, of course, was the same conclusion arrived at in the previous chapter after reviewing the results of previous follow-up studies.

Although the results of this study are consistent with the results of earlier investigations of the adjustment of the mentally retarded, generalizations from the findings are limited by the nature of the sample investigated and by problems in experimental design. Subjects represented only the upper intellectual range of mental retardation, with IQs between 50 and 80. The group was disproportionately represented by many borderline retarded (the mean IQ was 76 upon discharge, although it had been lower upon admission to the institution). The subjects were among the best within the institution, many of whom probably would not be institutionalized by today's standards.

It was not possible to compare subjects along the criterion measures used with comparable but nonretarded control populations. In addition, 50 percent of the group were lost as subjects. It is possible that the subjects located and willing to cooperate with the study represented a very different population than those who were "lost" as subjects. If this were true, it would represent a significant bias in the results and conclusions. An investigation of the differences in initial test characteristics of cooperative and noncooperative subjects suggests that such bias was minimal. For many noncooperative subjects for whom some information was available, community adjustment appeared quite favorable. For many of these persons, failure to cooperate was seen as an indication of better adjustment in the community and the desire to shed the image of mental retardation perpetuated by their association with the institution. However, this conclusion is inferential, and the possibility remains that many lost or noncooperative subjects were adjusting more poorly than those contacted.

Although the "failure" rate among the subjects of this study was very low according to such conventional criteria as reinstitutionalization, unemployment, and socially undesirable behaviors, there were nevertheless some persons who were leading very marginal existences.

One aspect of this project deserves special mention. The project results were extremely complimentary to the institution's habilitation programs. Since the project was federally funded (VRA Project No. 1275P), the final report and training manuals developed during the course of the funded project received national distribution and recognition. Over thirty research publications also helped to disseminate the findings and were beneficial to the public image of and awareness of the institution. This recognition by professionals outside the institution was extremely helpful in generating administrative support for the programs as well as in soliciting additional state and federal funds to perpetuate the programs, even after termination of the initial project. It would be an exaggeration to report that the project succeeded in transforming a traditionally custodial institution into a more active habilitation facility. A more accurate description was that these changes were already taking place at Elwyn at this time. The project itself represented a new habilitation philosophy that was gaining strength at Elwyn, as well as nationally. The project's results helped document these changes. By 1968, when the final report was written, Elwyn had undergone a drastic change to a comprehensive habilitation facility, emphasizing education, training, program evaluation, and research. Many students who had spent most of their lives within the institutional setting had been given the opportunity to function independently as responsible adults. More severely limited individuals were able to function at a higher and more dignified level within the institution. Staff members and professional workers were made more keenly aware of the habilitation potential of the mentally retarded. And certainly not least in importance, the stage was set for the development during the next few years of many outpatient and community services.

LITERATURE CITED

Carlson, R. E., Davis, R. V., England, G. W., and Lofquist, L. H. 1962. The measurement of employment satisfaction. Minnesota studies in vocational rehabilitation, XIII, Bulletin No. 35. University of Minnesota, Minneapolis.

Clark, G. R., Kivitz, M. S., and Rosen, M. 1968. A transitional program for institutionalized adult retarded. Project No. 1275-P. Vocational Rehabilitation Administration, Department of Health, Education, and Welfare, Washington, D. C.

Cohen, J. S., and Rusalem, H. 1964. Occupational values of retarded students. Amer. J. Ment. Defic. 69:54–61.

Davis, N. M. 1942. Attitudes to work among building operators. Occup. Psychol. 22:56–62.

Dipboye, W., and Anderson, W. F. 1959. The ordering of occupational values by high school freshman and seniors. Personnel Guidance Journal 38:121–124.

Harcourt, Brace, and World. 1959. Metropolitan Achievement Tests: Manual.

Hardin, E., Reif, H. G., and Heneman, H. G., Jr. 1951. Stability of job preferences of department store employees. J. Appl. Psychol. 35:256–259.

Jurgensen, C. E. 1947. Selected factors which influence job preferences. J. Appl. Psychol. 31:553–563.

Jurgensen, C. E. 1948. What job applicants look for in a company. Personnel Psychology 1:433–445.

Katz, M. M., and Lyerly, S. B. 1963. Methods for measuring adjustment and social behavior in the community: I. Rationale, description, descriminative validity and scale development. Psychological Reports, Monograph Supplement:4-V13.

McCarver, R. B., and Craig, E. M. 1974. Placement of the retarded in the community: Prognosis and outcome. *In* N. R. Ellis (ed.), International Review of Research in Mental Retardation, pp. 145–207. Academic Press, New York.

National Industrial Conference Board. 1947. Factors affecting employee morale. Studies in Personnel Policy No. 85. New York.

Rose, A. M. 1952. Union Solidarity. University of Minnesota Press, Minneapolis.

Rosen, M., Floor, L., and Baxter, D. 1974. IQ, academic achievement and community adjustment after discharge from the institution. Ment. Retard. 12:51–53.

Rosen, M., Halenda, R., Nowakiwska, M., and Floor, L. 1970*a*. Employment satisfaction of previously institutionalized mentally subnormal workers. Ment. Retard. 8:35–40.

Rosen, M., Kivitz, M. S., Clark, G. R., and Floor, L. 1970*b*. Prediction of post-institutional adjustment of mentally retarded adults. Amer. J. Ment. Defic. 74:726–734.

Scott, T. B., Davis, R. V., England, G. W., and Lofquist, L. H. 1960. A definition of work adjustment. Minnesota Studies in Vocational Rehabilitation: X. Bulletin No. 30. University of Minnesota, Minneapolis.

Wechsler, D. 1955. Manual for the Wechsler Adult Intelligence Scale. The Psychological Corporation, New York.

Windle, C. 1962. Prognosis of mental subnormals. Amer. J. Ment. Defic. Monograph Supplement 66:No. 5.

Chapter 11

Predicting Success in the Community

As previous chapters have indicated, a large proportion of the population classified as mildly mentally subnormal are capable of adequately coping with independent living. However, many such individuals must be considered habilitation "failures" in that they have either been reinstitutionalized or have encountered such problems in their economic, vocational, and social adjustment that they have become a severe burden to society. The fact that some retarded persons can succeed in the community while others fail suggests the need to determine, before their discharge from institutional or special school programs, which persons have the greatest potential for successful adjustment to independent living.

As Heber (1959) has noted:

> There is a great need for research directed toward a determination of the significant variables related to the ultimate personal, social, and vocational adjustment of the mentally retarded. Then, and only then, will we be in a position to carry out research evaluations of various kinds of educational treatments designed to accomplish favorable modifications on these significant variables (p. 1018).

A great number of prognostic studies have been directed toward this goal—i.e., to determine what variables are effective predictors of successful and unsuccessful habilitation outcomes for retarded persons entering the community.

Comprehensive reviews of these prognostic studies have been published by Windle (1962) and McCarver and Craig (1974). Both these reviews concentrate on studies of previously institutionalized retardates. As Windle points out, the reasons for selecting institutionalized persons for prognostic study are that these populations can be easily defined, and that the most serious adjustment problems are probably encountered by previously institutionalized populations.

LITERATURE REVIEW

Windle organized his review according to five general areas of predictive characteristics: demographic factors, individual abilities and disabilities, institutional experiences, family and community factors, and combination of factors. Studies bearing on each of these areas are described in terms of their effectiveness in relating such factors to outcome criteria directly relevant to post-institutional community adjustment. Such criteria include: avoidance of reinstitutionalization, vocational placement, salary, absence of aberrant or socially unacceptable behaviors, and interpersonal relationships.

McCarver and Craig's review follows a similar pattern of grouping prognostic studies in accordance with predictive variables. These variables include pre-admission factors such as home environment, history of delinquency, and sexual behaviors. Institutional variables include factors such as reasons for admission, age at admission, general behavior, training programs, work experiences, and length of institutionalization. Other variables include criteria for release from the institution, family interest, and type of community placement at discharge. In addition, studies are reported that have dealt with community attitudes toward, and with supervision of, mental retardates. Individual characteristics that have been related to post-institutional adjustment are listed as age at release, diagnosis, race, intellectual level, academic ability, personality, personal appearance, and physical handicaps.

Despite the large number of correlational studies that have been performed, the state of our knowledge concerning the prognosis of the mentally retarded discharged from institutions, based upon their personal characteristics, previous history, or institutional experience, is still quite poor. Windle offers a large number of tentative conclusions from the studies reviewed but emphasizes the methodological flaws in most studies, the discrepancies in their findings, and the poor generalizability of the evidence that particular predictor-criterion relationships exist. McCarver and Craig point out that despite the need to know which of the mentally retarded will benefit most from the increasing alternatives to institutional living, "placement is typically on a trial and error basis and evaluation is mainly subjective." Thus, if these reviews are accurate, the situation has not improved substantially from 1962 to 1974.

In reading these comprehensive reviews of prognostic studies involving such a wide variety of variables, one is struck by the number of times that contradictory results have emerged from different investigations, as well as the differing degrees of emphasis on certain factors as compared to others.

For example, as might be expected, intelligence (as measured by standard intelligence tests) has been one of the most widely used predictor variables, both for eligibility for release from institutions, and for community adjustment. McCarver and Craig cite 33 studies that produced findings on the relationship of IQ to adjustment success. Of these, 12 reported a positive relationship, and seven more provided suggestive evidence for such a relationship. On the other hand, 13 studies found no meaningful correlation between IQ and community adjustment, and one study is mentioned in which a negative relationship was reported (p. 171).

The discrepancy between verbal and performance IQ scores has also been investigated. For example, Ferguson (1958) indicates that sheltered workshop clients with performance superiority on the Wechsler Adult Intelligence Scale were more likely than those with verbal superiority to be able to obtain and hold a job outside of the institution. Several other studies, using different measures, also report that superiority on perceptual-motor tests over verbal or language tests is associated with favorable community outcomes. It may be that the performance-verbal discrepancy is more predictive of release than of success after release.

One reason for the failure of consistent prediction from IQ scores is the narrow range of IQs that are used in follow-up studies, usually between 50 and 80. In most studies this IQ range was representative of the majority of persons who left institutions or public school programs. Lower IQ populations remained within the institution or, if they lived at home, were often excluded from public school programs where they could have come to the attention of research investigators. With the advent of the deinstitutionalization trend and the burgeoning use of group homes for lower functioning mentally retarded persons, the entire concept of adjustment has been expanded. Outcomes in community living are no longer limited to employment stability, vocational competence, law-abiding behavior and the like for persons making their own way in the world. Adjustment for a moderately or severely retarded person today can mean maintaining a quiet existence within the group home in a manner that differs little from institutional living arrangements. It is clear, then, that a much broader dimension of community adjustment exists today than in previous years. When IQ is studies as a correlate of such a criterion of adjustment, there is likely to be a greater chance of demonstrating significant relationships.

Bell (1976) separated a group of former state school residents into those whose predischarge IQ was below 55 and those whose IQ was above 55. A questionnaire was mailed either directly to the resident (for the higher ability subjects) or to a parent or guardian (for the lower ability subjects). Substantial differences in life style were found to be related to IQ differences. The higher ability subjects appeared to be leading a more fulfilling life, were more involved in community activities, dated more often, and saw friends more frequently. Forty-seven percent of the high group and only 18 percent of the low group were competitively employed, either full or part-time. The author acknowledges, however, that the two ability groups were also different in environmental support factors such as institutional training, institution-initiated release, and agency assistance in the community. It is possible that differences in life style were affected by these factors rather than by IQ.

Evidence for predictor-criterion relationships for variables other than IQ, such as age or years of institutionalization, is equally inconclusive. Nor is predictability improved by studying noninstitutionalized populations (Phelps, 1956; Lee, Hegge, and Voelker, 1959; Kolstoe, 1961).

As if to remedy the problem of prediction from single variables, some investigators have studied a wide variety of predictive and criterion measures and attempted to organize their results by factor analyses. Stephens (1964), for example, identified 80 continuous and 61 dichotomous variables as measures of success in the community. These were broadly grouped into vocational, sociocivic, and personal types of success. However, when the continuous variables were resolved by factor analysis into 17 factors, these did not fall clearly into the initial three groupings. "Furthermore, just to emphasize complexity worse confounded, criterion variables combining positively to form a factor called 'success syndrome' did not combine negatively to form the factor 'failure syndrome' " (pp. 8–9).

Shafter (1957) identified 12 predictive characteristics that had some value for successful community placement. He formulated these into a predictive equation and found that the highest possible rated score on the 12 variables would yield a 66 percent probability of successful placement outside the institution. As Cobb and Epir (1966) point out, this is indicative of the limited prognostic value of even the best estimates.

Rosen, Kivitz, Clark, and Floor (1970) selected a battery of psychometric tests, behavioral ratings, and demographic indices to represent a wide spectrum of variables reported in previous studies as measures of social or vocational community adjustment. All together there were 29 predictor variables. Twenty-two criterion variables included measures of economic, vocational, and social adjustment. Economic adjustment included such things as amount of savings and monthly rents. Vocational adjustment included job stability, degree of unemployment, income, occupational level, employment satisfaction, and ratings of vocational functioning. Social adjustment included the management of personal affairs, interpersonal relationships, and subjective measures of personal happiness and satisfaction. The 65 subjects represented approximately one-half of the persons discharged from Elwyn Institute over a four-year period. Most subjects had IQs between 50 and 80, and all were discharged to independent living and competitive employment situations.

The number of statistically significant relationships obtained was approximately five times that expected by chance alone. However, the correlation coefficients were low, with only about 10 percent of the predictor variables explaining as much as 25 percent of the criterion variance. Because of the relatively low correlations and small number of subjects, generalizations from these data were considered tentative.

In general, tests contributing most to verbal IQ and scholastic achievement were relatively less important as correlates of post-institutional adjustment than were those tests reflecting perceptual-motor skills. Similar relationships have already been reported from other studies. The importance of nonverbal ability was further emphasized by the large predominance (almost 4 to 1) of subjects with high performance IQ relative to verbal IQ scores. Those having this IQ pattern tended to earn higher salaries.

Of the various behavioral ratings reflecting institutional adjustment, only those dealing with employability were significantly related to criterion variables. Ratings by community employers showed no significant relationships with criteria, nor did they relate to psychometric scores or ratings by institutional staff. Similarly, ratings of social adjustment within the institution did not relate to any of the social or vocational criteria of adjustment in the community. Job-related criteria showed the majority of predictive relationships; criteria of social adjustment were not readily predicted.

The 29 predictor variables and 22 criterion variables were subjected to a separate factor analysis to identify the minimum number of independent factors needed to account for the variance in the correlational matrices. Since verbal reasoning played a major role in both the IQ and achievement tests, it is not surprising that a verbal factor accounted for the largest proportion of the total variance. A second factor, perceptual-motor skill, showed no relation to staff ratings of institutional adjustment or community potential.

While the predictor factor labeled ''employability'' had no correlation with either demographic information or test scores, all employability ratings were strongly intercorrelated. It would appear that while raters' impressions of how well the individual is able to handle a vocational assignment is an important factor influencing his perceived suitability for discharge from the institution, it is also likely that ratings of employability involve considerably more than the ability to handle the physical demands of the job. Employability scales included many items devoted to social judgment and ability to engage in interpersonal relationships.

The factor contributing most to the total variance of criterion measures reflected a set of self-maintenance behaviors encompassing the handling of personal affairs and the demonstration of a minimal degree of personal responsibility. It included such things as housekeeping, the handling of medical problems, finances, transportation, and personal hygiene. The emergence of these areas of functioning as a unitary factor suggests that there may be some underlying trait or ability accounting for the specific areas rated. It is reasonable to believe that this characteristic could be measured directly during the training program and used in selection for discharge. Other interim factors reflected interview questions related to job satisfaction, job stability, and general adjustment.

In general, the factor analysis was a more productive facet of this study than were the predictor-criterion relationships. The emergence of specific clusters of both predictor and criterion variables provided a basis for interpretation of complex and sometimes seemingly contradictory findings and enhanced the meaningfulness of both predictor and criterion measures.

Few studies have attempted cross-validation of their initial findings. One investigation that did use this procedure was performed by O'Connor and Tizard (1951), who attempted to combine a variety of predictive indices. Some relationships with criteria were demonstrated but these results were not replicated in a second investigation. To explain this contradiction, the authors suggest that the difference in findings of the two studies was due to the unreliability of both the predictive tests used and of the measurement of their criterion, work success. However, regardless of the contradictory results, the sophisticated research methods of O'Connor and Tizard represented an advance over those previously employed by other workers in the field.

A few years after the first prognostic study was completed, two cross-validation studies were undertaken by Rosen, Floor, and Baxter (1972). Subjects for the first of these investigations were chosen in the same manner as those of the previous study—i.e., they were formerly institutionalized adults who had completed the habilitation programs, had been discharged for from six months to two years, and were actually or functionally orphaned. The second group of subjects numbered 60. They did not include any persons interviewed in the original prognostic study;

however, an analysis of relevant comparison variables showed no significant differences between the two subject populations, either in terms of original characteristics or in subsequent community adjustment. Measurement of predictor and criterion variables was accomplished in the same manner as in the original sample. Intercorrelations and factor analysis were repeated as before, using the same criteria of statistical significance.

It was found that the earlier relationships reported were not repeated in the replication study. While the predictor and criterion factors that emerged were similar to those found earlier, the relationships of perceptual-motor skills and employability ratings to indices of community adjustment were not substantiated.

A second replication study was performed with a group of 69 subjects, none of whom had participated in the other two studies. A more immediate, dichotomous criterion of success or failure was chosen. The transitional, community-work experience before discharge was selected to reflect competence at community functioning during the halfway house period. Twenty-nine persons who failed to adjust to the program and were withdrawn within a period of one month or less were designated as a ''short-term'' group. Forty others, who were able to remain in the program for four months or longer constituted the ''long-term'' group. (Most of these were later discharged, but this was not a criterion for inclusion in the group.)

T-test comparisons were performed for all original predictor variables between the short- and long-term groups. There were no significant findings to support those of the original prognostic study. However, it was found that age correlated with employment stability—older subjects and those with longer histories of institutionalization were more frequently found in the long-term group.

CONCLUSION

The problems that account for the absence of much solid prognostic data to support administrative decisions affecting parole and discharge from institutions include both methodological and practical considerations. The most obvious problem is the absence of reliable criteria of adjustment in the community to use as a basis for developing predictive variables. A step in developing programmatic research in this area would seem to be the construction or adaptation of existing scales of social, vocational, and personal functioning, and the collection of normative data in a variety of community settings. Such scales would be widely disseminated to those having interests in conducting predictive studies. This would provide a maximum amount of data in the shortest time possible and greater uniformity among the studies done in the future. Similarly, a cooperative effort among investigators could ensure that similar predictive and criterion measures were studied from one investigation to another. This would allow the collection of more reliable information that could be generalized to different populations.

The failure of research to establish valid predictor-criterion relationships casts doubt upon the efficacy of an empirical "shotgun" approach to predicting complex criteria of community adjustment. While meaningful guidelines for selection of candidates for training and discharge from institutions can probably be derived from future research studies, more sophisticated methods for identifying potential predictors and meaningful criteria are needed.

Except when extreme IQ comparisons are considered, there has been little in research to indicate the usefulness of cognitive-intellectual factors as determinants of community adjustment of retarded persons. For those persons being prepared for independent living arrangements and competitive employment, there is a need to consider personality variables as predictors (Skaarbrevik, 1971; Stephens, Peck, and Veldman, 1968; Zigler and Harter, 1969).

Despite the potential value of personality variables, little meaningful research has been done in this area. In his conclusions, Windle states that "Few investigators have had the temerity and determination to study the prognostic value of personality systematically. ...This lack is especially severe for the field of mental subnormality in which the verbal and self-reporting skills which most personality tests depend upon are deficient" (p. 138). McCarver and Craig point out that while personality factors have been stressed by many investigators, "little objective research has been conducted concerning the relationship between personality and outcome."

The use of personality rather than cognitive variables necessitates the development of a construct validity approach to prediction (Cronbach and Meehl, 1955). The first step in this process is to choose criteria of adjustment in the community that have more specific behavioral referents. Variables such as job stability, income, and job complexity, while having general interest as indices of adjustment, represent extremely complex variables. Income levels, for example, are determined by far more than the competence or training of the employee. The conceptual link between such variables and many of the psychometric predictor variables used in prognostic study is quite tenuous. By choosing narrower areas of community behavior, predictive efficiency should be increased.

The second step is to choose an intervening personality construct that might account for such criterion behaviors and that would also relate to measurable test constructs. Next, measures should be chosen that seem to have face validity in assessing this personality construct, and normative information should be obtained using relevant experimental and control populations. Once reliable measurement techniques have been established, it should be possible to conduct correlative studies to establish the predictive validity of such measures with previously developed criteria. Predictive studies of community adjustment following this plan have never been performed, and our own efforts described in succeeding chapters represent only a beginning.

LITERATURE CITED

Bell, N. J. 1976. IQ as a factor in community lifestyle of previously institutionalized retardates. Ment. Retard. 14:29–33.

Cobb, H. V., and Epir, S. 1966. Predictive studies of vocational adjustment. *In* S. G. DiMichael (ed.), New Vocational Pathways for the Mentally Retarded. American Personnel & Guidance Association.

Cronbach, L. J., and Meehl, P. E. 1955. Construct validity in psychological tests. Psychol. Bull. 52:281–302.

Ferguson, R. G. 1958. Evaluation of the potential for vocational rehabilitation of mentally retarded youths with muscular, orthopedic, and emotional impairments. Second annual report. Sheltered Workshop of the MacDonald Training Center, Tampa, Florida.

Heber, R. 1959. Promising areas for psychological research in mental retardation. Amer. J. Ment. Defic. 63:1014–1019.

Kolstoe, O. P. 1961. An examination of some characteristics which discriminate between employed and non-employed mentally retarded males. Amer. J. Ment. Defic. 66:472–482.

Lee, J. L., Hegge, T. G., and Voelker, P. H. 1959. A study of social adequacy and social failure of mentally retarded youth in Wayne County, Michigan. Wayne State University, Detroit.

McCarver, R. B., and Craig, E. M. 1974. Placement of the retarded in the community: Prognosis and outcome. *In* N. R. Ellis (ed.), International Review of Research in Mental Retardation, pp. 145–207. Vol. 7. Academic Press, New York.

O'Connor, N., and Tizard, J. 1951. Predicting the occupational adequacy of certified mental defectives. Occup. Psychol. 25:205–211.

Phelps, H. R. 1956. Post-school adjustment of mentally retarded children in selected Ohio cities. Except. Child. 23:58–62.

Rosen, M., Floor, L., and Baxter, D. 1972. Prediction of community adjustment: A failure at cross-validation. Amer. J. Ment. Defic. 77:111–112.

Rosen, M., Kivitz, M. S., Clark, T. R., and Floor, L. 1970. Prediction of post-institutional adjustment of mentally retarded adults. Amer. J. Ment. Defic. 74:726–734.

Shafter, A. J. 1957. Criteria for selecting institutionalized mental defectives for vocational placement. Amer. J. Ment. Defic. 61:599–616.

Skaarbrevik, K. J. 1971. A follow-up study of educable mentally retarded in Norway. Amer. J. Ment. Defic. 75:560–565.

Stephens, W. B. D. 1964. Success of young adult male retardates. Unpublished doctoral dissertation, University of Texas.

Stephens, W. B., Peck, J. R., and Veldman, D. J. 1968. Personality and success profiles characteristic of young adult male retardates. Amer. J. Ment. Defic. 73:405–413.

Windle, C. 1962. Prognosis of mental subnormals. Amer. J. Ment. Defic. Monograph Supplement 66:No. 5.

Zigler, E. F., and Harter, S. 1969. The socialization of the mentally retarded. *In* D. A. Goslin (ed.), Handbook of Socialization Theory and Research. Rand McNally & Company, Chicago.

Section V

Social and Emotional Factors

Chapter 12

Personality and Emotional Factors

The frontispiece of the revised ninth edition of A. F. Tredgold's monumental textbook on mental deficiency (Tredgold and Soddy, 1956) depicts a most unusual photograph. Standing in the foreground is the late Tredgold, holding a small notepad and interviewing an elderly lady. The woman, apparently mentally retarded, has a happy, almost beatific expression on her face. Far in the background, and almost unnoticed at first, stands another lady, younger, more sullen in appearance, intently observing the other two. The photograph's caption reads: "The doctor (right) is the late A. F. Tredgold in 1900 or thereabouts, aged 30, very likely collecting notes for the first edition of this book. The expressions of the two aments are interesting, showing clearly doubt and some jealousy (left) and happy self-importance (centre)."

It is of interest that the authors acknowledge at the beginning of their book the importance of emotional life of their subjects. Surprisingly, little else in the book is devoted to personality of the mentally retarded. Tredgold's text and other sources deal with emotional components in the etiology of mental retardation or focus upon more extreme cases of emotional dysfunction such as autism, psychosis, the "idiot savant," or the "moral imbecile," but minimize the issue of personality development or structure. More recent writers have attempted to apply to the mentally retarded theoretical formulations developed for normal intelligence populations (Cromwell, 1963; Woodward, 1963) in order to describe personality assessment procedures (Cromwell, 1967), and to study empirically personality characteristics of the mentally retarded (Turnure, 1971; Zigler, 1967). Despite these positive changes, there have been few attempts to apply personality constructs specific to mentally retarded populations to their education, training, or social habilitation.

This chapter summarizes early and more recent formulations about the emotional life of the mentally retarded. It suggests some new directions for the exploration of personality and for applying these constructs in habilitative efforts.

Tredgold and Soddy (1956) define mental deficiency as arrested development of the "mind," which includes not only areas of cognition, but also a lack of instinctual drive and a poverty of affect. They describe the compliant and sluggish behavior of mentally retarded infants and their focus upon objects that are immediate, near at hand, and narrow in range as evidence of "instinctual weakness." They point out an apparent paradox between the "weak instincts" of the retarded and the fact that they may sometimes become aggressive and violent. The latter observation is seen as a problem of control rather than of excess energies. The feeble-minded or higher level retarded are described in similar terms:

> Like imbeciles, only less so, they need fairly direct satisfaction of their instinctual drives; they can tolerate only limited diversion of impulse and postponement of their rewards. Like children of their mental age, their morality will continue to depend on their personal relationships, for they are incapable of regulating their conduct by abstract principle. This failure results both from a cognitive incapacity to select, discriminate, make judgments, generalize and abstract; and from a conative-affective failure to identify themselves strongly with a loved adult and so to modify the satisfaction of their instinctual drives. It is not difficult, on such a basis, to work out in detail the likely behaviour patterns of the feeble-minded.
>
> In many respects the behavior of the feeble-minded shows considerable advance on that of imbeciles. Very many feeble-minded, for example, can be gainfully employed, under suitably protected circumstances. In their social relationships they often manage to work through their infantile dependence on their mothers and enter into stable relationships with their siblings and contemporaries. On the whole, the feeble-minded make good club members; they are gregarious, usually friendly, but not capable of forming those deep individual attachments that sometimes wreck club life. Their lack of instinctual drive leaves them with little incentive to compete and their quarrels are superficial and short-lived. They normally develop sufficiently to make good, though over-dependent, substitute relationships with other adults. They, therefore, will adapt well to an institutional life provided that their instinctual needs are met. In considering the characteristics of institutionalized defectives, however, it should be remembered that good superficial sibling relationships, gregariousness and lack of quarrelling, combined with inability to abstract, to form deep personal relationships and to develop responsibility are features not only of feeble-mindedness but of institutionalization itself. It is

possible that much of what we regard as typical of institutionalized defectives is due to the institution rather than the deficiency (p. 73).

Another concept pertaining directly to the emotional or temperamental qualities of the retarded was borrowed from a prevailing notion in psychiatry during the late 19th century. Kerlin (1889) describes the condition of "moral imbecility" as one in which "there is a loss of control over the lower propensities, or in which the moral sentiments rather than the intellectual powers are confused, weakened, or perverted." This condition was interpreted to be an inherent fault associated with organic damage to the nervous system and irreversible regardless of training or education. Kerlin described four classes of moral imbeciles: the alcoholic, the tramp, the prostitute, and the habitual criminal. He believed that most such cases were intellectually feeble and of generally bad heredity. "To constitute a case of moral imbecility we must have badness without reason, violence without motive, deception without purpose, thieving without acquisitiveness, brutality inspired by a fiendish love for inflicting pain." Many writers of this era understood such characteristics as a throwback to more primitive behaviors of primordial man.

By the turn of the century the concept had already undergone some change. Fernald (1909) believed all imbeciles to be potential criminals but acknowledged that such tendencies may be "suppressed" by environmental conditions. He seemed to endorse the concept of moral imbecility but indicated that such persons were cases of "true imbecility," exhibiting intellectual impairment as well as moral degeneracy.

Goddard (1910) examined so-called moral imbeciles with the Binet intelligence scale and described the condition as an arrest in development at about the nine-year-old level, at a time when impulses for lying and stealing have come into full maturity, but reasoning, judgment, and other faculties that might control those instincts have not.

Tredgold and Soddy treat the problem of "moral deficiency" as part of a general issue of psychological instability and the regulation of conduct among the mentally retarded. They point out that the British Mental Deficiency Act of 1955 retained a section devoted to moral deficiency first drafted in 1927 when *moral defectives* were defined as "persons in whose case there exists mental defectiveness coupled with strongly vicious or criminal propensities, and who require care, supervision, and control for the protection of others." The authors debunk earlier conceptions of a throwback to precivilized behaviors in favor of a combination of genetic and environmental factors. Because of its existence as a legal entity, Tredgold and Soddy suggest it is convenient to retain the designation. The term "moral imbecile" was awkward because of cases that fit the description without also showing gross intellectual impairment. It was dropped in 1927 in favor of the more workable term "moral defective."

Masland, Sarason, and Gladwin's (1958) authoritative account of the biological, psychological, and cultural factors associated with mental subnormality emphasizes the importance of personality factors in predicting nonacademic problem-solving behavior. The authors discuss the possibility that personality or emotional factors rather than intellectual deficiencies may be the primary determinants of social and behavioral maladjustment. They note that despite the fact that numerous sources call for investigations of emotional factors in the mentally retarded, little systematic research has been undertaken.

> What is the nature and role of emotions and feelings in the (mentally retarded) individual's adjustment and thinking?...What may be inferred about the role and adequacy of the defensive reactions associated with strong feeling and emotion?
>
> What light is shed on the above questions from an examination or reconstruction of the life history? What are the experiences (e.g., separation, trauma, failure) or types of relationships (e.g., social class, ethnic) which influenced the development of the individual and are reflected in his current life adjustment?
>
> The above are certainly not all the questions that are asked when one is faced with the diagnostic problem of psychosis or, for that matter, understanding the personality of *any* individual. But we think we have listed enough of the questions to substantiate the conclusion that the diagnostic process is a searching comprehensive investigation which has the understandably ambitious aim of attaining understanding of another person's 'psychology'—*that* individual's way of thinking, feeling, and acting. *Rarely, if ever, is the mentally defective individual studied or viewed in this light* (pp. 312–313).

The authors call for a national effort in developing longitudinal research dealing with the development of mentally retarded children at selected child research centers.

It is not our intention to convey the impression that interest in personality structure or dynamics in mental retardation has been entirely lacking or that Masland, Sarason, and Gladwin's challenge has gone completely unheeded. A few stalwart investigators have risen to this challenge and have produced a set of theoretical constructs and empirical findings that have potential for greater understanding of the personality development of mentally retarded persons. Some of these findings have been applied in therapeutic efforts that will be discussed in a later chapter. However, these efforts have been isolated and without a great deal of impact upon persons who deal with the mentally retarded in a professional or service capacity. The school or institutional psychologist continues to cling to intellectual or other cognitive constructs in diagnosis and evaluation and to rely upon the old assessment warhorses of Wechsler and Binet. The habilitation counselor may use work samples or vocational aptitude tests; he may be expert in a variety of vocational training alternatives; and he may fully appreciate the necessity to teach the retarded to count change or to orient him to the "world of work." Yet how often does he ask how a history of failure may have conditioned the mentally retarded to accept lower aspiration levels; how often does he speculate about the effect of limited intellect or physical stigmata upon self-concept; how often does he wonder about how the regimentation within the institution conditions patterns of helplessness or dependency?

Four major theoretical models have been applied to clarify personality development and dynamics in the mentally retarded. Of these, three have been productive of empirical research, one has not. The models derive from the social learning theory of Rotter (1954), the developmental theory of Piaget (1960, 1962), the psychoanalytic theory of Freud, and the motivational-cognitive position of Zigler (1969).

SOCIAL LEARNING THEORY

Probably the most well-researched and thoroughly developed conceptualization of the personality of mentally retarded persons derives from social learning theory. This body of research stems from the conceptual framework of Julian Rotter (1954). The constructs of this model are offered by their investigators, not as proven facts, but as useful constructs to handle what empirical information is currently available and as self-correcting when new research ideas are generated. The approach and its major constructs are presented briefly here in the same spirit.

Rotter focuses on interaction of the individual and his meaningful environment, i.e., the goal objects that determine the direction of behavior. Two major factors that determine the potential for an individual to behave in a given situation and in relation to a specific goal are the value or importance of that goal to the individual, and his expectancy of achieving that goal.

Investigations applying this model to understanding the mentally retarded have built upon each other and resulted in a gradual evolution of a more sophisticated theoretical network. The original notions stemmed from the assumption that the mental retardate experiences more failure experiences than the normal child and, therefore, develops a lower generalized expectancy of success. It would then follow that his potential is lowered for goals that had resulted in failure as well as for goals in general. This lowered potential to behave would produce further failures and further lowering of expectancies of success, and the cycle would be repeated.

It is not our intention here to review the numerous studies that have been conducted to test these assumptions. As in most behavioral research associated with theory building, the results have not always been confirmatory. The interested reader is directed toward Cromwell's comprehensive chapters (Cromwell, 1963, 1967) and to Heber's (1964) review of personality research and mental retardation for a survey of this literature and the development of the theory.

Initial studies of expectancy generated by social learning theory were conducted by Heber (1957). He reasoned that mentally retarded children equated on initial task performance with normal controls would have a higher potential for performance under conditions in which they encountered success experiences. This reasoning was based upon the assumption that the retardates have an initially lower generalized expectancy of success than the normal intelligence children. Success experiences, therefore, should increase expectancies more for the retarded than the normal children. Failure experiences, on the other hand, should produce less decrement in performance with retarded children than with normal children since the failure would not be discrepant with the expectancies of success already held by the retarded children. The results of the Heber study and of a later study by Gardner (1958) were generally supportive of this position.

The next step was an extension of the model by the formulation of two types of behavioral tendencies to deal better with directionality. The success-striving individual was described as one with a high generalized expectancy for success who responded primarily to cues pointing the way to continued success. The failure-striving person was described as one having a very low generalized expectancy for success who responded primarily to negative environmental cues that would lead to the prevention of additional failure. At this point in the development of the theory the failure-avoiding tendency was associated with mental retardation.

Again empirical results were not completely supportive of the theoretical postulates and again the theory was modified. The possibility was suggested that many of the mentally retarded subjects in the experiments being conducted were too young or too retarded to conceptualize success or failure. Such a conceptualization requires that the individual attribute the outcome of his efforts to his own effectiveness. In cases where the individual did not conceptualize the attainment or non-attainment of the goal as due to his own efforts, the constructs of success or failure-striving could not be used to predict results. It was postulated that not all avoidant behavior was caused by failure avoidance. Some aversive objects or situations might be avoided even when the individual assumed no responsibility for nonattainment of the goal. Similarly, not all goal attainment would be assumed to be owing to personal effectiveness by the individual but might be perceived as owing to chance or to the efforts of others.

Developmental evidence was accumulated to demonstrate that in young children experiences are viewed by them as being externally controlled, i.e., imposed by some outside agency. Such experiences may be perceived by the child as pleasant or unpleasant but not related to his own behavior. As development progresses the child learns that he is able to influence the outcome of events by his own actions. This shift in conceptualization by the child from external to internal locus of control parallels the development by the child of the ability to categorize the outcomes of goal-directed behavior as success or failure. If a goal is attained by the child, not only is it perceived as pleasant, but also as a success caused by his own ability. Likewise, an unfavorable outcome is not only unpleasant to the child, it is also a failure. Development of the ability to internalize locus of control for goal-directed behavior is necessary for the ability to respond to certain situations as ego-involving and also to learn to delay gratification.

The locus of control formulation assumes that there exist two motivational systems: 1) a hedonistic pleasure-approach and pain-avoidance system based upon primary and secondary reinforcement and operating in the younger child; and 2) a success-approach and failure-avoidance system operating in the older child. The second system does not replace, but supplements, the earlier one. It probably does not develop in the absence of language.

Three methods have been used to evaluate these motivational systems. The first is a puzzle situation in which the child is given the opportunity to return to a puzzle he has previously failed. It is assumed that a child operating under a hedonistic system would choose to return to a previous successful experience because of its pleasant, reinforcing qualities. A more mature child will return to a failed puzzle in an attempt to succeed. A second evaluation strategy allows the individual to choose between an immediate lesser reward and a delayed larger reward. The third approach is the use of a series of questions in a locus of control questionnaire in which the individual is asked whether he sees himself in control of events or whether he sees them as externally controlled.

In general, each of these measures was found to relate positively to age. Older children were more likely to have an internal locus of control, to choose the previously failed puzzle, and to delay gratification in order to receive a larger reward. As expected, the measures related more closely to mental age than to chronological age. The latter finding, of course, is the important theoretical and empirical link with mental retardation. Although research findings with the retarded are not always consistent in supporting the theory, evidence has accumulated that suggests that mentally retarded individuals often perform in novel situations below their ability levels, conceptualize and react to failure less than normal intelligence groups, and are less likely than normals to increase their goal-striving efforts after a mild failure experience.

The extension and modification of social learning theory on the basis of research results is a good example of the application of the hypothetico-deductive method in studying personality characteristics of the retarded. The utility of the approach is found not only in its contribution to theory building but also in its flexibility as a clinical evaluation method. The constructs of expectancy, reinforcement value, behavior potential, and locus of control may prove to be important in conceptualizing how mentally retarded persons behave. The approach provides a plethora of concepts for both research and clinical use. The locus of control construct should potentially add to the clinician's armamentarium. Unfortunately, it has not yet been developed as a psychometric instrument.

Cromwell (1967) makes an initial stab at applying these constructs clinically in a chapter dealing with personality evaluation. He provides an interesting discussion dealing with the heightened potential for personality problems that may be associated with the development of the more mature success-failure motivational system. A child who perceives himself as a failure may regress to more hedonistically determined behaviors, may show decreased effort, may avoid goal-striving situations, may show excessively high or low levels of aspiration, or may develop strong feelings of inadequacy. On the other hand, a person who develops unrealistically high feelings of internal control may abandon caution and subject himself to danger. If he becomes excessively responsible for the outcome of events, he may become worried and depressed or hostile toward those blocking his progress toward a goal.

DEVELOPMENTAL LEARNING THEORY OF PIAGET

A second theoretical approach derives originally from the theory of intellectual development and moral development of Piaget (1960, 1962; Woodward, 1963). Piaget postulates a sequence of developmental steps that are consistent for all individuals although the time sequence of development may vary. The theory traces the evolution of abstract reasoning from its origins in the sensorimotor behavior in infancy to the stage of formal operations that typically develops around the age of eleven. The types of thinking characteristic of each developmental stage are analyzed in terms of the logical operations involved. The "schema," Piaget's basic structural unit of intelligence, is described as a response pattern that has both behavioral and physiological referents. It is a biological system with certain functions. Piaget does not consider structure and function independently. More complex schemata develop and are progressively organized from simpler ones. Schemata develop through the child's interaction with physical objects so that experience and the child's exploratory activities are given a significant role in the development of intelligence.

The stages of Piaget's developmental sequence progress from simple reflex activities such as kicking and sucking to abstract and logical thinking, including the formulation of hypotheses, deductive reasoning, and checking solutions. The theory has been well elaborated (Piaget and Inhelder, 1947) as well as attacked (Birch, 1966), and no further discussion of developmental stages will be provided here. Instead, our interest is in the implications of the theory for personality and emotional development. Unfortunately, Piaget does not deal directly with emotional development per se. Relevant aspects of the theory derive from those aspects of the theory pertaining to moral judgment and moral conduct and from research investigations that have attempted to relate developmental stages of moral development to stages of intellectual development that may be requisite for such moral growth. Our discussion here, therefore, is limited to those aspects of emotional, social, and personality development that determine moral reasoning and conduct. Other aspects of personality may only by implication be related to Piaget's developmental theory.

Studies of moral development of the mentally retarded have dealt primarily with three research issues. The first concerns the differences between mentally retarded children and normal intelligence children of equivalent mental age. This question touches upon a more general issue concerning whether the mentally retarded are qualitatively different from normal intelligence groups or whether differences that exist can be understood entirely on the basis of overall developmental delays. The second issue concerns the relationship between cognitive and moral development. Kohlberg (1969) has defined a sequence of stages of moral development and has demonstrated that it is positively correlated with age. He has hypothesized that a particular stage of cognitive development constitutes a necessary but not sufficient condition for each stage of moral growth. The third issue concerns the logitudinal development of moral reasoning and conduct. Longitudinal studies of the same individuals over time can provide more definitive answers to such questions as the interrelation between various measures of moral development, the generality of such traits as honesty, responsibility, and self-control, and the degree to which later behaviors of a moral or nonmoral nature can be predicted from earlier evaluations of moral reasoning and behavior.

In general, research (Kohlberg, 1958) has confirmed the developmental nature of moral judgment although age changes do not always conform to Piaget's expectations. Retarded and nonretarded children who differ in chronological age but are matched on mental age tend not to differ in level of moral judgment (Taylor and Achenbach, 1975) or moral conduct (Moore and Stephens, 1974). The studies of moral conduct are most relevant to the interest in personality factors since they deal specifically with situations of temptation and situations in which behaviors of self-restraint and self-control are evaluated. Structured situations employed in these studies included observations of behaviors such as stealing cigarettes or candy from a dish when the subject believed he was not being observed, pocketing an attractive ball point pen "found" by the subject as opposed to returning it to the experimenter, returning money allegedly given to him in error, reporting or concealing a mishap that had been contrived by the experimenter, and cheating when there was an opportunity to do so. Moore and Stephens (1974) report that their findings destroy the myth that retarded persons are more prone to misconduct than nonretarded persons.

In general, moral judgment does show weak correlative relationships with cognitive development, but such relationships seem to be accounted for by mental age rather than by specific cognitive operations (Taylor and Achenbach, 1975).

Longitudinal studies at Temple University (Mahaney and Stephens, 1974; Moore and Stephens, 1974) support the contention that moral judgment and conduct are developmental and improve with increased mental age and chronological age.

In outlining the present chapter, the authors were undecided about including the research deriving from Piagetian theory. The developmental model for moral judgment and behavior seems only tangentially related to personality and emotional factors. Nor has the expansion and validation of the model by American researchers sufficiently advanced the state of knowledge that we can speak definitively about those aspects of personality structure of the mentally retarded that relate to characterological traits described by Piaget. The decision to include this area stems more from its potential contribution to our knowledge of mental retardation than from its present accomplishments. During the past two decades, professional attitudes have undergone a drastic change. The so-called "menace of the mentally retarded'' is seldom discussed, and the term ''moral imbecile'' has all but disappeared from the literature. Normalization, deinstitutionalization, and community programs for the mentally retarded are now accepted as alternatives to demands for segregation and control previously advocated by dedicated professionals. The decision to pursue community alternatives to institutionalization for the retarded rests squarely upon assumptions about social and emotional capacities of the retarded, i.e., upon a confidence that their moral behaviors, self-control, and other characterological traits are at least no worse than other populations for whom alternatives to community living were never considered. Despite the importance of these assumptions, they are seldom verbalized in evaluating the retarded for community placement, in counseling the retarded, or in personal adjustment training programs. Yet the development of behaviors of self-control and socially appropriate judgment would seem to be crucial in the social learning and habilitation process. Reiss (1967) has pointed out the importance of adapting Piaget's developmental model to methods of assessment of the mentally retarded and the need to integrate Piaget's theory with more comprehensive theories of personality. As Reiss indicates, the ultimate value of Piaget's model rests upon how useful it will prove when measured against the needs in specific education, training, and life situations of the mentally retarded. If the model provides a means and a impetus to examine areas of emotional and personality development that have heretofore been ignored by the habilitation specialist, then the model is valuable.

PSYCHOANALYTIC THEORY OF FREUD

A third major theoretical orientation derived from psychoanalytic theory (Chidester and Menninger, 1936) is mentioned only in passing since it has contributed little toward education or treatment approaches and has not generated meaningful research.

Clark (1932*a*, 1932*b*) presented what he considered to be the essential tenets of the psychoanalytic approach to mental retardation before the American Association for the Study of the Feeble-minded. The essence of this model is a dynamic conception of personality with intellectual function energized by instinctual forces. The stages of psychosexual development of the child are described as most relevant to the learning process, particularly the change from primary narcissism to secondary narcissism. This stage of development witnesses the shift in the attachment of libidinal energies from the ego to external objects, which begins at the time the infant first recognizes his mother as separate from his own ego. Subsequent stages of identification represent the ego's attempt to incorporate the mother symbolically by adapting her mannerisms, attitudes, and ways of understanding. Learning is also seen as a "taking in" or oral incorporation symbolizing the need to make mother a part of the ego.

> That which seems to characterize mental arrest is a failure of the instinctual energy to be applied to these processes. Either there is some barrier against the forming of identifications or there are elements in the personality which interfere with the digesting and using of what is taken in...The lower grades of amentia seem to include those who are unable to form identifications and to ingest knowledge from the environment. Their primary narcissism is found to be one of the chief obstacles against maintaining a receptive contact with the outer world. As one approaches slightly higher levels of mentality, it appears that the secondary narcissism has developed and there are capacities for 'taking in' reality; but these ingestions are unusually dependent upon auto-erotic and narcissistic accompaniments that there is little absorption of the required material within the ego.... (Clark, 1932, pp. 321–322).

Clark suggests that psychoanalytic treatment may offer a "loosening" of fixations in emotional development so energy may be more freely applied to learning. He also suggests the "giving of libido" by the teacher in the form of love and encouragement, more permissive attitudes toward the discharge of destructive impulses, and the need for greater self-understanding by teachers (perhaps by psychoanalysis) to avoid excessive involvement in the pupils' regressive trends.

It is perhaps unfair to criticize 1932 psychoanalytic dogma in light of today's understanding and experience. Suffice it to say that the mentally retarded have rarely been judged acceptable for psychoanalytic treatment and the vague recommendation about freeing libidinal energies in and of themselves are virtually useless as education, training, or even therapeutic recommendations. The approach shares with the models presented previously in pointing out the contribution of personality, temperamental, and developmental factors in influencing mental growth and learning activities.

MOTIVATIONAL-COGNITIVE POSITION OF ZIGLER

The theoretical orientation of Edward Zigler originated from a cognitive theory of Kurt Lewin (1936) but developed along independent lines when empirical results suggested new directions. It concerns motivation, learning, and performance of the mentally retarded as much as it does personality variables. While Zigler has been misinterpreted as espousing a motivational explanation for mental retardation, he has denied that this was his intent. Rather, Zigler's developmental position can best be described as a motivational-cognitive approach.

Zigler believes that many of the behavioral differences between familial retardates and normals of the same mental age are a result of differences in the motivational systems of the two types of individual rather than a result of the intellectual factor alone. Zigler attacks what he terms a "difference orientation" of those theorists who believe that differences in performance between the familial retarded and normals of comparable mental age are due to differences in their cognitive structure. Rather, he sees such differences as determined by differences in the environmental and experiential histories of the two groups, differences in the way in which reinforcers are effective and valued by the groups, and differences in their expectations of success and failure. The latter difference is one which, as we have already seen, is the same focus of Cromwell and his colleagues.

One example of what Zigler calls a difference position is found in the early work of Lewin (1936) and Kounin (1941). Lewin suggested that mental retardates, compared to normal children of similar mental age, are characterized by a degree of "cognitive rigidity." This concept derives from Lewin's dynamic view of personality as consisting of differentiated "regions" representing need or tension systems. Mental retardation was characterized as a condition in which the boundaries between such regions were less permeable than those of normals so that the degree of communication or "fluidity" between regions was lessened. Lewin and Kounin offered as evidence their findings that the mentally retarded were more persistent on a task than normal mental age (MA) controls who tended to "satiate" faster. The retarded showed less transfer of learning from one task to another, and demonstrated greater difficulty in switching from one concept to another when it was required that they do so. Stevenson and Zigler (1957) tested the Lewin-Kounin hypothesis using a reversal problem and found greater similarities than differences in groups of mentally retarded and normal intelligence subjects matched on mental age. They interpreted the differences between their results and those of Kounin on the basis of differences in the motivation to comply with instructions given by the experimenter rather than to differences in cognitive ability. This explanation was based on the assumption that the mentally retarded have been relatively deprived of adult contact and approval and have a higher motivation to obtain such contact than do normal children.

This "social deprivation hypothesis" was confirmed by later studies demonstrating the greater reinforcement value of supportive instructions to retarded subjects than to normals (Zigler, Hodgden, and Stevenson, 1958) and the positive relationship between the degree of pre-institutional social deprivation and the amount of time the child spent playing a monotonous game that was being socially reinforced. Zigler concluded that the persistence of the mental retardate is not a function of cognitive rigidity but a manifestation of his heightened motivation to secure attention and approval. The greater his social deprivation, the higher the need of the mental retardate for social reinforcement. In a study already referred to in Chapter 7, Butterfield and Zigler (1965) found that differences in social climate between two residential institutions, one repressive and depriving, the other relatively more open and supportive, were sufficiently powerful to produce differences in motivation for social reinforcement among children residing at these facilities.

More recent findings by Zigler and Williams (1963) suggest that the effects of institutional climate depend upon more than the social and physical structure of the institution. The general effects of institutional experience upon motivation for social reinforcers also depend upon the preinstitutional history of the individual. Those persons coming from more socially depriving homes showed a smaller increase in motivation for social reinforcement within the institution than those coming from relatively good homes. Thus, institutionalization apparently does not represent the same psychological situation to all mental retardates. For persons accustomed to more supportive and nurturing home environments the institution may represent a cultural shock that has important repercussions in their relationships with other persons in their environment. Those coming from more limited and restrictive environments may not be so adversely affected within the institution. This finding is reminiscent of results of studies investigating IQ change within the institution. It will be recalled that Clarke and Clarke (1953) reported that persons coming from poor homes were more likely to show IQ increments than decrements within the institution while persons coming from homes rated less poorly showed no differences between the frequency of IQ increment and decrement. The Clarkes interpret these findings on the basis of the "fading of intellectual scars" in the more deprived persons. Parallel factors may operate in the area of social and motivational variables within the institution.

Zigler (1966) believes that the mentally retarded are characterized by a heightened motivation to interact with supportive adults but are also wary about doing so. The need for social reinforcement from adults may sometimes result in behaviors that are antagonistic to learning or performance or at least that appear that way. One example is in the realm of distractibility or short attention span. Mentally retarded persons often show a lack of attention toward tasks that teachers or supervisors consider to be important. Turnure and Zigler (1964) have suggested that such "nonorienting behavior" in the mentally retarded may actually represent an information-seeking behavior. In one of the studies reported, familial retarded children were exposed to a success or a failure experience while playing games with the experimenter. Following this they were tested on two imitation tasks. The retarded children were found to be more imitative than normals matched on mental age and sex. All the children were found to be more imitative following failure than following success on the games. The results were interpreted as supporting the view that the mentally retarded show an oversensitivity to external models that may sometimes be detrimental to their performance on problem-solving or learning tasks. Their "outer-directedness" is an outgrowth of life histories characterized by an inordinate amount of failure. Rather than utilize his own resources, which he learns to mistrust, the mentally retarded individual relies upon cues from others. This would account for his greater distractibility. However, distractibility does not represent a disinterest in the task. It merely represents a style of problem-solving, rooted in his history of failure experience. The findings of Turnure and Zigler (1964) and later confirmations (Achenbach and Zigler, 1968; Turnure, 1970*a*, 1970*b*, 1970*c*, 1971, 1973) substantiate the outer-directedness hypothesis and provide evidence for a developmental change in attentional strategy by retarded children from outer-directed to inner-directed styles.

In concluding his chapter dealing with personality factors and mental retardation, Heber (1964) points out the absence of substantiation for the numerous references to personality attributes of the retarded in the literature. The most striking evidence, he reasons, concerns the importance of motivational variables, such as expectancy of success and failure, in influencing behavior. He points to the lack of clearly defined terms and constructs in studying personality variables and urges a research strategy that would abandon attempts to discover personality characteristics that are universally descriptive of the mentally retarded: "...a more profitable approach would focus on those aspects of the life experience of a retarded child which may be expected to produce deficits in personality development" (p. 170).

Heber emphasizes that research should proceed in two directions:

> "(1) toward the development of techniques, both observational and standardized, for more effective assessment of various aspects of personality and (2) toward the initiation of comprehensive, longitudinal studies of personality development in retarded children" (p. 170).

The task at hand is to question the relevance of all the preceding research and theory to the habilitation of mentally retarded adults. Specifically, we need to know whether the constructs and variables postulated as influencing the behavior of mentally retarded children, and examined from an etiological and developmental orientation, extend into adulthood and continue to influence adjustment and coping in meaningful life situations. Heber's proposed strategy for progress in studying personality in children could easily be extended to the study of adult personalities. It will not suffice merely to study the development of personality; rather, the choice of variables for scrutiny should originate in the role of those variables in the day-to-day living of the mentally retarded. The observational techniques suggested by Heber should be applied in occupational and social situations representative of the daily living of the mentally retarded. Such an approach was initiated in the follow-up studies at Elwyn Institute described in previous chapters.

The research originated with the failure to identify variables related to outcome in post-institutional studies of adjustment (Chapter 9, 10, and 11). Because psychometric tests of cognitive and motor abilities had proven to be such poor predictors (see Chapter 11), it was reasoned that greater success might accrue from the use of personality variables as predictors. It was also apparent that criteria of adjustment would need to be less global than variables such as income, employment stability, and work satisfaction. It was necessary to develop criteria of adjustment bearing some conceptual relationship to predictor variables. Demonstration of predictive validity of personality variables would necessitate the establishment of construct validity of intervening personality dimensions linking test behaviors to community coping behaviors.

An initial approach was an analysis of the difficulties encountered by mentally retarded adults leaving the institution and their methods of resolving such problems. Identified behavioral deficiencies and strengths in coping with the community were to be analyzed in relation to institutional training and experiences. Hopefully, this analysis would result in a set of hypotheses about the effects of institutions in conditioning behavior and personality traits that could be empirically tested.

This strategy resulted in speculation about what the authors initially described as the "institutional personality" (Rosen, Floor, and Baxter, 1971). Individual case studies of approximately 200 "graduates" of Elwyn Institute were analyzed to discover some underlying commonalities about their personalities gleaned from their experiences in the community. Five personality traits were described: lowered self-esteem and related motivational deficits, conditioned helplessness, acquiescence to authority, inappropriate behavior, and sexual inadequacies. Each of these variables was studied individually with the intention of finding ways to measure the construct, relating it to community adjustment, and finding ways of remediating these deficiencies if this were possible. As we shall see in later chapters, the concept of an institutional personality did not stand up to empirical tests. In most cases studied these traits were found in both institutional and noninstitutional populations and were more pronounced in both populations than in normal controls. The investigation of these variables and their relation to habilitation of the mentally retarded is treated in subsequent chapters.

SUMMARY AND CONCLUSIONS

1. Observations about the emotional constitution of the mentally retarded, repeated in most earlier textbooks, had little basis in empirical research and probably cannot be verified because of their generality and anecdotal nature.
2. Nineteenth century conceptions regarding the moral nature of the mentally retarded gave way after the turn of the century to a greater acknowledgment of the effect of environment and experience in determining behavior and a greater appreciation of conduct, judgment, and control as developmental traits, and a greater awareness of the effect of motivation upon behavior.
3. Social learning theory approaches to mental retardation have emphasized the importance of failure experience in influencing motivation to succeed and the development of a conceptualization of success and failure as due to one's own efforts or ability. Research deriving from the theory has confirmed that the mentally retarded do perform below their ability levels, that they internalize responsibility for the outcomes of their efforts later than normal intelligence populations and that they are less likely than normal groups to try harder after a failure experience.
4. Research deriving from Piaget's development theory has had much more limited applicability than social learning theory. It focuses exclusively on aspects of moral judgment and conduct and their relation to levels of intellectual and cognitive development. This research has emphasized the importance of longitudinal studies of the mentally retarded. In general this research has served to document the developmental nature of these characteristics and has helped to destroy the myth of the "menance of mental retardation." The mentally retarded seem no more prone to misconduct than do normal populations of comparable mental age.
5. Psychoanalytic reasoning shares with other theoretical conceptions in emphasizing the importance of temperamental factors in learning but offers no unique contributions to education or training.

6. Like social learning theory, Zigler's motivation-cognitive model has stressed motivational factors. Specifically, Zigler explains performance deficits in the mentally retarded on the basis of a heightened motivation to secure attention and social reinforcement, both of which are needs arising from the retardates' histories of social deprivation. He has stressed the significance of the institutional and pre-institutional environment in the learning of these attention-seeking behaviors. The oversensitivity of the mentally retarded to external models, which Zigler labels as outer-directedness, is reminiscent of Rotter's external locus of control. While Cromwell describes this characteristic as a more infantile stage preceding the ability to conceptualize success and failure, Zigler describes outer-directedness as a result of failure experience. The mentally retarded individual learns to distrust his own judgment and relies on external sources for information. This behavior, frequently interpreted as a cognitive defect, is regarded by Zigler merely as a different problem-solving strategy.
7. The state of the field of mental retardation today does not include an integrated and comprehensive understanding of personality that may be applied by clinicians, teachers, and habilitation workers. Despite the availability of the major theoretical models described above, there is little evidence that such models are well known to professional workers in the field, let alone used by them. Yet such models seem to have a great deal of potential for application in evaluation, counseling, and social habilitation efforts.
8. An integrated personality model of mental retardation having this type of applicability should have the following characteristics:
   a. It should derive from and relate to day-to-day functioning of the mentally retarded individual in school, workshops, residential situations, community work, and living environments.
   b. It should take into account developmental aspects and relate to stages of intellectual and cognitive development.
   c. It should relate to the unique experiential histories of the mentally retarded.
   d. It should include the same subjective areas of emotional functioning (affect, attitudes, motives, etc.) that are applied to normal populations.
   e. It should incorporate not only indices of adaptive behavior but also measures of personal adjustment.
   f. It should incorporate the use of longitudinal methods of study.
   g. It should allow for the dynamic understanding of the interaction of

personality traits, needs, and motives in a single individual, i.e., the idiographic study of personality.

LITERATURE CITED

Achenbach, T., and Zigler, E. 1968. Cue learning and problem learning strategies in normal and retarded children. Child. Dev. 39:827–847.

Birch, H. G. 1966. Remarks in discussion. Amer. J. Ment. Defic. Monograph Supplement 70:84–105.

Butterfield, E. C., and Zigler, E. 1965. The influence of differing institutional climates on the effectiveness of social reinforcement in the mentally retarded. Amer. J. Ment. Defic. 70:48–56.

Chidester, L., and Menninger, K. A. 1936. The application of psychoanalytic methods to the study of mental retardation. Amer. J. Orthopsychiatry 6:616–625.

Clark, L. P. 1932*a*. Psychoanalysis and mental arrest. J. Psycho-Asthenics 37:316–327.

Clark, L. P. 1932*b*. The psychology of idiocy. Psychol. Rev. 19:257–269.

Clarke, A. D. B., and Clarke, A. M. 1953. How constant is the IQ? Lancet, pp. 877–880.

Cromwell, R. L. 1963. A social learning approach to mental retardation. *In* N. R. Ellis (ed.), Handbook of Mental Deficiency, pp. 41–91. McGraw-Hill Book Company, New York.

Cromwell, R. L. 1967. Personality evaluation. *In* A. A. Baumeister (ed.), Mental Retardation: Appraisal, Education and Rehabilitation. pp. 66–85. Aldine Publishing Company, Chicago.

Fernald, W. E. 1909. The imbecile with criminal instincts. *In* M. Rosen, G. R. Clark, and M. S. Kivitz (eds.), The History of Mental Retardation: Collected Papers, pp. 165–184. Vol. 1. University Park Press, Baltimore, 1976.

Gardner, W. 1958. Reactions of intellectually normal and retarded boys after experimentally induced failure. Unpublished doctoral dissertation, George Peabody College for Teachers.

Goddard, H. H. 1910. Four hundred feeble-minded children classified by the Binet method. *In* M. Rosen, G. R. Clark, and M. S. Kivitz (eds.), The History of Mental Retardation: Collected Papers, pp. 355–366. Vol. 1. University Park Press, Baltimore, 1976.

Heber, R. 1957. Expectancy and expectancy changes in normal and mentally retarded boys. Unpublished doctoral dissertation, George Peabody College for Teachers.

Heber, R. 1964. Personality. *In* H. A. Stevens and R. Heber (eds.), Mental Retardation: A Review of Research, pp. 143–174. University of Chicago Press, Chicago.

Kerlin, I. N. 1889. Moral imbecility. *In* M. Rosen, G. R. Clark, and M. S. Kivitz (eds.), The History of Mental Retardation: Collected Papers, pp. 303–310. Vol. 1. University Park Press, Baltimore, 1976.

Kohlberg, L. 1958. The development of modes of moral thinking and choice in the years 10–16. Unpublished doctoral dissertation, The University of Chicago.

Kohlberg, L. 1969. The cognitive developmental approach to socialization. *In* D. Goslin (ed.), Handbook of Socialization: Theory and Research. Rand-McNally Book Company, New York.

Kounin, J. 1941. Experimental studies of rigidity. I. The measurement of rigidity in normal and feebleminded persons. Charac. Personal. 9:251–273.

Lewin, K. 1936. A Dynamic Theory of Personality. McGraw-Hill Book Company, New York.

Mahaney, E. J., Jr., and Stephens, B. 1974. Two-year gains in moral judgement by retarded and non-retarded persons. Amer. J. Ment. Defic. 79:134–141.

Masland, R. L., Sarason, S. B., and Gladwin, T. 1958. Mental Subnormality: Biological, Psychological, and Cultural Factors. Basic Books, New York.

Moore, G., and Stephens, B. 1974. Two-year gains in moral conduct by retarded and non-retarded persons. Amer. J. Ment. Defic. 79:147–153.

Piaget, J. 1960. Psychology of Intelligence. Littlefield, Adams & Co., Patterson, New Jersey.

Piaget, J. 1962. The Moral Judgment of the Child. Collier Books, New York.

Piaget, J., and Inhelder, B. 1947. Diagnosis of mental operations and theory of intelligence. Amer. J. Ment. Defic. 51:401–406.

Reiss, P. 1967. Implications of Piaget's developmental psychology for mental retardation. Amer. J. Ment. Defic. 72:361–369.

Rosen, M., Floor, L., and Baxter, D. 1971. The institutional personality. Brit. J. Ment. Subnormal. 17(2):2–8.

Rotter, J. B. 1954. Social Learning and Clinical Psychology. Prentice Hall, Englewood Cliffs, New Jersey.

Stevenson, H., and Zigler, E. 1957. Discrimination learning and rigidity in normal and feebleminded individuals. J. Personal. 25:699–711.

Taylor, J. J., and Achenbach, T. M. 1975. Moral and cognitive development in retarded and non-retarded children. Amer. J. Ment. Defic. 80:43–50.

Tredgold, R. F., and Soddy, K. 1956. A Text-Book of Mental Deficiency. 9th Ed. The Williams & Wilkins Company, Baltimore.

Turnure, J. E. 1970*a*. Children's reactions to distractions in a learning situation. Dev. Psychol. 2:115–122.

Turnure, J. E. 1970*b*. Distractibility in the mentally retarded: Negative evidence for an orienting inadequacy. Except. Child. 37:181–186.

Turnure, J. E. 1970*c*. Reactions to physical and social distractors by moderately retarded institutionalized children. J. Spec. Ed. 4:283–294.

Turnure, J. E. 1971. Control of orienting behavior in children under five years of age. Dev. Psychol. 4:16–24.

Turnure, J. E. 1973. Outerdirectedness in EMR boys and girls. Amer. J. Ment. Defic. 78:163–170.

Turnure, J., and Zigler, E. 1964. Outer-directedness in the problem solving of normal and retarded children. J. Abnorm. Soc. Psychol. 69:427–436.

Woodward, M. 1963. The application of Piaget's theory to research in mental deficiency. *In* N. R. Ellis (ed.), Handbook of Mental Deficiency, pp. 297–324. McGraw-Hill Book Company, New York.

Zigler, E. 1966. Motivational determinants in the performance of retarded children. Amer. J. Orthopsychiatry 36:848–856.

Zigler, E. 1967. Familial mental retardation: A continuing dilemma. Science 155:292–298.

Zigler, E. 1969. Developmental versus difference theories of mental retardation and the problem of motivation. Amer. J. Ment. Defic. 73:536–556.

Zigler, E., Hodgden, L. and Stevenson, N. 1958. The effect of support on the performance of normal and feebleminded children. J. Personal. 26:106–122.

Zigler, E., and Williams, J. 1963. Institutionalization and the effectiveness of social reinforcement: A three-year follow-up study. J. Abnorm. Soc. Psychol. 66:197–205.

Chapter 13

The Acquiescent Personality

The assumption that mentally retarded persons show excessive degrees of gullible, compliant, and acquiescent behaviors has long been a part of the popular image of this disability group. Concern over the susceptibility of the retarded to exploitation or abuse has been as prevalent as concern over the possibility of their antisocial inclinations (Coleman, 1950; Floor et al., 1971). With increasing likelihood that mentally retarded adults will live and work within the community, such concerns are more relevant than when institutionalization and segregation were accepted as desirable treatment measures. In the search for meaningful personality constructs for evaluating the mentally retarded, acquiescence as a personality variable represents a dimension that has both theoretical importance and practical significance.

To the theorist, the questions of generality and consistency of acquiescence as a personality trait or behavioral predisposition are most important. Does acquiescence occur with sufficient frequency to be regarded as a characteristic of the retarded? Does it represent a general dimension of personality expressed in a variety of acquiescent behaviors? Is it consistent over time in the same individual? What factors in the unique experience of the retarded determine the acquisition of this trait? How does it relate to a history of failure and rejection already described as characteristics of the mentally retarded and to personality constructs such as expectancy of success and locus of control?

To the clinician, more practical concerns are paramount. Is acquiescence a dimension that can be reliably assessed? Is it a behavior that can be modified? What are the implications of acquiescence for counseling and therapy?

To the habilitation counselor, acquiescence poses important questions about vocational and social adjustment. Does an acquiescent individual become a steady and reliable employee who shows up for work on time, does as he is told, and obeys the company rules? Does he become a good citizen who stops at red lights, does not litter, and pays his rent? Or does acquiescence imply potential for exploitation? Is the acquiescent retarded individual led easily into trouble, an easy prey for unscrupulous persons?

It must not be assumed that concern over acquiescent behavior is unique to the field of mental retardation. In recent years, educators and social scientists have expressed concern about scholastic, parental, and societal norms that serve to condition submissive, uncritical, and compliant behaviors in children (Friedenberg, 1963). Social conformity and submissive behavior have also been central issues of social psychology for many years (Asch, 1956; Cartwright and Zander, 1960; Crutchfield, 1955; Sherif, 1935). Acquiescence and social conformity have not been defined as completely congruent behaviors. While the former usually refers to a personality trait, the latter describes behavioral adaptation to a perceived norm of a relevant reference group. Social conformity has been considered a correlate of affiliation needs (Berkowitz and Lundy, 1957; McGhee and Teevan, 1967; Mehrabian and Ksionzky, 1970; Schacter, 1959; Sistrunk and McDavid, 1965) and may also be related to independence training (Winterbottom, 1953), birth order (Sampson, 1962), and volunteering behavior (Capra and Dittes, 1962).

Cronbach (1946; 1950) has studied acquiescent behavior as a "response set." Bentler, Jackson, and Messick (1971) have suggested that acquiescent responses on personality questionnaire items may reflect a consistent individual style or personality trait, an assumption that has been challenged by Foster and Grigg (1963).

Perhaps the most explicit statement of a model of acquiescent behavior derives from Helson's adaptation level theory (1959). Blake has investigated a series of artificial social situations in which an attempt is made to influence the behavior of an individual in an acquiescent direction. These have included petition-signing (Blake, Mouton, and Hain, 1956), volunteering (Rosenbaum, 1956; Rosenbaum and Blake, 1955), contribution or gift-giving (Blake, Rosenbaum, and Duryea, 1955), and disobeying rules (Freed et al., 1955; Lefkowitz, Blake, and Mouton, 1955). Blake analyzes the subject's response in such situations as a resultant of three forces: "(a) the central stimulus . . . that defines the *type* of response for the situation; (b) the background or context . . . represented . . . by reactions of *others;* and (c) personality factors, including individual differences in past experiences and physiological states (Blake, 1958, p. 229)." Helson et al. (1956) were able to show that all three factors were related to the social influence phenomenon.

If, as Friedenberg (1963) asserts, schools are capable of shaping acquiescent personalities in normal children, then home environments, special classrooms, and residential environments may be even more powerful agents of social conformity in the mentally subnormal. A series of research findings led the present writers to consider acquiescence as a personality variable in mildly retarded persons discharged from the residential institution.

In the follow-up study of persons discharged from Elwyn Institute (Clark, Kivitz, and Rosen, 1968), loss of subjects for research purposes was a consistent problem. Fifty percent of potential subjects in the study were unavailable for interviews. Most of these persons refused to be interviewed by project staff. An investigation of the reasons for this refusal was undertaken (Floor, Baxter, and Rosen, 1972). It was discovered that older persons, with longer years of institutionalization, tended to cooperate with research procedures (i.e., a one- to three-hour interview in their homes). Younger persons, on the other hand, were much more likely to refuse. This was true even when subjects were paid for their time. The interview, which included inspection of savings account books, rental receipts, W-2 forms, and other personal documents, was often of no direct benefit to the subject. Thus, refusal to participate was not inappropriate from the subject's point of view. Persons who refused the interviews had been judged before their discharge from the institution as being more employable than acceptors and intended to have higher academic achievement. Males were more cooperative than females and single persons more cooperative than married persons. Married females were most likely to refuse completely.

Additional data related to acquiescence is provided by studies of job stability, unemployment, and sociosexual problems in the community. Older persons were more likely to maintain their community jobs longer (Rosen, Floor, and Baxter, 1972), while older females experienced fewer sexual problems (Floor et al., 1971).

The authors reasoned that consenting to follow up contacts after discharge may be an example of continued acquiescence to authority. Traits of conformity and acquiescence, conditioned within the institution, may be instrumental to good institutional adjustment. This behavior may also be a significant determinant of job stability in the community. Along with lowered occupational level and limited income, constriction in social experience is characteristic of the life style of many discharged graduates of the institution. An acquiescent personality may be conducive to coping with these conditions without rebellion. However, to the extent that the environment requires assertive, independent functioning and decision making, the acquiescence engendered by institutional living or oversheltering in the home is probably detrimental.

However, not all retarded persons studied were compliant. Those individuals who refused to be interviewed may be demonstrating a need for independence that distinguishes them from their more compliant counterparts. Refusers may wish to indicate their freedom from institutional control. On the other hand, subjects who cooperate may do so partly from a sense of inadequacy and a need for affiliation and contact with the institution as a supportive element.

As mentioned in a previous chapter, the likelihood of identifying meaningful predictors of community adjustment by means of a shotgun approach to prognosis is small. However, the chance of identifying such predictors should increase if both predictor and criterion variables are selected to reflect some intervening theoretical construct related to both types of variable. It is also likely that the successful identification of predictors will be found in the realm of personality, rather than in cognitive-intellectual measures (Sarason, 1959; Windle, 1962). Because of the paucity of reliable personality tests for mentally subnormal populations, the measurement of personality variables should proceed in the direction of situational tests or behavioral measures.

This reasoning launched the authors on a research program that was designed to explore the utility of the acquiescence concept as a meaningful variable in the understanding and training of mentally retarded persons. The overall plan was to: 1) develop a theoretical model of acquiescence as a personality dimension; 2) construct a reliable test of acquiescence; 3) collect normative information for groups of institutionalized and noninstitutionalized retarded persons; 4) study the relationship between acquiescence as a personality characteristic and institutional experience; 5) relate acquiescence to criteria of community adjustment, particularly to those variables that bear some theoretical or common-sense relation to acquiescence; and 6) develop and evaluate remedial procedures for deconditioning acquiescent behaviors where they are considered inappropriate. This general plan was adopted for the investigation of several personality variables. The results of initial efforts to accomplish the first four steps in this program in studying acquiescence are reported in this chapter.

THEORETICAL CONSTRUCT

Before inaugurating a research program it was necessary to develop a theoretical model of acquiescence that would guide research efforts. This model was developed as a jumping-off point in our thinking, with the understanding that the model was subject to modification of the basis of empirical findings. The various facets of the model are discussed below:

1. Acquiescence is defined as an enduring predisposition to comply or submit to persuasive or coercive attempts by others, even when such attempts are contrary to the best interests of the individual. This definition implies that acquiescence is a consistent personality characteristic for a given individual, and that it represents a general dimension of personality that accounts for the occurrence of a variety of acquiescent or compliant behaviors in many different situations.
2. As a personality dimension acquiescence will vary in strength in different individuals, and these differences may be reliably measured. This assumption implies that acquiescent behaviors may vary from one individual to another in the likelihood of their occurrence or in the manner in which they occur. In other words, it is assumed that individual differences in acquiescence exist and are subject to measurement.
3. Acquiescence is defined as mutually exclusive to independent coping behaviors, i.e., to the degree that the individual has learned to cope independently with situations and to trust his own solutions to problems, he is less likely to be acquiescent.
4. Acquiescence is a learned behavior. To the extent that the individual has been exposed to situations providing the opportunity for independent behavior and has been reinforced for independent decision making and coping efforts, he will not demonstrate acquiescent behaviors. To the extent that he has been exposed to situations that demand and provide reinforcement for compliance, he will develop acquiescence as a personality trait.
5. Acquiescence is similar, but not identical to "locus of control" and "outer-directedness." Locus of control refers to the individual's subjective evaluation of whether or not he is responsible for his behavior. It is likely that a person oriented toward an external locus of control would be more likely to demonstrate acquiescent behaviors too. How-

ever, locus of control bears more directly upon whether the individual internalizes responsibility for his behavior and whether he experiences success or failure. Persons who do not assume that the outcome of their efforts is due to their own resources will not accept these efforts as successful or unsuccessful.

Outer-directedness refers to the problem-solving strategy of the individual. Mentally retarded persons are more likely to reply on external cues provided by models in their environment than to use their own ideas in solving a problem.

Acquiescent behavior requires not only an acquiescent personality but also an external source who serves as a persuasive or coercive influence. It is likely that both the individual who maintains an external locus of control and is outer-directed in his problem-solving efforts will also prove to be a more acquiescent personality. However, this is an empirical question, and the necessary research studies have not been performed. Furthermore, it is possible that in a more sheltered setting the acquiescent personality will have little opportunity to demonstrate acquiescent behavior.

ACQUIESCENCE TEST—STUDY 1

The next step was to assemble a series of measurement techniques designed to elicit various aspects of what was considered to be acquiescent behavior (Rosen, Floor, and Zisfein, 1974). The plan was to explore the use of many procedures and instruments suggested by the available literature, to test their utility with the mentally retarded, and to select those that proved to discriminate best between retarded and nonretarded populations.

Test procedures were derived in large part from research studies and tests of related personality variables among normal intelligence subjects. Because mentally retarded persons are often characterized by poor verbal and reading skills, many of the procedures selected represented behavioral or situational tests. In two of the social influence procedures it was necessary to use a confederate who posed as a "student."

Ten assessment techniques were initially chosen for testing. They represented four general types of items: tests of social conformity reminiscent of those used by Asch (1956), self-evaluation, acquiescence response set, and behavioral compliance. In the social conformity situation the subject was asked to make a judgment after first witnessing another "student" responding in a predetermined manner. The degree to which the subject's response conformed to the model was observed. The self-evaluation measures utilized direct questions to the subject about how he would respond in certain situations where compliance was one of the response options. The acquiescence response set tested the tendency to answer ''yes'' to a ''yes-no'' type of question. Tests of behavioral compliance exposed the subject to a direct command or suggestion, often to behave in a manner that was aversive or foolish, assessing the degree of his compliance to this pressure. Several of these procedures could also be described by other conceptualizations (e.g., suggestibility; outer-directedness). Considered together, the group of ten measures appeared to be measuring what we had defined as acquiescent behavior.

The notion that a tendency to answer ''yes'' rather than ''no'' indicates compliance stems from research pertaining to acquiescence response set (Cronbach, 1950, 1946; Foster and Grigg, 1963). Ideas for measuring varying degrees of assertion versus submission were drawn in part from the MMPI (Hathaway and McKinley, 1951) and the Kessler Passive-Dependency Scale (Kessler, 1953). Various studies by Asch (1956) and others suggested test procedures in which a confederate was used to influence the subject's judgment or behavior. Studies of petition signing (Blake et al., 1956) suggested the use of spurious documents. The specific procedures are described briefly below:

Picture Judgment

In this situation the subject was asked to make a judgment about three pictures. He made his judgment in the presence of another ''student'' (really a confederate of the experimenter). First the confederate was asked his opinion and gave an erroneous judgment. Next, the subject was asked his opinion. The pictures included the Müller-Lyer illusion in which two lines of equal length appear in juxtaposition. Because of the nature of the extraneous lines on the drawing, one of the lines appears longer than the other. Confederate and subject were asked ''Which line is longer?'' The confederate always chose the line that appeared shorter. Two other pictures were situation drawings in which the confederate and subject were asked to choose the instigator of an ''accident.'' In all three situations the number of agreements with the confederate were scored.

Drawing Replication

The subject was asked to draw a house and a person. Stylized drawings of both were conspicuously displayed nearby but were not acknowledged by the tester. Both the subject and the confederate were instructed to make the drawings any way they wished. The confederate was obvious in copying the stylized drawings. The number of similarities between the subject's drawings and the prototype were scored according to a predetermined rating procedure.

Yea-Saying—Part I

The subject was asked to answer "yes" or "no" to 21 relatively ambiguous questions, i.e., "Winter is more fun than summer." The item was scored by tabulating the number of "yes" responses.

Assertion-Submission

The subject was asked to judge himself using a scale of twelve items selected to reveal his impression of himself as assertive or submissive, i.e., "If I were on a team, I would be the captain." The scale was scored by tabulating the number of submissive responses.

Pill-taking

The tester withdrew a small red pill from a medicine vial. The pill, which was actually candy, was treated by the tester as if it were a drug. The subject was asked to take the pill because "it will make you feel good." Since the tester was not a physician, the testing situation was neither a hospital nor dispensory, and the subject was not referred for medical reasons. Acceptance of the pill (swallowing) was scored as acquiescence.

Electric Device

An ominous-looking (but actually innocuous) electrical apparatus was turned on. The device had many knobs, tubes, and coils that made it appear powerful. It emitted a loud, raucous, and mildly aversive buzz. Protruding from one end of the apparatus was a single wire. The subject was informed that the wire produced an electric shock and was told to grasp the bare end of the wire. If he complied he was asked: "Did you feel anything?" The subject's behavior and his response were noted.

Document-signing

Two spurious legal documents were produced by the tester. The documents had been drawn up in legal terminology and were affixed with impressive seals. Actually they indicated that the signer was surrendering many rights or possessions. The subject was asked to sign the documents. No explanation was offered concerning the meaning of the documents.

Yea-Saying—Part II

The yea-saying scale was readministered. The same items used in Part I were presented but were reversed as to content, i.e., "I like summer better than winter." Scoring was based not only on the number of "yes" answers, but also on the number of contradictions of statements made on Part I.

Clerical Task

The subject was told that he had finished the test and could leave the testing room. As he exited he was asked if he would be willing to stay a little longer and do the tester a "favor." This involved the performance of a simple, repetitive task of filling in Xs on lined pages. The subject was asked to indicate how long he was willing to work at this task and was told that he could leave whenever he wished. The tester left the room but first turned on the raucous buzzer allegedly to "test this apparatus." The actual amount of time spent by the subject and the number of Xs completed determined his score. No subject was allowed to remain more than twenty minutes.

Trash Can

When the subject voluntarily left the room or was interrupted after twenty minutes by the tester, he was asked to empty the contents of a full trash can into an identical trash can standing next to it. The subject's compliance or refusal of this request was noted.

For research purposes, raw scores were obtained for each of the ten items. A value of 1 or 0, indicating an acquiescent or nonacquiescent response, was assigned according to each dichotomous item. For non-dichotomous items, this value was assigned according to whether the raw score was above or below the combined median for that item for the three groups tested in the original study. Individual items were added to yield a total score, with a possible range from 0 to 10. Although these items were studied under formal research conditions, the ultimate goal was to develop measures for evaluating the mentally retarded that would have utility for the clinician and habilitation counselor. At their present stage of development, the measures have not been sufficiently validated to pass as standardized assessment procedures. However, the construct of acquiescence as a clinical tool is offered as a measure that will prove useful for counseling and education of mentally retarded persons and will, it is hoped, supplement available methods of evaluating this population.

NORMATIVE INFORMATION

Once the procedures were assembled it was necessary to try them out with mentally retarded and nonretarded persons. Initially three groups of 25 subjects each were tested. The first group consisted of mentally handicapped residential students at Elwyn Institute. These students were all enrolled in habilitation programs that included vocational training and community preparation classes. Eight of these students were already working daily in the community in preparation for their ultimate discharge from the institution. The second group, 25 day students, were also receiving social and vocational training at the Institute. All of these subjects lived at home with their families and attended daily classes at the Institute. None had ever been institutionalized. These students were matched as closely as possible with the residential group according to sex and IQ. Unfortunately, the day students tended to be somewhat younger than the residential students. The third group consisted of seventh-grade students from two public junior high schools. They were chosen so that their mental age roughly matched that of the two retarded groups.

Group Differences

Significant group differences were found for yea-saying I, contradictions, drawing replication, pill-taking, electric device, and total score. Three of the items (pill-taking, electric device, and document-signing) measure behaviors that can be considered potentially harmful to the subject. Both the handicapped day students and the junior high students were significantly less compliant than institutional residents on the pill-taking and electric device, but did not differ significantly from each other. While only 48 percent of the junior high subjects and 44 percent of the day students were willing to take the pill, 80 percent of the residents complied with this request. The electric device was touched by 36 percent of junior high subjects, 44 percent of day students, and by 68 percent of the residents. Although document-signing did not significantly differentiate the three groups, it did, nonetheless, reveal results similar to those found on the other two items. The documents were signed by 76 percent of the junior high subjects, 84 percent of the day students, and 92 percent of the residents. When yea-saying, self-contradictions, drawing replication, and total score are considered, however, the junior high group differed significantly in a nonacquiescent direction from both handicapped groups.

The most extreme total acquiescence scores for both retarded groups were signifcantly higher than the most extreme scores for the controls. Among the residents, IQ significantly differentiated the extreme high and low acquiescers with low acquiescers having superior IQs. The same trend held for day students, but the difference did not reach statistical significance. Age was not a significant correlate of acquiescence among the two handicapped groups. However, when all subjects were considered, there is a weak positive correlation (r = .44) between age and acquiescence.

Item Analysis

The internal consistency of the acquiescence test was assessed by intercorrelation of the items, and correlation of each item with the total score. With the exception of yea-saying II, picture judgment, and trash can, all items were found to relate significantly to the total score. A constellation of three items, yea-saying I, pill-taking, and electric device, all related to each other as well as to one or two other items; pill-taking and electric device both related to document-signing. No other items showed a significant pattern of interrelationship.

There were marked differences among specific items in the degree to which subjects acquiesced. Since approximately half the subjects refused to take the pill or touch the electric device, and since these items also discriminated significantly among the three groups, it was felt that these were powerful discriminators of acquiescent behavior.

Using total score as the criterion for subject selection, responses were analyzed to identify those items that consistently discriminated between high and low extremes. Yea-saying I, document-signing, and assertion-submission all met this criterion.

SIGNIFICANCE OF FINDINGS

The length of the acquiescence test and the overlap between items suggest the need for a shorter measurement procedure. Redundant items and those that discriminate poorly between groups may be eliminated without sacrificing effectiveness.

The most powerful and meaningful measures appear to be drawing replication, yea-saying I, assertion-submission, pill-taking, electric device, and document-signing. These six items represent the four basic components of the original item pool. It would appear that a test composed of these six items would be an adequate measure of acquiescent tendencies.

One of the limitations of the present study is the lack of normative data derived from relatively nonacquiescent groups. The use of a mental age control group was intended to provide a stable reference point for better evaluating acquiescent behavior as a function of mental retardation and/or institutional experience. Despite the group differences pointed out, normal and retarded groups were remarkably similar. A group of chronological age controls with normal IQ remains to be tested in order to assess the significance of mental age in determining acquiescent behavior. Similarly, the effect of chronological age is still not clear. The differences between the mental age controls and the handicapped groups suggest that acquiescence may increase with age. However, the relationship does not hold in handicapped groups, and the effect of age in normal intelligence persons is unknown. Thus, the present data must be interpreted in light of limitations imposed by the subject populations used in developing the acquiescence scale. Distinctions between high and low ratings may be relevant only to a retarded or relatively young population. We are not yet in a position to determine whether low scores are objectively low in relation to older, nonretarded populations.

As has been pointed out in studies of social conformity with normal subjects, specific measures of acquiescence cannot always be equated. In order to test the agreement between verbalized response to a hypothetical acquiescence situation and behavior in the actual situation, 23 residential retarded subjects were asked, "What would you do if . . . (1) someone whom you do not know asked you for money; and (2) a stranger asked you to sign a paper you could not read or understand?" Eighty-eight percent of the subjects indicated that they would not give money, and 100 percent maintained that they would not sign the paper. When actually confronted with these situations, however, 75 percent of those who previously said they would not, did give the experimenter money, and 96 percent signed the document. Similarly, in the initial study, post-test interviews revealed discrepancies between the subjects' concept of appropriate behavior and the actual behavior in the test situation. For example, several residential subjects indicated that they had known it was unwise to take the pill, touch the wire, or sign the document, but did so anyway because "you told me to." This discrepancy between saying and doing emphasizes the necessity of teaching behaviors along with information in institutional training programs.

The degree of compliance demonstrated by the junior high school students indicates that even among normal persons there is a tendency to acquiesce to rather bizarre requests from authority figures. Whether these students would have reacted differently in a test situation conducted elsewhere than the familiar, trusted environment of their school is an important question. The handicapped students might also have displayed different behaviors in a test administerested in unfamiliar surroundings. Until such testing can be carried out, perhaps outside the institution and by experimenters totally unknown to the subject, it is unwise to overgeneralize from the test results to potential behavior in other situations.

Institutionalization may contribute to acquiescent behavior although not as strongly as had been originally suspected. The residential students were significantly more compliant on two of the crucial test items than the retarded day students. In all other respects, however, the two groups were remarkably similar. Since greater differences exist between both retarded groups and the normal controls than between the two retarded groups, retardation and its social implications upon personality, rather than institutionalization, may be the key factor contributing to compliant behavior. Furthermore, length of institutional experience for the residential group did not relate to total acquiescence score when the effects of IQ or age were partialled out of the correlation.

Group differences, especially on the potentially "harmful" items, suggest that retarded persons, both within and without institutions, are potentially vulnerable to manipulation by others, and that this vulnerability may have serious consequences. Their greater tendency toward self-contradiction also suggests a lack of conviction or ambiguity of opinion among retardates that could lead to other kinds of susceptibility. It is of interest, however, that residential and day students differed most on the potentially harmful items (pill-taking, electric device, and document-signing). On these three items, day students were more like the normal mental age controls. It may be that where personal threat or danger is involved, experience in the community is important in teaching noncompliant responses.

The subject's perception of both the examiner and the test situation appear to influence test performance. For example, in the junior high school situation, the two female psychologists administering the test differed markedly from each other. One was older, more maternal in appearance, and was assigned in one school to a testing room adjoining the office of the school nurse. While this experimenter attained 76 percent compliance on pill-taking from her subjects, only 17 percent of the subjects tested by the younger psychologist complied with this item. This finding led to a second study investigating the effects of situational variables on acquiescent behavior.

SITUATIONAL DETERMINANTS—STUDIES 2 AND 3

It was assumed that retarded day students and normal seventh graders are sophisticated about the dangers of accepting drugs and therefore less compliant to pressures to do so. Retarded residents of an institution, on the other hand, are accustomed to receiving various medications from institutional personnel and are therefore more compliant in an office setting. It was questionable, however, whether institutionalized retardates would show as high a degree of compliance were the pill offered by a non–authority figure in a less traditional setting. Differences between experimenters in the junior high situation suggested that the subjects' perception of the experimenter was an important variable in producing compliance. Accordingly, two additional studies (Rosen, Floor, and Zisfein, 1975) were devised to explore the effect of situational factors upon acquiescent behaviors. These studies were conducted in natural settings in order to ensure credibility.

Pill Study

In this study, a male and female confederate were used to simulate institutional residents. Twenty-four day students and 24 residents, roughly matched for age and IQ and equally divided according to sex were chosen as subjects. The male and female confederates were each used for four groups of males and four groups of females. Characteristics of the subjects are included in Table 1.

Subjects were administered a standard achievement test. Upon completion of testing, the subject left the test office via a designated stairway and encountered the confederate, who asked directions for finding the Psychology Department. The confederate then produced a bottle of "pills" from his pocket and offered them to the subject, saying, "Hey, I got these great pills—make you feel great—want one?" If the subject refused, the confederate was to try again; if refused again, he asked, "Hey, why not?" If the subject took the pill, the confederate then asked, "Isn't that the greatest? How do you feel?" In order to explore their perceptions of and reactions to the incident, subjects were interviewed three weeks later.

Table 1. Comparison of subjects from two studies

Characteristics of subjects	Pill study	Petition study
Number of subjects	48	94
Mean age and (S.D.)	22.7 (4.9)[a]	22.7 (11.5)[a]
Mean Full Scale IQ and (S.D.)	72.7 (9.2)[a]	69.8 (14.4)[a]
Percent male	50[b]	78[b]
Percent residential	50	60
Percent acquiescent	6	88

[a]Variances are significantly different. Petition study subjects are more variable than pill study subjects ($p < .001$). S.D. = standard deviation.

[b]Petition signers are more predominantly male ($p < .05$).

Of 48 subjects, only one day student (male) and two residents (one male, one female) actually took the pill. The female resident accepted the pill from the female confederate; the male students from the male confederate.

Twelve residents and five day students are known to have reported the "pill-pusher" to staff. In addition, the female confederate was challenged about her identity by several subjects; the male confederate, who was known in another context to some students, found himself being decisively snubbed by such former acquaintances. All in all, subjects' reactions were strongly disapproving. Typical comments were: "I can't take anything unless the nurse tells me to . . . No thanks, I don't take pills . . . Hell, no . . . No, I'm already taking medicine . . . You're going to get into trouble doing that." Day students were more able to verbalize their refusal definitively than residents, who tended more often to say, "no," and go rapidly on their way without further comment.

Forty-one of the original 48 subjects were later interviewed. Of these subjects, 54 percent had perceived the confederate (male or female) as a student, and 22 percent had thought he or she was a counselor (attendant); 24 percent said they did not know the identity of the confederate. There were no significant differences between residential and day students or between males and females in their perception of the confederate. Forty-nine percent of the subjects admitted having been afraid at the time of the encounter. Subjects were more often afraid of the male than of the female confederate ($p < .05$), and female students more often showed fear than males ($p < .05$). Sixty-eight percent of the subjects indicated they had reported the incident either to staff, other students, or (in the case of day students) to their parents. Females were significantly more likely to make such reports than males ($p < .05$).

Of the three students who accepted the pill, one had been confined to a mental hospital and was not available for interview. Another only reluctantly admitted having taken the pill, and the third completely denied her previous behavior.

When asked if they knew what the pill was, 95 percent of the subjects reported that they thought it was dope or drugs. A few indicated that they had been approached by others pushing drugs outside the institution. Many subjects said that their knowledge of drugs had come from television commercials, information that was spontaneously given and not solicited in the interview. Typical comments indicating why they had refused the pill included, "I guess I'm too smart for them. . . They're not my things, there are other ways to kill yourself . . . You don't know what they could do to you, your baby could be deformed." Once again, day students were more explicit in their statements than residential students. Finally, when asked how they would handle the situation if it recurred, several subjects indicated that they would take more assertive action, i.e., "I'd shove him away, tell him to get lost . . . I wouldn't panic next time . . . I would try to talk her out of doing that."

Petition Study

In this study, students were asked to comply with a neutral-appearing request having few, if any, connotations of institutional approval or disapproval. Their signatures on a meaningless "petition" were requested by a young, casually dressed female who appeared to be another student or a visitor, with no outward characteristics of an "authority figure." Students were encountered at one of two sites on the grounds of the institution. They were approached at random with no attempt made to control for age, sex, IQ, or day versus residential status. The random selection procedure generated a sample that was comparable in age but lower and more variable in IQ than subjects in the pill study and contained a greater proportion of males. In contrast to the pill study, the encounters took place in public settings, and the confederate, although possibly perceived as a fellow student, had an open, rather than furtive, approach. She asked for signatures "to help me win a prize. If I get 100 names, I win a color TV."

At the two sites, 88 percent of the students signed the petition. Roughly equal proportions of day and residential students comprised the signers. Of the 83 signers, ten had also participated in the pill study, and all had refused to take the pill. Five signers had participated in the original acquiescence test and had signed the "documents" at that time. Four signers had completed a personal adjustment group counseling program in which the signing of ambiguous documents had been emphasized as an undesirable behavior. Of the eleven nonsigners, one is known to have signed the documents in the original acquiescence test. Very few subjects even attempted to read the petition. Many signed after being encouraged to do so by other students or after seeing others sign. Social pressure thus appears to have been a determinant in this situation. Some subjects signed under the misapprehension that they could win the prize.

IMPORTANCE OF SITUATIONAL VARIABLES

The degree to which a mentally handicapped individual will demonstrate compliant behavior may depend upon a combination of factors. The most obvious possibilities are: 1) a previous history of reinforcement for acquiescent response patterns, either within the institution or at home; 2) sex and age, which may relate to the frequency of such social reinforcement; 3) intellectual limitation, which probably encompasses gullibility and helplessness; and 4) various situational variables.

Findings in both the original and present acquiescence studies emphasize the importance of situational variables in influencing acquiescent behaviors. Such variables might include the type of task the subject is asked to perform, the degree of fear involved in compliance, the amount of coercion or social pressure applied, the physical surroundings, and the sex and apparent identity of the person making the request.

Comments and behaviors exhibited in the pill study were in marked contrast to those observed during the administration of the acquiescence test when subjects were also asked to take an unidentified pill. Evidently, a peer on a stairway is quite differently perceived than a known staff member in a testing room. In the latter situation, institutionally fostered acquiescence apparently led subjects to accept the pill from staff members. When approached by a presumed "peer," on the other hand, subjects responded by refusing the pill and by reporting the "pusher." Although there was also an age difference between subjects in the two situations, it was judged to be negligible in relation to the effect of physical setting and perception of the confederate. Apparently a powerful situational variable had been manipulated.

It should be noted, however, that while radical differences in acquiescent response occurred in the two situations, both behaviors may be interpreted as compliance to institutional norms. A subject who accepted the pill in the office setting and another who refused it on the staircase were both behaving in accordance with expectations of the institution. Acquiescence and compliance may not be congruent concepts in all instances.

Furthermore, it is obvious that pill-taking and petition-signing are not comparable. Even in the office situation, nearly twice as many subjects signed a fictitious document as took a pill. The petition study supported this finding with regard to the willingness of subjects to sign unhesitatingly an unknown document. Substitution of peer pressure for authority pressure and alteration of physical setting did not affect results as they did in the pill study. The key factor appears to be the fear element that is associated with drugs but not evidently with signatures. Even persons who had had training in the inadvisability of signing without understanding did not transfer what they had learned to this new situation.

In summary, acquiescence does not appear to be a trait that generalizes to all situations, nor in response to all persons who attempt influence or coercion. Measurement of acquiescence as a personality factor is meaningful only when situational variables are also considered.

IMPLICATIONS FOR THE CLINICIAN AND HABILITATION WORKER

It will be recalled that exploration of acquiescence as a personality dimension in the mentally retarded had its roots in the need for the identification of meaningful prognostic indices of community adjustment. Specifically, it was anticipated that acquiescence could be related to the likelihood of exploitation in persons trained for independent community living. As yet, the critical studies have not been performed. Our research plans include investigations that will attempt to relate results on the most meaningful acquiescence measures to objective criteria of exploitation in the community. If the reasoning has been accurate, we would anticipate finding that subjects who can be classified as relatively high and low in their potential for acquiescent behaviors will also sort themselves according to known histories of having been subjected to exploitation.

Hopefully, these procedures can add to the armamentarium of those evaluating the mentally retarded. The provision of meaningful constructs and measures of personality and emotional functioning should expand the scope of such evaluations beyond mere classification. New dimensions of assessment can provide the clinician with useful means of selection of candidates for specific teaching or therapeutic programs and for the identification of areas requiring remediation. Information derived from such procedures may suggest areas of need, therapeutic techniques, and remedial programs designed to decrease self-defeating behaviors and to promote a healthy degree of independence. An attempt to develop such a program is presented in a later chapter. The findings presented here, tentative as they may be, have implications not only for the mentally retarded, or for institutional residents, but for public schools and other agencies that may be, to varying degrees, encouraging compliance that is detrimental to the development of a mature personality.

LITERATURE CITED

Asch, S. E. 1956. Studies of independence and conformity: 1. A minority of one against a unanimous majority. Psychology Monographs 70, No. 416.

Berkowitz, L., and Lundy, R. M. 1957. Personality characteristics related to susceptibility to influence by peers, or authority figures. J. Personal. 25:306–316.

Bentler, P. M., Jackson, D. N., and Messick, S. 1971. Identification of content and style: A two-dimensional interpretation of acquiescence. Psychol. Bull. 76:186–204.

Blake, R. R. 1958. The other person in the situation. *In* R. Tagiuri and L. Petrullo (eds.), Personal Perception and Interpersonal Behavior, pp. 229–242. Stanford University Press, Stanford.

Blake, R. R., Mouton, J. S., and Hain, J. D. 1956. Social forces in petition signing. Southwest. Soc. Sci. Quart. 36:385–390.

Blake, R. R., Rosenbaum, M. E., and Duryea, R. A. 1955. Gift-giving as a function of group standards. Hum. Relat. 8:61–73.

Capra, P. C., and Dittes, J. E. 1962. Birth order as a selective factor among volunteer subjects. J. Abnorm. Soc. Psychol. 64:302.

Cartwright, D., and Zander, A. 1960. Group Dynamics: Research and Theory. 2nd Ed. Row, Peterson & Company, Evanston, Ill.

Clark, G. R., Kivitz, M. S., and Rosen, M. 1968. A transitional program for institutionalized adult retarded. Research and Demonstration Project No. 1275P, Vocational Rehabilitation Administration, U.S. Department of Health, Education, and Welfare, Washington, D.C.

Coleman, J. C. 1950. Abnormal psychology and modern life, p. 477. Scott, Foresman & Company, Chicago.

Cronbach, L. J. 1946. Response sets and test validity. Ed. Psychol. Meas. 6:475–494.

Cronbach, L. J. 1950. Further evidence on response sets and test design. Ed. Psych. Meas. 10:3–31.

Crutchfield, R. S. 1955. Conformity and character. Amer. Psychol. 10(5):191–198.

Floor, L., Baxter, D., and Rosen, M. 1972. Subject loss in a follow-up study. Ment. Retard. 10:3–5.

Floor, L., Rosen, M., Baxter, D., Horowitz, J., and Weber C. 1971. Socio-sexual problems in mentally handicapped females. Train. Sch. Bull. 68(2):106–112.

Foster, R. J., and Grigg, A. E. 1963. Acquiescent response set as a measure of acquiescence. J. Abnorm. Soc. Psychol. 67, No. 3:304–306.

Freed, A., Chandler, P. J., Blake, R. R., and Mouton, J. S. 1955. Stimulus and background factors in sign violation. J. Personal. 23:499.

Friedenberg, E. Z. 1963. Coming of Age in America: Growth and Acquiescence. Vintage Books, New York.

Hathaway, S. R., and McKinley, J. C. 1951. The Minnesota Multiphasic Personality Inventory Manual. (Revised Edition). Psychological Corporation, New York.

Helson, H. 1959. Adaptation level theory. *In* S. Koch (ed.), Psychology: A Study of a Science, pp. 565–621. Vol. 1. McGraw-Hill Book Company, New York.

Helson, H., Blake, R. R., Mouton, J. S., and Olmstead, J. A. 1956. The expression of attitudes as adjustments to stimulus, background and residual factors. J. Abnorm. Soc. Psychol. 52:314–322.

Kessler, S. 1953. Kessler Passive-Dependency Scale. Los Angeles.

Lefkowitz, M., Blake, R. R., and Mouton, J. S. 1955. Status factors in pedestrian violation of traffic signals. J. Abnorm. Soc. Psychol. 51:704–705.

McGhee, P. E., and Teevan, R. C. 1967. Conformity behavior and need for affiliation. J. Soc. Psychol. 72:117–121.

Mehrabian, A., and Ksionzky, S. 1970. Models for affiliative and conformity behavior. Psychol. Bull. 74(2):110–126.

Rosen, M., Floor, L., and Baxter, D. 1972. Prediction of community adjustment: A failure at cross-validation. Amer. J. Ment. Defic. 77:111–112.

Rosen, M., Floor, L., and Zisfein, L. 1974. Investigating the phenomenon of acquiescence in the mentally handicapped: I—Theoretical model, test development and normative data. Brit. J. Ment. Subnormal. XX, 39:58–68.

Rosen, M., Floor, L., and Zisfein, L. 1975. Investigating the phenomenon of acquiescence in the mentally handicapped, II. Situational determinants. Brit. J. Ment. Subnormal. XXI, 40(1):6–9.

Rosenbaum, M. E. 1956. The effect of stimulus and background factors on the volunteering response, J. Abnorm. Soc. Psychol. 53:118–121.

Rosenbaum, M. E., and Blake, R. R. 1955. Volunteering as a function of field structure. J. Abnorm. Soc. Psychol. 50:193–196.

Sampson, E. E. 1962. Birth order, need achievement and conformity. J. Abnorm. Soc. Psychol. 64:155–159.

Sarason, S. B. 1959. Psychological Problems in Mental Deficiency. Harper & Row, New York.

Schacter, S. 1959. The Psychology of Affiliation. Stanford University Press, Stanford.

Sherif, M. 1935. A study of some social factors in perception. Arch. Psychol. No. 187.

Sistrunk, R., and McDavid, J. W. 1965. Achievement motivation, affiliation motivation and task difficulty as determinants of social conformity. J. Soc. Psychol. 66:41–50.

Windle, C. 1962. Prognosis of mental subnormals. Amer. J. Ment. Defic. Monograph Supplement 66, No. 5.

Winterbottom, M. R. 1953. The relation of childhood training in independence to achievement motivation. University of Michigan Abstract on University Microfilms, Publication No. 5113.

Chapter 14

Helplessness

The mental retardation literature includes many reports of the failure of mentally retarded persons to cope with problem situations arising in their daily lives (Cohen, 1960; Edgerton, 1967; Floor et al., 1971; Mattinson, 1970). It has been hypothesized that while inertia and inability to act may reflect intellectual deficits, they may also represent personality deficits developed during years of overprotection and oversheltering (Rosen, Floor, and Baxter, 1971). Although the relatively low intellectual levels of the mentally retarded could certainly be a factor in limiting their coping ability, the bulk of the evidence, as reviewed by Windle (1962) and McCarver and Craig (1974), has indicated that, for this population, IQ differences among individuals are not significantly related to their success in the community. As we have suggested in the previous chapter, personality factors would appear to be more important than intellectual level in determining successful community adjustment, at least for those mentally retarded persons who achieve the opportunity for independent living status.

The personality dimension we are interested in studying here is a pattern of inertia, passivity, or "helplessness" that has been observed in many mentally retarded adults. Like acquiescence, discussed previously, helplessness is conceptualized as a learned behavior. Helplessness may be conditioned over a period of years by the circumstances associated with experience as a mentally retarded individual. These circumstances include the perception of the individual by significant persons in his home and in the surrounding community as incompetent and incapable of independent functioning. This situation may exist at home, at school, or within the residential institution. The result may be the absence of a response set to take effective action in a problem situation.

Helplessness involves an apparent inability to act in a manner necessary to extricate oneself from economic and social crises. For example, a discharged "graduate" of an institution for the mentally retarded has been making an adequate social and vocational adjustment in the community. Because of circumstances totally unrelated to his situation, he must vacate his living quarters and find new accommodations. He is given three months notice but makes no effort to move until the last moment when a counselor from his home institution "rescues" him. Another person, unemployed for some time, runs completely out of funds before he takes any steps toward applying for a job or for welfare support.

In some instances a helpless person may avoid disaster only by the intervention of a well-meaning neighbor, employer, landlord, or other advocate who provides the needed assistance. However, unless the individual actively seeks such assistance, his behavior is still considered ineffective. Overdependence on others is not identical with helplessness. A dependent person may actually have found a way of coping by manipulating others to gain his ends. A truly helpless person, on the other hand, has no systematic way of meeting his needs. Similarly, helplessness differs from what Zigler has termed outer-directedness. While the latter describes what may be a problem-solving strategy that involves relying upon external cues, helplessness is a broader concept encompassing the effect of the behavior as a social phenomenon. Outer-directedness describes how the individual behaves. Helplessness includes the concept of social maladjustment. A helpless person cannot adequately cope with his environment. Helplessness and acquiescence are defined separately and may or may not characterize the same individual. Helplessness, as we have conceived it, appears to involve both behavioral-motivational and competence factors. The institution or the overly sheltering family may play a role in establishing helpless behaviors by influencing both factors. In both situations there may be little or no relationship between behavior and consequence in terms of important need-fulfilling responses of the environment. Within the institution, for example, punishment and restrictions may follow disciplinary breaches, but the individual always receives food, shelter, and clothing. There may be little in the institutional regime that allows for the learning of basic coping mechanisms necessary for self-sufficiency. All environmental occurrences, positive or negative, must often seem beyond the control or influence of the student. As with the weather, he may complain but probably will do nothing about it. Denied the opportunity to deal with problems by himself, the individual never learns to make decisions or solve problems. On the contrary, he learns not to try to deal with problems when they do present themselves. We believe that such learning may also take place at home when parents and family regard and respond to the mentally retarded person as if he were unable to learn basic coping behaviors.

Our interest in helplessness as a behavior among mentally retarded adults was inspired by some animal research that was originally conducted at The University of Pennsylvania (Seligman and Maier, 1967). In these studies dogs are exposed to an inescapable electric shock in a Pavlovian harness. Unlike a more typical conditioning procedure in which the dog can learn to scramble over a barrier in order to escape or avoid the shock, the noncontingent shock procedure allows the animal no way to avoid or even predict the onset of the shock. Dogs exposed to this training regime seem to ''give up'' and passively accept the shock, remaining motionless until it terminates.

This shock treatment produces a lasting behavioral abnormality in the animals. If they are later exposed to situations in which they can avoid the shock at a signal by making appropriate escape responses, they typically cower and make no effort to escape the aversive stimulation. Normal dogs, on the other hand, unexposed to such prior conditioning, learn in one or two trials to escape the shock. The investigators concluded that the dogs who received inescapable shock learned that responding was useless. This learning interfered with the likelihood of learning an appropriate avoidance response in a new situation where such escape behavior would have been adaptive for them. In contrast, dogs who were allowed to escape shock in the harness learned that responding produced relief from the shock. When placed into a new shock situation, they were able to generalize this learning by initiating responses to escape normally. Interestingly, a behavior modification strategy of treatment with helpless dogs (by calling them or pulling them across the barrier to safety in the face of shock) was totally successful (Seligman, Maier, and Greer, 1968). Thus, the chronic failure of dogs to escape shock (a response that, once learned, is strongly resistant to extinction) can be eliminated by physically compelling the dogs to respond in a way that terminates shock.

Mentally retarded persons living in overly protective settings may also be exposed to conditions of noncontingency. Our studies of adults in the community revealed few instances of independent action and exploratory searching for solutions to problems. There was a seeming inability to cope with emergency situations or reversals. The analogy may be limited due to the absence of a strong aversive stimulus in the real-life situation comparable to the shock in the animal studies. However, the absence of contingencies for predicting and controlling behavior may have parallel effects with positive reinforcements. Seligman (1973) draws this conclusion in applying the helplessness model to an explanation of depression. ''Rewards as well as punishments that come independently of one's own efforts can be depressing'' (p. 44). Where Seligman accounts for the passivity of the depressive in terms of learned helplessness, we speculate as to whether the same behavior in the mentally retarded originates in similar ways.

Like acquiescence, helplessness may also be related to locus of control. As Lefcourt (1973) has pointed out, the perceived freedom or power to control aversive stimuli in the environment may function as a major determinant of a variety of behaviors. Persons with a relatively high internal locus of control may be better able to cope with their environment and hence be less helpless than persons who feel externally manipulated or see themselves as victims of fate. This interpretation is substantiated by Shipe (1971), who showed a significant relationship between internal locus of control and ratings of personal and social adjustment among mentally retarded community residents.

In a recent study (Floor and Rosen, 1975) helplessness was operationally defined and investigated as a personality dimension in mentally retarded and nonretarded control subjects.

Three groups of adult subjects were given the helplessness test (described below). The first group, consisting of 20 mildly retarded residential students, were all enrolled in habilitation programs, including vocational training and adult education classes. The second group, composed of 20 retarded day students, were enrolled in similar programs but lived at home with their families and attended the institution on a daily basis. All students were attending special group counseling sessions in personal adjustment training, and all were considered as having potential for eventual independent living. The day students were matched as closely as possible to the residents according to age, sex, and IQ.

The third group, chosen as chronological age controls, consisted of 16 college students, most of whom were working as volunteers at the institution. All control subjects participated voluntarily, and none knew in advance about the purpose of the test. While this group was matched in age to the retarded subjects, it proved impossible to approximate the sex distribution of the first two groups.

HELPLESSNESS TEST

A helplessness test, consisting of five behavioral items and three questionnaires, was developed. The behavioral items were designed to assess coping ability in simple problem-solving situations in which intellectual capacity would not be a dominant requirement. Items were devised that would not harm or frighten the subject but would require him to take action to solve a problem or extricate himself from mildly aversive circumstances.

Care was taken to select low-key situations that would not result in "grapevine" descriptions by participants to future subjects.

The questionnaires included a passive-dependency scale, adapted from Kessler (1953), that was intended to measure the subject's concept of himself as an action-oriented and independent or a passive and dependent personality. A coping behavior questionnaire was constructed to assess subjects' ability to verbalize solutions to problems they might encounter in daily living. These problems were similar to those actually encountered by retarded persons interviewed in previous community follow-up studies.

The locus of control questionnaire was adapted in entirety from the Bialer-Cromwell Children's Locus of Control Scale (Gozali and Bialer, 1968) but converted to a forced choice between pairs of opposing statements in the manner of Rotter's (1966) Internal-External Scale.

The items in the order presented are described briefly below:

Phone

The subject arrived at the testing offices and was asked to hang his coat on a rack in the lobby. He was then seated in a room with a one-way observation window and was given a nut and bolt assembly task to complete. He was left alone for five minutes at a desk with a telephone on it. After the experimenter's departure, a confederate made a call to the experimenter's phone and allowed it to ring ten times. The subject was scored on whether he answered the phone, how many rings elapsed before he answered, and whether he later relayed to the experimenter either the message or the fact that the phone rang.

Buzzer

The subject was asked to disassemble the nuts and bolts. While the experimenter was explaining this task, a loud buzzer was turned on by remote control. The experimenter turned it off, indicating that the buzzer sometimes goes on inadvertently. The experimenter later left the subject alone; after a few minutes the buzzer again was turned on. The subject was scored on whether he turned off the buzzer and how many minutes elapsed before he did so.

Passive-Dependency Questionnaire

The subject was administered a ten-item passive-dependency scale that contained such questions as: "Do you prefer to start something yourself rather than wait and let someone else do it?" and "Do you wish you were still a child?'' The subject was required to answer ''yes'' or ''no'' to each question.

Coping Behavior Questionnaire

The subject was asked a series of eight questions designed to determine his ability to cope with such problems as: ''What would you do if your wallet were stolen?'' and ''If you had to find a job by yourself with no one helping you, what would you do?'' Answers were scored according to the degree of positiveness and appropriateness of the subject's statement.

Pencil

On the table near the subject were several unsharpened pencils, a hand sharpener, and two nonworking ball-point pens. The experimenter (who had earlier demonstrated the use of the sharpener on his own pencil) then asked the subject to draw pictures of a house, a tree, and a person. He handed the subject some paper and one of the nonworking pens and then left the room. In order to comply the subject would have had to sharpen one of the pencils without specific instructions to do so. The subject was scored on whether he used the pencil sharpener and how long it took him to do so; he was also given credit if he carried, and used, his own pen or pencil.

Locus of Control Questionnaire

This consisted of 23 forced-choice alternatives. The subject was asked to choose the more appropriate statement from such pairs as: ''When nice things happen to you it is only good luck,'' or ''When nice things happen to you it is because of something you did,'' and ''A person can be whatever he wants to be when he grows older,'' or ''A person has no choice of what he will be when he grows older.'' The subject's responses were scored according to the number of choices indicating a self-determination or personal (internal) control versus domination by others and resignation to the whims of fate or external control.

Departure

At the conclusion of the third questionnaire, the experimenter left the room. Just as he went out the door he said, ''We're finished now,'' and closed the door behind him. The subject was scored on how long he remained in the testing room without either leaving or seeking someone to ask if he was permitted to leave.

Coat

When the subject was ready to leave, he discovered that his coat was missing from the rack where he had left it. (A confederate had hidden the coat in a nearby office.) The subject was scored on how long he took to find his coat and whether or not he made inquiries or took other constructive action to locate it.

At the conclusion of the test, subjects were asked to explain why they had performed as they did on the behavioral measures. A raw score was obtained for each item as indicated. Individual items were added to yield a subtotal (for behavioral items only) and a grand total (behavioral items and questionnaires). Higher scores indicated a greater degree of helplessness.

The duration of the test was approximately 40 minutes. Test procedures and questionnaire wording were slightly modified for the control group, but the number and type of procedures were not altered.

The data were analyzed to allow comparison among all three groups on each of the eight helplessness measures as well as on a total helplessness score reflecting all items combined. On most measures, differences between the two retarded groups were negligible. However, both retarded groups differed significantly from the normal control group on almost all items in a helpless direction.

Another approach to analyzing results compared high- and low-scoring persons in all three groups. To accomplish this, the upper and lower quartiles of each group were determined, omitting the middle group, in order to select only extreme scorers on the helplessness measures. The mean of the extreme "highs" on the control subjects was similar to that of the extreme "lows" of the mentally retarded groups, with almost no overlap.

Only three (7.5 percent) of the mentally retarded subjects answered the telephone while eight (50 percent) of the control subjects did so. Sixty percent of the retarded subjects and 87 percent of the control subjects turned off the buzzer in less than one minute. Thirty percent of the retarded subjects and 57 percent of the control subjects sharpened the pencil in less than one minute. Seventy-two percent of the retarded and 81 percent of the control subjects left the testing room in less than one minute after the experimenter said, "We're finished now." Seventy-five percent of the retarded subjects and 85 percent of the control subjects found their coats without difficulty.

On the passive-dependency questionnaire, 17 percent of the retarded and 81 percent of the control subjects answered all items in a nonpassive manner. All but one question (of a total of ten) were answered in a positive direction by the majority of all subjects. The question most often answered in a passive direction was, "Do you like to rest and relax most of the time?" (Yes.) However, this was often contradicted by the retarded subjects who also answered "yes" to the question, "Do you like to keep busy most of the time?"

Seven percent of the retarded and 37 percent of the control subjects gave entirely satisfactory answers to all eight items on the coping behavior questionnaire; only one control subject had more than two points scored against him out of a possible 16. The questions causing the most difficulty for the retarded subjects were, "If you had to find an apartment (or job) by yourself with no one helping you, what would you do?" and "What would you do if you had a dentist's appointment and after you waited a long time, the dentist didn't show up?"

Items on the locus of control scale were answered in a predominantly internal direction by all students. However, 36 percent of the total responses of the retarded subjects were in an external direction while only 12 percent of the control group's responses were external. The items that were most likely to be answered in an external direction were, "People will do what they want no matter what you do," "Only certain people can have their own way," "You can be friends with someone only if he wants to," and "When you get in an argument it is seldom your fault." (The internal responses to these items implied that the subject could affect the actions or feelings of others by something he himself could do.) Several items on the scale appeared to be getting at the same point, e.g., "A person can be whatever he wants to be," and (later) "A person can be whatever he wants to be when he grows older." The retarded subjects often gave contradictory answers to these and other paired items.

Among the retarded groups, persons with higher IQs performed less helplessly on the buzzer, passive dependency, coping behavior, and the overall total helplessness score. There was no relationship between the length of time of institutionalization of the residential students and their helplessness score.

The various items of the helplessness assessment tended to correlate with the total score. Behavioral and questionnaire items also intercorrelated with each other. The passive dependency and pencil measures consistently discriminated "highs" from "lows" between the two retarded groups.

Further analysis attempted to obtain some clinical evidence concerning the validity of the indices. Without identifying their score, the names of the extreme high and low scorers were given to the leaders of the counseling groups in which the subjects had participated. Staff were asked to comment on the degree of competence or helplessness that they had observed in these persons over a period of several weeks. The evaluations of the group leaders did show considerable (although not perfect) correspondence with the actual performance of the subjects. Examples of comments on "high" scorers include: "He takes no initiative... and nebulously drifts.... He fails to see the implications of his actions;" "She takes no action unless being led by the hand;" "He is a very dependent, insecure boy.... He is actually fairly capable, but not really convinced of that." Comments on "low" scorers include: "He demonstrates spontaneous, self-initiative type behaviors... acts independently... definitely a leader;" "He would rather do things for himself... ;" "She is independent in her actions, fulfilling external demands as she sees fit."

In general, the results of the study supported the hypothesis that helplessness is a meaningful personality variable among retarded populations and that it can be studied objectively. Measures of helplessness discriminate between retarded and nonretarded groups of the same age, there is internal consistency among various test items, and there is consensual agreement among clinicians concerning the generality of the findings for subjects identified independently as helpless or nonhelpless.

Although the test items were devised to require as little intellectual functioning as possible, the relationship of IQ to coping ability was apparent for the retarded subjects on a number of items. For the control subjects, however, a negative relationship was obtained between IQ and passive dependency score, indicating that the brighter subjects gave relatively more passive answers. Such a finding may reflect a more self-critical and insightful approach on the part of intelligent control subjects.

It is possible that the substitution of different items might produce a test that was less contaminated by intelligence factors. However, because our initial definition of helplessness included both motivational and competency dimensions, it would seem that our present test would be adequate for measuring helplessness among mildly retarded persons if it were reduced to the pencil item and three questionnaires.

The failure of any item on the test to discriminate between institutionalized and noninstitutionalized groups suggests that the test is measuring something other than the effects of institutionalization in producing helplessness. Retardation, as such, would appear to be a more important factor than institutionalization. Day students often have extremely over-protective families and lead quite sheltered lives. Thus, decision-making and the experience of initiating action may be denied to this population in the home as well as to their counterparts in the institution. Similarly, a broken home and weak parental identification (noted among some high-scoring day students) coupled with sporadic confinement in orphanages and other institutions are also factors that may extinguish initiative by rendering the individual too insecure to trust his own actions.

It seems likely, therefore, that helplessness is a personality dimension compounded of relatively low IQ and overly sheltered experience at home or within an institution. If helplessness is a pervasive problem among mildly retarded persons, the next step would be to develop remedial procedures to encourage independent decision-making and behavior and to test their effectiveness.

LITERATURE CITED

Cohen, J. 1960. An analysis of vocational failures of mental retardates placed in the community after a period of institutionalization. Amer. J. Ment. Defic. 65:371–375.

Edgerton, R. B. 1967. The Cloak of Competence. University of California Press, Berkeley.

Floor, L., and Rosen, M. 1975. Investigating the phenomenon of helplessness in mentally retarded adults. Amer. J. Ment. Defic. 79:565–572.

Floor, L., Rosen, M., Baxter, D., Horowitz, J., and Weber, C. 1971. Socio-sexual problems in mentally handicapped females. Train. Sch. Bull. 68(2):106–112.

Gozali, J., and Bialer, I. 1968. Children's locus of control scale: Independence from response set bias among retardates. Amer. J. Ment. Defic. 72:622–625.

Kessler, S. 1953. The Kessler passive-dependency scale. Unpublished scale. (Available from S. Kessler, Encino Counseling Center, 18075 Ventura Blvd., Encino, California 91316.)

Lefcourt, H. M. 1973. The function of the illusions of control and freedom. Amer. Psychol. 28:417–425.

Mattinson, J. 1970. Marriage and Mental Handicaps. University of Pittsburgh Press, Pittsburgh.

McCarver, R. B., and Craig, E. M. 1974. Placement of the retarded in the community: Prognosis and outcome. *In* N. R. Ellis (ed.), International Review of Research in Mental Retardation. Academic Press, New York.

Rosen, M., Floor, L., and Baxter, D. 1971. The institutional personality. Brit. J. Ment. Subnormal. 17(2):2–8.

Rotter, J. B. 1966. Generalized expectancies for internal versus external control of reinforcement. Psychol. Monogr. (General and Applied) 1:80.

Seligman, M. E. P. 1973. Fall into helplessness. Psychology Today. June: 43–108.

Seligman, M. E. P., Maier, S. F., and Geer, J. 1968. The alleviation of learned Exp. Psychol. 73:1–9.

Seligman, M. E. P., Maier, S. F., and Geer, J. 1968. The alleviation of learned helplessness in the dog. J. Abnorm. Soc. Psychol. 73:256–262.

Shipe, D. 1971. Impulsivity and locus of control as predicators of achievement and adjustment in mildly retarded and borderline youth. Amer. J. Ment. Defic. 76:12–22.

Windle, C. 1962. Prognosis of mental subnormals. Amer. J. Ment. Defic. Monograph Supplement 66, No. 5.

Chapter 15

Self-Concept

The question of the need for self-concept as an explanatory psychological construct is a controversy that still rages. Epstein (1973) has pointed out that, while disagreement about the value of self-concept still exists, "... there can be no argument but that the subjective feeling state of having a self is an important empirical phenomenon that warrants study in its own right." The relevance of self-concept to performance decrements in mentally retarded populations has also been well recognized. The most productive research dealing with personality variables of the retarded (Cromwell, 1963; Zigler, 1966) bear upon a subjective awareness of one's capabilities, expectancies for success, internalized responsibility for behavior, and other indices of self-perception and self-evaluation. Most models of psychotherapy and habilitation developed for mentally retarded populations (Bialer, 1967; Hannon, 1968; Sternlicht, 1966) have alluded to changes in self-concept as desirable outcome criteria.

A significant obstacle to the more general acceptance of self-concept as a useful clinical construct is the diversity of procedures that have been developed for measuring this phenomenon. Operational definitions of self-concept vary from study to study, and instrumentation has been so diverse as to make generalizations difficult (Schurr, Joiner, and Towne, 1970). Moreover, self-concept research in mental retardation has been limited almost exclusively to studies seeking to derive nomothetic statements and to build theories.

A handful of investigators have attempted to develop clinically useful assessment procedures. Guthrie, Butler, and Gorlow (1961), for example, published a more sophisticated attempt to develop a system of personality assessment based upon the retardate's conceptualization of himself and his world. The basic assumption of the Laurelton Self-Attitude Scale was that "... a retarded person learns a set of attitudes, favorable or unfavorable, about himself, his worth, his talents, his threat to others, and these reflected appraisals influence many aspects of his behavior'' (p. 223).

The scale contains 150 items that are read to each subject and can be answered ''Yes'' or ''No.'' The scale is scored by counting the number of negative characteristics that are accepted and positive characteristics that are rejected by the subject. The instrument includes such items as ''I always do what I am told,'' ''The teacher thinks I'm sort of jittery,'' ''People think I get upset too easily at work,'' ''I am as smart as most girls.'' Responses to these items from fifty mildly retarded girls were subjected to an inverse factor analysis. The seven resulting factors represented seven groups of subjects or seven different outlooks. Three of these were generally favorable outlooks: There's nothing wrong with me; I do as well as others do; I don't give trouble. Four themes emphasized feelings of failure: I act hatefully; I am shy and weak; I am useless; Nobody likes me. The authors suggest that differential programs of treatment and training should take into account the specific pattern of self-attitude characteristic of the individual.

A follow-up study of the correlates of the Laurelton Self-Attitude Scale (Guthrie, Butler, and Gorlow, 1963*a*) revealed ''small but significant'' positive correlations between self-acceptance and measures of intelligence, school achievement, success in institutional training programs, and success on parole. Subjects separated from their parents at an early age expressed more negative self-attitudes than those separated later. Another study by the same authors (Guthrie, Butler, and Gorlow, 1963*b*) reports that the scale also differentiates between institutionalized and noninstitutionalized retardates matched on age and IQ. However, only eight of the 150 items demonstrate statistically significant group differences.

Although the authors of the Laurelton Self-Attitude Scale have done a commendable job in attempting to establish the reliability, validity, and clinical utility of their instrument, results with the scale are disappointing in terms of predictive validity and practical usefulness for the clinician.

A shortened version of the Self-Attitude Scale was used by Kniss et al. (1962) to assess ideal self-attitudes of retardates. This interest stems from Rogers' (1951) view that psychological adjustment derives from discrepancies between a *real* self and an *ideal* self. To each of 50 items selected from the original scale, subjects were asked to decide, ''How good or how bad is it to be like this?'' Subjects responded by choosing one of five categories ranging from Very Good to Very Bad. They were able to conceptualize ideal self in terms of a general factor of personal worth and physical health as well as specific factors that represented getting along with other people by social conformity, emotional control, physical assertiveness, or fearfulness and deception. It was not possible to demonstrate significant correlations between these patterns of ideal self with age, IQ, or length of institutionalization.

Brodsky et al. (1970) suggest that self-evaluative responses may function as conditioned reinforcers necessary for generalization and maintenance of behavior. In this case the individual would match his behavior to the criteria or standards specified by contingencies of reinforcement. An accurate evaluative conclusion by the individual that his behavior has reached required standards should have reinforcing qualities that aid in the maintenance and generalization of behavior. Retarded adolescents initially tended to over-evaluate the accuracy of their performance in a matching-to-sample task. When experimental subjects were given precise feedback about the accuracy of their responses, there was an increase in the accuracy of their own performance. While the study does not demonstrate the authors' speculations about the role of self-evaluation in maintaining behavior, it does indicate that self-evaluation can be manipulated and made a more realistic self-monitoring process in retarded persons.

Using the Tennessee Self-Concept Scale, Collins, Burger, and Doherty (1970) compared the self-concept of a group of educable mentally retarded adolescents with a group of nonretarded adolescents attending a public high school (Fitts, 1965). This instrument is composed of 100 self-report items grouped into ten different scales. Significant differences were found on only four of these scales, with both groups showing relatively negative self-concepts. The failure of global measures of self-concept to reveal significant group differences indicates that specific dimensions of self-concept should be investigated in future research. The four scales yielding significant between-group differences included Self-Criticism (the mentally retarded groups were less self-critical than controls), Identity, Social Self, and Moral-Ethical Self scales. The lack of more definitive results with the Tennessee Scale raises considerable doubt about the value of this instrument, or this type of self-report technique, with mentally retarded populations.

SELF-CONCEPT AND INSTITUTIONALIZATION

Methodological problems notwithstanding, the importance of motivational factors in determining performance deficits in the mentally retarded continues to interest psychologists in the investigation of self-concept. If histories of failure, rejection, and atypical learning experiences are as important as theorists such as Cromwell (1963) and Zigler (1966) have suggested, it should be possible to link estimates of self-concept to significant experiential variables. The relation between institutionalization and self-concept is intriguing for this reason.

Ideally, a major goal of any special training or habilitation program is to improve the skills of the trainees so that they can live and work with no more assistance than the community customarily provides for its "ordinary" citizens. Put another way, the aim is to enable the individual to satisfy his needs and achieve his goals within the framework of local norms of conduct. The more-or-less independent citizen analyzes his situation to discover the means-end relations it contains; he also evaluates himself, whether consciously or unconsciously, with respect to whether his skills, ability, and information are adequate "equipment" to ensure a reasonably high probability of success in his desired activities (Diggory, 1966). In the specific case of the institutionalized mentally retarded individual, protection, supervision, and financial support exceed that available in the workaday world of the larger community. Therefore, it is natural to ask whether the experience of the sheltered institutional setting affects the individual's adequacy in the performance of purposive activity, including his evaluation of himself as a purposive agent and of the situation in which he must operate.

The research literature suggests at least two different viewpoints concerning the effects of long-term institutionalization on levels of motivation and self-evaluations of the mentally subnormal. The first of these assumes that institutional experience reduces motivation and performance by depriving the individual of social stimulation (Zigler, Hodgden, and Stevenson, 1958). The alternative view maintains that the institution reduces failure experiences and thereby enhances self-confidence and motivation to succeed (Green and Zigler, 1962; Turnure and Zigler, 1964). This assumes that a history of failure is a significant factor in the personality development of mental subnormals. Cromwell (1963) predicts that retarded children will have a lower generalized expectancy of success than normals as a result of having had fewer successes in past situations. This is substantiated by studies demonstrating differential effects, in normals and retarded subjects, of failure in experimental situations (Gardner, 1958; Heber, 1957).

The level of aspiration procedure (Lewin, 1935) has a long history as a method of evaluating motivation toward a goal and for more general assessment of goal-striving patterns (Rotter, 1954). Diggory (1966) has modified the level of aspiration procedure utilizing a laboratory analogue of a goal-striving situation in which the subject is presented with an externally imposed fixed performance goal and a temporal limitation or deadline on his attempts to achieve the required level of performance. He finds that, in situations where a specified level of performance must be achieved within a fixed time period, the estimated probability of success is better than the level of aspiration as an indicator of subjective feelings of success and failure. Furthermore, this course of changes in successive estimates of probability of success is rather closely paralleled by the course of changes in direct self-evaluations.

Rosen, Diggory, and Werlinsky (1966) explored the use of level of aspiration and probability of success measures in comparing institutionalized and noninstitutionalized retarded adolescent boys. In this study, trial-by-trial levels of aspiration and expectancies of success on a nut and bolt assembly task (Roberts, 1945) were studied in two matched groups of mentally retarded students. Time allowed for each trial was manipulated without the subject's knowledge so that a rigged performance curve could be shown to each subject on a large Masonite pegboard.

Two groups of mentally subnormal subjects (Institutional and Noninstitutional) and two treatment conditions (Performance Prediction and Level of Aspiration) were used in a treatment by levels design. All subjects were male; none was orphaned. The two groups were matched for age and IQ.

Each subject performed ten trials of a nut and bolt assembly task (Roberts, 1945), with instructions to try to complete 40 assemblies in at least one of the ten two-minute trials. Though the experimenter pretended to time the subject, he actually manipulated his performance by stopping each trail after a predetermined number of units had been assembled, rather than after two minutes. The number of completed units was counted after every trial and plotted by inserting colored golf tees in a perforated Masonite board. This was open to the subject's inspection throughout the experiment and enabled him to see his trial-by-trial progress towards the goal and deadline. All subjects received the same false performance information.

Before every trial, the subject was asked two questions. The first required him to state an expectancy of success for the assembly task. To answer the question, "How sure are you that you will do 40 before you finish all your tries?", the subject moved a wooden slider along an 11-point scale representing a graduated dimension. The only labels on the scale were the words "WILL" and "WILL NOT," the two end points of the dimension.

The second question reflected the treatment condition to which the subjects had been assigned. In the Level of Aspiration treatment, the subject was asked, "How many will you try to do on your next try?" The Performance Prediction question was, "How many do you think you will do on your next try?"

A measure of Actual Performance was obtained by recording the number of seconds the subject required for every trial. The number of completed assemblies per trial was divided by the time spent on the trial.

The results of this study were generally consistent with the Green and Zigler (1962) contention that residential care is more conducive to optimism and self-confidence than is nonsheltered school and community experience. Institutionalized subjects set higher goals, predicted higher performance for themselves, and actually produced more than their noninstitutionalized peers. This effect was comparable to results obtained with two groups of chronic schizophrenics (Manasse, 1965). Self-regard, as measured by Q-sorts, was found to be higher in a group of hospitalized schizophrenics than in schizophrenics attending a day treatment center. This suggested that optimism and self-esteem are related to the degree to which a person is able to meet the demands of his social situation. Institutions for the mentally retarded, like those for the mentally ill, provide a set of demands and expectations that differ from those provided by a noninstitutional environment. Protection, encouragement, training, more realistic standards for performance, and more realistic conditions of competition may well serve to heighten optimism and self-evaluation.

Rosen et al. (1971) attempted to replicate the earlier findings in comparing institutionalized and noninstitutionalized retarded males on measures of goal-setting and expectancy of success. This study also attempted to measure self-evaluation directly. Comparative data were obtained from normal control groups of comparable mental age and chronological age. In addition to the goal-setting and expectancy procedures used originally, subjects were orally administered a Self-evaluation Questionnaire (Cutick, 1962) as modified for children by Farnham-Diggory (1966). This consisted of eight questions in which the child is asked to rate his capacity for doing things, (e.g., "When you are doing something you love to do, show me how good you think you are at it;" "When you try to do something that is important to you, show me how often you succeed.") The subject responded by moving a wooden slider along a scale representing a dimension from zero (lowest self-evaluation) to 100 (highest self-evaluation).

The results of this study clarify the relationship between self-evaluation and goal-setting or expectancy of success measures. They also provide a proper frame of reference for interpreting the earlier results of Rosen, Diggory, and Werlinsky (1966). In the replication study, institutionalized and noninstitutionalized retarded groups showed more striking similarities than differences. All retarded groups set substantially lower expectancies of success and actually performed more poorly on the task than normal chronological age controls. Both these measures were more closely related to mental age than IQ, suggesting that performance decrements among mentally retarded persons reflect developmental lags rather than qualitative differences. It suggests that the differences between institutionalized and noninstitutionalized groups, found in the original study to be statistically significant, may not have been of sufficient magnitude to have practical significance. The most important finding for the purposes of this chapter concerned the relationships between the goal-striving and expectancy measures to self-evaluation. These relationships were most striking with the institutionalized retarded group and the normal controls of the same chronological age. Self-evaluation scores were most closely related to stated expectancies of success, with high self-evaluators setting high, and low self-evaluators setting low expectancy levels. This finding lends support to the assumption that measurement of stated expectancy of success for reaching important goals is a valid index of self-confidence and self-regard.

The findings of these studies have important implications for the habilitation counselor. While numerous studies suggest group differences between handicapped and nonhandicapped persons along important personality dimensions, interpretation of these findings for any given individual is hazardous. It may well be that low levels of aspiration, fear of failure, outer-directedness, or poor self-concept are traits more prevalent among the mentally retarded than among normally intelligent populations, or that significant differences in these variables occur between institutionalized and noninstitutionalized groups. However, such traits represent a considerable amount of individual variation within these groups. Measurement of goal-setting or expectancy of success appears to be a highly relevant tactic in evaluating the mentally retarded and would seem to have potential as part of the standard assessment battery of psychologists and habilitation counselors. The assessment of self-concept by these measures should allow the clinician to incorporate these constructs in his thinking about the mentally retarded as a meaningful correlate of actual performance.

It was with this intent that Zisfein and Rosen (1974) set out to demonstrate that self-concept could be objectively assessed in mentally retarded populations and that the findings would have clinical utility. The authors accepted an operational definition of self-concept as one's perceived capacity to achieve important goals. The study examined the relationship among four measures of self-concept as well as the relationship between these measures and more broadly defined indices of functioning. The measures were chosen to represent a broad spectrum of procedures involving the evaluation of one's own capacities. These included: (a) a general self-evaluation questionnaire; (b) a level of aspiration procedure; (c) a risk-taking choice; and (d) a self-comparison scale on which the subject rated himself in comparison with a reference population of "other people."

The subjects were 56 day and residential students at a treatment center for the mentally retarded. All were adults enrolled in more advanced vocational training programs geared toward independent living and work situations in the community. The students were each tested individually with all four procedures administered consecutively. The evaluation was explained to the students as being relevant to their training and preparation for community living.

SELF-EVALUATION SCALE (SE)

This procedure, adapted from Diggory (1966), requires participants to respond by moving a wooden sliding arrow along a scale numbered from 0 to 100, with demarcations at 5-point intervals. They were instructed to respond to "how good you are at certain things." Eight questions were used, and included such items as: "When you try to do something that is important to you, show me how often you succeed." Responses were made by moving a wooden slider along the scale representing a dimension from 0 (lowest SE) to 100 (highest SE). Practice trials in moving the slider were given until it was clear that each participant understood the task. The task was scored as the average SE for the eight items.

LEVELS OF ASPIRATION (LA)

Using a simple nut and bolt assembly task, each student was asked after every trail, "How many will you try to do this time?" Each performed ten trials of the nut and bolt assembly task (Roberts, 1945). Two practice trials were given and were unscored; each trial was one minute in duration. A "D" score was computed for each trial by subtracting the immediate task performance (P) from the subsequent level of aspiration. The "D" score could be positive, negative, or zero. The algebraic mean of the ten trials was computed.

RISK-TAKING TASK

The evaluator read these directions: "I have two puzzles here which will tell me how smart you are. This one is easy; almost everyone can do it. It is worth two points. I am sure that you can do it. This puzzle is much harder and only the smartest people can do it. It is worth ten points. If you choose the hard puzzle and cannot do it, you cannot change to the easy one and you will get zero points. Which puzzle will you try?'' As he read, the evaluator displayed the two puzzles with cards indicating two points on the easy puzzle and ten points on the hard puzzle respectively. The easy puzzle consisted of six large pieces, while the hard puzzle contained 60 smaller pieces. The puzzles, similar to those sold in dime stores, depicted children and animals.

SELF-COMPARISON SCALE

A series of 22 questions to which each participant was asked to respond ''true'' or ''false'' was read. He was instructed that he was to be asked questions about himself. All the questions dealt with comparing oneself to ''others,'' e.g., ''I have more problems than most people; I can take care of myself as well as other people; I can hold a job as well as other people.'' Self-comparison scores were computed by adding the number of ''true'' responses. The scale was scored in such a way that a high self-comparison score represented a positive self-concept.

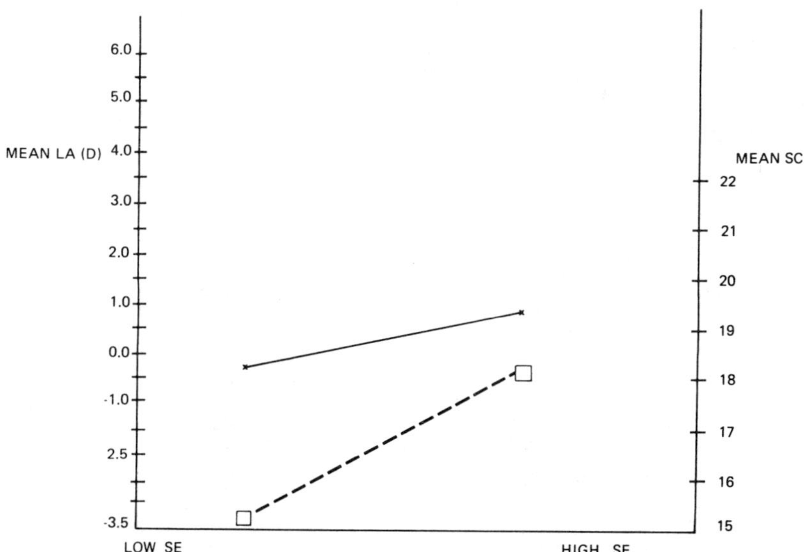

Figure 1. Mean difference between D score (× ——— ×) and self-comparison score (□——□) of high and low self-evaluators. LA = level of aspiration; SE = self-evaluation; SC = self-comparison.

In general, the four measures were readily comprehended by subjects and yielded normal distributions. Results on the four measures demonstrated small, statistically significant correlations with each other, suggesting that to some degree they were measuring the same personality dimension. Performance on the measures showed few significant relationships with IQ or years of institutionalization. The relationships between self-evaluation, "D" score, and self-comparison are illustrated in Figure 1. On this graph participants in the study were divided into first and fourth quartiles according to their score on the self-evaluation measure. Fourteen subjects fell within each category; the 28 persons falling within the second and third quartiles were omitted from this analysis. The average "D" score for the level of aspiration procedure and self-comparison score were graphed for the two extreme groups. Those who rated themselves relatively high on the self-evaluation scale also tended to set levels of aspiration that were higher than their actual performance and to rate themselves highly on the self-comparison scale.

Figure 2 depicts a breakdown of the frequency of high and low risk-takers for the two self-evaluation groups. Those individuals with a high

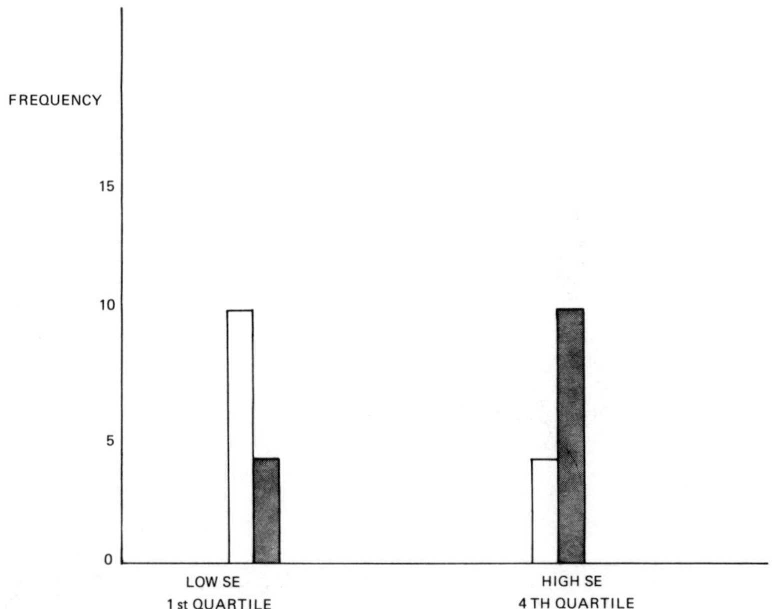

Figure 2. Frequency of risk-taking of high and low self-evaluators. *Shaded columns* indicate high risk, *plain columns* indicate low risk. SE = self-evaluation.

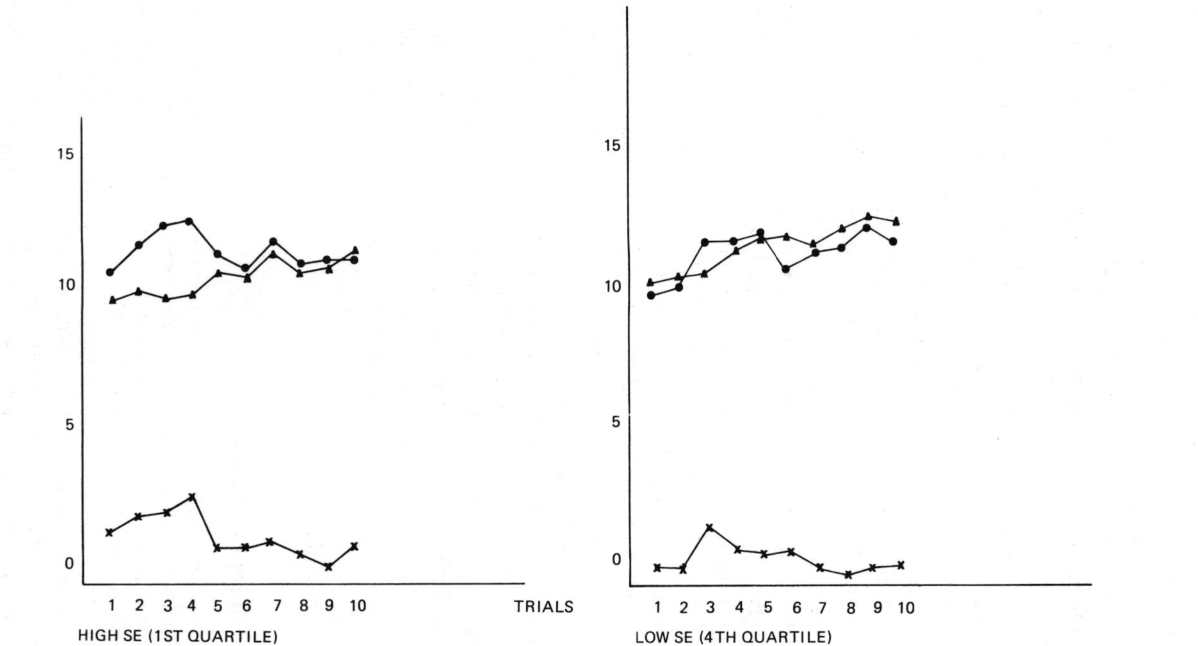

Figure 3. Level of aspiration (LA), immediate task performance (P), and D score trends of high and low self-evaluators (SE). LA = ●———●, P = ▲———▲, and D = ×———×.

self-evaluation were more than twice as likely to assume a high risk than a low risk with the puzzle task, while those with a low self-evaluation were more than twice as likely to assume a low risk than a high risk.

Figure 3 presents the ten-trial LA, P, and D trends for the highest and lowest quartile subjects according to SE. High self-evaluators initially set high and somewhat unrealistic LAs even following performance decrements. By the fifth trial, however, high self-evaluators learned to lower their aspirations to approximate more closely their actual performance. Low self-evaluators, on the other hand, were initially cautious and, by the sixth trial, tended to consistently underestimate their next performance. Performance of high SEs was actually lower than that of low SEs, but LAs of the two groups had a reverse relationship to each other.

There were no significant differences between high and low SE groups in IQ, reading, arithmetic, or spelling achievement, a finding suggesting that self-concept may be shaped by factors other than intellectual functioning or academic achievement.

From the 56 students, those with the two highest and two lowest scores were chosen so that the utility of the four measures could be examined more closely. Interest lay in discovering the relationship between the objective measures and subjective, clinical, or qualitative analyses of the personalities involved. Each of the four persons chosen was interviewed by a psychologist who had no prior knowledge of the study or the self-concept scores of these persons, nor was he previously acquainted with the students. A Thematic Apperception Test and Sentence Completion Test were administered. Information about the person was also obtained from his dormitory supervisor, vocational counselor, and from case records. The following case study material was abstracted from summaries written by the psychologist, dormitory supervisor, and vocational counselor, as well as from case records.

High Self-Concept—Student 1

> "... has a very high opinion of himself ... liked by others ... seems to be aware of his deficits and assets and deals with them appropriately ... proud of his work skills and does not belittle himself nor become overly frustrated at those things which he cannot do ... able to form meaningful interpersonal relationships ... does not seem to think of himself as handicapped ... vocationally reliable and consistent ... able to take on responsibility ... to do various tasks with only minimal supervision ... efficient ... quit a previous community job because of menial demands placed upon him ... TAT and Sentence Completion Tests have optimistic, future-oriented quality ... refers repeatedly to what he hopes to accomplish and expresses confidence in his ability to do so."

High Self-Concept—Student 2

"... basically quiet, stable, consistent... well-liked by the other men... confident in competitive game skills... enjoys winning... reacts appropriately to others' behaviors, becoming angry when warranted... vocationally he has been a late bloomer... recently placed on a trial basis in a sheltered workshop... demonstrated very high productivity... transferred to custodial training where he has proven himself capable and reliable... new vocational plans for him include community employment in the near future... he expresses confidence in his ability to get a job."

Low Self-Concept—Student 1

"... childish, completely dependent... over-extends herself to peers and adults to the point of irritation... totally compliant... having little, if any, concept of herself as an individual... interacts with others as child-to-parent... calls all female adults 'mom'... constantly asks how much she is loved... gleams at praise and encouragement... takes no action without being led by the hand... bobs her head in agreement to anything said... judges personal behaviors according to availability of affection and attention... speaks of herself as 'low-grade,' as unattractive and helpless... seems that there is virtually nothing she will not do to evoke approval... totally obedient and predictable... main concern is to do what she is told... needs constant praise and reinforcement... conception of work unrelated to work itself, bearing more upon the feedback which it evokes... no job preferences for the same reason."

Low Self-Concept—Student 2

"... nervous, highstrung, argumentative with peers... behaves helplessly, asking for assistance and reassurance in an excited manner... refuses to make decisions... describes herself as ugly... must be reassured of her capability before doing anything... has a very low opinion of herself... extremely nervous, self-conscious... afraid to express herself for fear of disapproval... speaks in a 'woe is me' fashion... a large discrepancy between her attractive appearance and personal competence vs. her self-descriptions... extremely anxious... virtually a 'wreck' when first placed on a job... flustered... expresses fear of making mistakes and being reprimanded... any changes in routine cause her great upset and she begins to doubt and criticize herself... actually a capable girl but no confidence in her ability to perform... TAT and Sentence Completion contained numerous references to loneliness for the purpose of avoiding teasing, and hurt feelings coming from others' making fun... themes of dissatisfaction and depression over present circumstances."

These results suggest that self-concept can be measured meaningfully in the mentally handicapped, and that it varies independently of IQ. The interrelationship between the four measures chosen indicates that it is possible to achieve reliable measurement using a variety of objective measures. Students designated as "high" or "low" via LA procedures, global self-evaluation ratings, risk-taking procedures, or self-comparison procedures with reference to a norm will have a reasonable probability of being classified consistently. More important, perhaps, is the finding that the measures appear to have clinical utility in terms of common sense impressions of personality performed by nonbiased raters.

The measures chosen for the present study derive from experimental research formulations of self-evaluation. In general, they agree with conclusions drawn from traditional projective tests of personality as well as with impressions of less psychologically sophisticated observers. The procedures, therefore, appear clinically useful for detecting individual variation in personality functioning in a mentally retarded population.

LITERATURE CITED

Bialer, I. 1967. Psychotherapy and other adjustment techniques with the mentally retarded. *In* A. A. Baumeister (ed.), Mental Retardation: Appraisal, Education, and Rehabilitation. Aldine Publishing Company, Chicago.

Brodsky, G., LePage, T., Quiring, J., and Zeller, R. 1970. Self-evaluative responses in adolescent retarded. Amer. J. Ment. Defic. 74:792–795.

Cromwell, R. L. 1963. A social learning approach to mental retardation. *In* N. R. Ellis (ed.), Handbook of Mental Deficiency, pp. 41–91. McGraw-Hill Book Company, New York.

Collins, H. A., Burger, G., and Doherty, D. 1970. Self-concept of EMR and non-retarded adolescents. Amer. J. Ment. Defic. 75:285–289.

Cutick, R. A. 1962. Self-evaluation capacities as a function of self-esteem and the characteristics of a model. Doctoral dissertation, University of Pennsylvania, Philadelphia.

Diggory, J. C. 1966. Self-evaluation: Concepts and Studies. John Wiley & Sons Inc., New York.

Epstein, E. 1973. The self-concept revisited: Or a theory of a theory. Amer. Psychol. 28:404–416.

Farnham-Diggory, S. 1966. Self, future and time: A developmental study of psychotic, brain-damaged, and normal children. Child Dev. Monogr. 31:1.

Fitts, W. H. 1965. Tennessee Self-Concept Scale, Manual. Counselor Recordings and Tests. Nashville Mental Health Center, Nashville, Tennessee.

Gardner, W. I. 1958. Reactions of intellectually normal and retarded boys after experimentally induced failure—a social learning theory interpretation. University Microfilms, Ann Arbor, Michigan.

Green, C., and Zigler, E. 1962. Social deprivation and the performance of retarded and normal children on a satiation type task. Child Dev. 33:499–508.

Guthrie, G., Butler, A., and Gorlow, L. 1961. Patterns of self-attitudes of retardates. Amer. J. Ment. Defic. 66:222–229.

Guthrie, G., Butler, A., and Gorlow, L. 1963*a*. Correlates of self-attitudes of retardates. Amer. J. Ment. Defic. 67:549–555.

Guthrie, G., Butler, A., and Gorlow, L. 1963*b*. Personality differences between institutionalized and noninstitutionalized retardates. Amer. J. Ment. Defic. 67:543–548.

Hannon, R. W. 1968. A program for developing self-concept in retarded children. Ment. Retard. 6:33–37.

Heber, R. F. 1957. Expectancy and expectancy changes in normal and mentally retarded boys. University Microfilms, Ann Arbor, Michigan.

Kniss, J. T., Butler, A., Gorlow, L., and Guthrie, G. M. 1962. Ideal self-patterns of female retardates. Amer. J. Ment. Defic. 67:245–249.

Lewin, K. 1935. A Dynamic Theory of Personality. McGraw-Hill Book Company, New York.

Manasse, G. 1965. Self-regard as a function of environmental demands in chronic schizophrenics. J. Abnorm. Psychol. 70:210–213.

Roberts, J. R. 1945. Pennsylvania Bi-manual Work-sample. Educational Test Bureau, Philadelphia.

Rogers, C. R. 1951. Client-centered Therapy. Houghton Mifflin Company, Boston.

Rosen, M., Diggory, J. C., Floor, L., and Nowakiwska, M. 1971. Self-evaluation, expectancy and performance in the mentally subnormal. J. Ment. Defic. Res. 15:81–95.

Rosen, M., Diggory, J. C., and Werlinsky, B. E. 1966. Goal-setting and expectancy of success in institutionalized and noninstitutionalized mental subnormals. Amer. J. Ment. Defic. 71:249–255.

Rotter, J. B. 1954. Social Learning and Clinical Psychology. Prentice-Hall, Englewood Cliffs, New Jersey.

Schurr, K. T., Joiner, L. M., and Towne, R. C., 1970. Self-concept research on the mentally retarded: A review of empirical studies. Ment. Retard. 8:39–43.

Sternlicht, M. 1966. Psychotherapeutic procedures with the retarded. *In* N. R. Ellis (ed.), International Review of Research in Mental Retardation. Vol. 2. Academic Press, New York.

Turnure, J., and Zigler, E. 1964. Outer-directedness in the problem solving of normal and retarded children. J. Abnorm. Psychol. 69:427–436.

Zigler, E. 1966. Motivational determinants in the performance of retarded children. Amer. J. Orthopsychiatry 36:848–856.

Zigler, E., Hodgden, L., and Stevenson, H. 1958. The effect of support on the performance of normal and feebleminded children. J. Personal. 26:106–122.

Zisfein, L., and Rosen, M. 1974. Self-concept and mental retardation: Measurement and clinical utility. Ment. Retard. 12:15–19.

Chapter 16

Psychosexual Adjustment

Recent trends toward normalization practices for the mentally retarded and concerns about human rights of disadvantaged populations have awakened an interest in the sexuality of the mentally handicapped. Acknowledgment that injustices have existed in suppressing the rights of the mentally retarded to enjoy sexual expression is found in the platforms of numerous legal advocacy groups. The 1973 "Conference on the Mentally Retarded Citizen and the Law" and the "Declaration of General and Special Rights of the Mentally Retarded" prepared by the International League of Societies for the Mentally Handicapped both support the principle of equal rights for all and pay special attention to the questions of marriage and child rearing. A "Rights of Mentally Retarded Persons" official policy statement of the American Association on Mental Deficiency includes the right to marry and to have a family as one of the specific rights of the mentally retarded.

In keeping with this new interest in the mentally retarded as sexual organisms, there has been a proliferation of resource materials for sex education of the retarded as well as for training professionals and parents to accept and deal with sexual behavior of handicapped populations (Gordon, 1973; Kempton, 1975; Kempton and Foreman, 1976). There has also been an increasing emphasis on research dealing with the sexual adjustment and behavior of mentally retarded persons. The authoritative text of de la Cruz and LaVeck (1973) and the review chapter of Hall (1974) deserve special mention as comprehensive summaries of available knowledge in this area.

This chapter summarizes research findings in key areas of sexual adjustment. It presents our own findings and experience and concludes with a workable model for understanding such adjustment in mentally retarded populations and for designing programs of remediation. As in previous chapters, because excellent comprehensive reviews in this area already exist, the major findings are presented without detailed elaborations of the research.

SEXUAL DEVELOPMENT

As with other indices of physical development, there is a relationship between the development of sexual characteristics and degree of mental retardation. Flory (1936) reported that mentally retarded boys classified as "idiots" were significantly more delayed in the development of secondary sexual characteristics than those classified as "morons." Kugel and Mohr (1963) demonstrated that the degree of physical impairment in the mentally retarded is related to the severity of their retardation. Mosier, Grossman, and Dingman (1962) examined a group of 653 males and females at the Pacific State Hospital for the presence or absence of pubic and axillary hair and for breast development and menstruation in females. The results were compared with available statistics for populations of normal intelligence. With almost every index utilized in the study, the mentally retarded were significantly delayed with respect to their development of secondary sex characteristics when compared with a cross-section of the normal population. The greater the degree of retardation, the greater the retardation in sexual development. However, even mildly retarded groups were significantly delayed in rate of development when compared with norms. With the possible exception of a Down's syndrome group, it was not possible to demonstrate differences among the four diagnostic categories of the mentally retarded.

Mosier et al. point out that at present there is no explanation of the reason for this delay. Delay is not correlated with length of institutionalization or nutritional factors. Since physical stature is also related directly to the degree of retardation, it may be that the same explanation also accounts for delayed sexual development.

The validity of these findings seems to be undisputed. It is reasonable to expect that such delays in sexual development be considered in designing programs of sex education and sex counseling for the retarded. Yet to the authors' knowledge none of the manuals and curricula developed for this purpose have come to grips with this issue.

SEXUAL KNOWLEDGE AND ATTITUDES

There is evidence (Hall, Morris, and Barker, 1973) that educable mentally retarded adolescents are lacking in basic knowledge concerning conception, contraception, and venereal disease. Little sex education is offered to the mentally retarded at home (Hammer, Wright, and Jensen, 1967; Goodman, Budner, and Lesh, 1971). Parents can fairly accurately perceive the extent of their adolescent child's sexual knowledge but judge their sexual attitudes to be more "puritanical" with regard to sexual behavior codes than they actually are (Hall, Morris, and Barker, 1973).

The results of a survey administered to a small number of institutionalized males and females at Elwyn Institute suggest that the sexual knowledge available to the institutionalized retardate is either inadequate, distorted, or both. In studying sexual knowledge of retardates, it is necessary to distinguish between knowledge of sexual terms and knowledge of concepts to which they refer. Despite marked deficiencies in terminology, subjects are not quite as naive as they might at first seem. Although they are involved in classes dealing with "sex education," the retardates in this population have little understanding of the more polite, socially acceptable sexual terms of our culture. Labels such as puberty, nocturnal emissions, reproduction, veneral disease, and contraception are for the most part without meaning. Slang terms seem to be fairly accessible to males but not to females (despite the fact that like-sex interviewers were used to elicit this information). Both sexes were well aware of the gross anatomical differences between sexes, but both were equally vague about internal organs. Body parts such as stomach, ovary, and womb were usually equated. It seems reasonable to conclude that retardates are slow learners of sexual physiology and anatomy just as they are of reading, writing, and arithmetic.

Major concern over the abuses of sex by mentally subnormal populations has often been expressed. However, we find this population to be more impressed with the inhibitions and prohibitions of sexuality than with sexual expression. They generally accept an extremely moralistic view, namely, that the purpose of sex is procreation, and then only through the bonds of marriage. Consequently, they exhibit naivete about contraception and birth control. Sex is viewed as purely functional rather than pleasurable in nature. Ask our subject: "Can an unmarried woman have a baby?" and he is likely to respond: "No, the baby needs a father." The interrogative verb "can," meaning in this case "physically able to" is misinterpreted to connote "may" or "is it permissible?" The physical sensations associated with sex seem misunderstood and are confused with emotional terms such as "liking" or "feeling for" a person.

Misconceptions still abound. Masturbation is often perceived as dangerous. Menstrual periods produce "bad blood." Words themselves, as well as the actions they connote, are construed as "dirty."

Sex roles in marriage seem to be defined purely in terms of parenthood rather than in terms of husband and wife functions. "Good" parents mean that they do not desert their child. A good father is one who provides financial support. The sample showed little understanding of the emotional or sexual roles marriage partners perform for each other or of their parental role beyond provision of food and shelter.

SEX EDUCATION

Despite almost unanimous agreement by parents and educators about the need for sex education programs for the mentally retarded (Hathaway, 1947; Meyen and Retish, 1971), adequate sex education programs do not exist on a large scale, and available curricula, which are now appearing with increasing frequency, do not provide data regarding their effectiveness in imparting information or changing behavior. All too often sex education programs focus upon cleanliness, morality, and good health habits (Gordon, 1972) or are geared toward teaching inhibition rather than reducing anxiety and increasing the repertoire of heterosexual behaviors (Rosen, 1970, 1972). Few materials exist on the reading level of the mentally retarded.

MARRIAGE

There is an increasing tendency to advocate marriage for the mentally retarded as a stabilizing influence (Edgerton, 1973; Mattinson, 1970) and as a right rather than a privilege granted to mentally retarded persons. Others (Bass, 1963, 1964) advocate marriage only for higher functioning mentally retarded with protection against child-bearing by sterilization accomplished with informed consent. In general, those advocating marriage confine this endorsement to those persons above an IQ of 50. Studies of the incidence of marriages among previously identified retarded populations vary greatly in their estimates of the frequency of such marriages. Older studies suggest the incidence of marriage is lower for the mentally retarded than for populations of normal intelligence, a finding perhaps reflecting the effect of many state laws prohibiting marriage for the mentally retarded. The incidence for males is consistently below that for females, while previously institutionalized persons seem to marry less frequently than persons identified in special classes in the community. Those persons who do marry often meet with far greater obstacles than those met by the general population (Bowden, Spitz, and Winters, 1971). Some of the problems include lower than average income and job status, minimal social skills and experience, the absence of a family model or family support, day-to-day existence levels, and lack of foresight in future planning. Peck and

Stephens (1965) confirm the inability of a small group of retarded males to successfully assume the responsibilities of fatherhood, at the same time citing evidence that marriage may be handled successfully by reasonably well-adjusted retardates. In an intensive follow-up of 32 previously institutionalized couples, Mattinson (1970) provides a wealth of anecdotal material concerning both successful and unsuccessful marriages. Nineteen out of 32 of the couples rated their marriage as a supportive and affectionate partnership and indicated that they felt better off married than single. Andron and Strum (1973) report on the overall adjustment of twelve married couples in which at least one partner was mentally retarded and had received services from a social agency because of his or her retardation. All but one individual reported that married life was better than single life. Seven of the couples had been sterilized, and only one couple had children. Many of the couples expressed bitterness about their inability to have children.

Floor et al. (1975) report on the marriages of 80 persons out of a total sample of 214 persons who were previously institutionalized. All of the subjects represented mild or borderline cases of mental retardation. Thirty-one percent of males and 52 percent of the females had married. Of the 80 married persons, 65 percent had married persons who were also former residents at the same institution. In many of these cases the relationship, although hampered by many restrictions, was initiated within the institution. Despite limitations imposed upon heterosexual socialization, the institution provides an opportunity for socializing somewhat analogous to that of the neighborhood, school, or college for noninstitutionalized persons. Forty-one percent of the males entered into marital relationships with (nonretarded) persons who had not been previously institutionalized ("mixed couples"). This was true for only 16 percent of the females. The males tended to have somewhat higher IQs, enjoyed greater mobility while they were residing within the institution, and may also have experienced greater social mobility in the community. At the time of the study, the couples had been married for an average of 3.5 years. During this time period, the 54 couples had produced a total of 32 known children. Eighteen children were produced by couples in which both members had been institutionalized and 14 children were produced by "mixed" couples. Only one couple had more than two children. Several of the couples were using birth control methods and two women had been voluntarily sterilized. These data suggest that the married couples were not reproducing at a rate in excess of the general population.

Of the 54 couples in the total sample, eight couples (15 percent) are known to be divorced or separated. (Only one legal divorce is confirmed;

four of the separations are of several years' duration but are not ascertained as having ended in divorce.)

Couples were categorized according to current marital status in a manner described by Mattinson (1970). Two independent raters, both of whom had sufficient information about the present circumstances of these marriages, rated them as "maintained satisfactorily" according to the criterion that both partners were living together with minimal economic, personal, or legal problems. "Symptoms of stress" applied to marriages with serious problems but in which the couple were nonetheless making an attempt at coping and were remaining together. "Unsatisfactory" referred to marriages characterized by violent fighting, promiscuity, or serious child neglect.

A chi-square analysis comparing institutional and "mixed" partnerships revealed no significant difference in patterns of stability. Further analysis revealed no significant differences in marital stability among those couples with children versus those with no children.

While some marriages seemed to be running smoothly, others were beset with various difficulties. Some of the more frequent problems included chronically poor health of one partner, money management, over-indebtedness, erratic employment, legal difficulties, and involvement with difficult or demanding relatives. While these problems occur in many marriages in the general population, whether or not the couples in the sample will be able to handle them sufficiently well to keep the marriage intact is as yet unknown. Positive influences on these marriages were noted when at least one partner had a virtually normal IQ, and when a relative, landlord, employer or other person in the community served supportively as an advocate for the couple.

Another consideration in the assessment of the socioeconomic and personal adjustment of the married couples in the sample was their comparison to unmarried graduates. Despite similarities between married and single persons in IQ, age, and length of institutionalization, they differed in other respects. While salaries for males were comparable regardless of marital status, the additional income of the few working wives made a substantial difference. Married persons saved significantly less and owed significantly more. They tended to live in apartments rather than rooming houses, thus paying higher rent. They had also changed jobs more often since entering the community.

Single persons tended to show a greater frequency and variety of social and personal problems than did married persons. These included vocational difficulties, lawbreaking, and drug- or drinking-related incidents. A number of individuals whose premarital lives had been characterized by a long series of such problems appeared to have "straightened out" since and to have assumed more responsible behaviors. This was particularly true of graduates who had entered into "mixed" marriages. In a few cases, on the other hand, persons who were functioning quite well on their own had become overly dependent on the marriage partner and regressed to a level of semi-helplessness.

The survey indicates that about 50 percent of the couples studied can sustain a marriage for several years with a reasonable degree of competence and that children do not, at least in the first few years, serve as an overwhelming burden.

While it might be supposed that prolonged institutionalization would extinguish the incentive to marry, this does not necessarily seem to be the case; several persons in the sample, institutionalized for over 20 years, married within a few years of discharge.

However, the numerous difficulties encountered by many of these couples emphasized the importance of preparing institutional residents for assuming the responsibilities of marriage. In addition to practical training in budgeting and money management, habilitation programs should include basic sex education, premarital counseling and contraceptive information for students contemplating marriage soon after discharge, increased experience in heterosexual social contacts, and, perhaps, the provision of a community advocate trained by the institution and available to the couple for advice and aid on various problems.

Personnel involved in training programs must be aware of the potential sources of social handicap that may be imposed by an institution on its residents. For example, institutional experience may encourage or reinforce homosexuality, a factor preventing some persons from marrying or causing difficulties for those who do marry. Those who fail to marry, even as long as ten years after discharge, may be manifesting their inability to make heterosexual social contacts. For some individuals, long years of sexual segregation may have lasting effects, leaving them incapable of initiating such relationships. Lack of knowledge, or sexual misinformation acquired during the institutional experience, may also deter some graduates from marrying or serve as a source of adjustment problems for those who do. Another problem inherent in many institutions is their failure to provide an adequate model of family life. Females, in particular, have little opportunity to identify with a "father figure," and there is virtually no contact for students of either sex with family units. In addition, the pre-institutional experiences of the graduates with often less than adequate parents may have served only to instill a negative perception of marriage and parenthood.

With the provision of new and enlightened community preparation methods, there is no apparent reason at this stage of the study to prevent any once-institutionalized retardates from taking on the responsibilities of marriage and parenthood. However, it must be emphasized that the marriages investigated here have been of a relatively short duration. Future research is needed to assess the long-term status and desirability of these partnerships, as well as the development and potential of their offspring.

SOCIOSEXUAL PROBLEMS

Brown and Courtless (1969) report a higher incidence of mentally retarded persons within penal and correctional institutions than would be expected from incidence figures within the general population. Results from a questionnaire study reporting IQs for over 90,000 inmates revealed that 9.5 percent of the reported cases had recorded IQ scores of 69 or less. Rape and sexual offenses were the crimes least frequently reported among the mentally retarded incarcerated. However, the incidence of crimes against persons among individuals with IQs lower than 55 (57 percent) was more than twice as high as the incidence of similar crimes among the total population of these prisons. Brown and Courtless point out the deficiencies in this data, particularly in the lack of knowledge about the patterns of sexual offense and the need for epidemiological research.

The fact that there is a higher incidence of the mentally retarded within prisons is only part of the story. It may be that mentally retarded persons convicted of crimes are more likely to be apprehended and sentenced to correctional institutions than are persons of normal intelligence who commit the same crimes. The other side of the coin is the incidence of mentally retarded persons who show records of criminal or antisocial behavior. This question has been reviewed in earlier textbooks by Davies (1930) and Wallin (1956).

Davies' (1930) treatise *Social Control of the Mentally Deficient,* by no means a completely negative book, expressed the prevailing feeling of the time with a strong social indictment of the "mentally deficient." Davies cites statistics of the percentage of "feebleminded" in New York's State prisons, reformatories, workhouses, and industrial training schools. In the Glueck (1918) study of Sing Sing Prison, for example, 28 percent of 600 consecutive prisoners admitted were "intellectually defective," and the recidivism rate in this group was over 80 percent. Davies has little to say about sexual offenses, however, seeming less concerned about this problem since many mentally retarded persons do not reach an adult level of sexual behavior. The author rejects general measures of sterilization of the retarded for this reason and because of the lack of understanding of the hereditary mechanisms of mental deficiency. Rather, Davies expresses hope about the value of special education and training within institutions, colonies, and the community in accomplishing the socializing process with the mentally retarded.

Wallin (1956), reviewing dozens of studies of the association between criminality and sex delinquency, concludes that the high percentages of mental deficiency among delinquents were caused by inadequate standards of diagnosis based solely on intelligence testing. As standards of diagnosis became more conservative, the percentage of reported mental retardates among delinquent populations dropped precipitously. While studies still show that higher percentages of mentally retarded can be found in delinquent than in nondelinquent populations, the incidence is not greatly different from populations with similar socioeconomic backgrounds.

> Most mentally deficient delinquents are not delinquent because of aggressive criminal tendencies, but because of their deficiencies, weaknesses, and gullibility, and because of the incentives and opportunities afforded by the environment in which they live . . . Mentally deficient girls become sex offenders not primarily because they are oversexed (many, in fact, are undersexed), but because of lack of protection and because of their weaknesses—lack of judgement and control, and because of inability to resist victimization. Adequate supervision will prevent such immorality and illegitimacy (p. 99).

According to the findings of follow-up investigations (Baller, 1936; Baller, Charles, and Miller, 1967; Charles, 1953; Kennedy, 1948, 1966; and Miller, 1965), the incidence of antisocial behavior of any kind, and sexual offenses in particular, has been very low for mentally retarded persons and does not differ significantly from normal control groups, even when matched according to social and economic background.

Floor et al. (1975) studied a group of 49 mentally retarded females specifically for the incidence of sex-related problems. The study examined the relationship between sex-related problems in the community and sex-related infractions recorded while the individual was still a student at the institution.

The subjects were divided into two groupings—those with known sociosexual problems after discharge (''high problem'' group) and those with little evidence of such problems (''low problem'' group). The criterion for defining the ''high problem'' group required that the individual's sexual activity in the community had resulted in severe economic, employment, or personal difficulties to the point of dysfunction. To be so classified the individual must have sought help from some outside source, either institutional or private. For example, one woman gave birth to an illegitimate child and was forced to seek assistance from a public agency for placement of the child. Other cases of nonmarital sexual relationships, when known, were not classified as problems if no outside assistance was required to help the subject deal with the situation. Using this criterion, 15 subjects were classified as having major sociosexual problems in the community. Their behaviors ranged from indiscretions with men to living with men, premarital pregnancies, and illegitimacies. The consequences were such things as eviction from living quarters, loss of job, and financial exploitation by men. Frequently this resulted in the girl being left without money for food or lodging for a significant period of time. Such situations often continued until aid was provided by other institutional graduates, relatives, or concerned individuals.

It was not possible to distinguish between the high problem and low problem groups on the basis of IQ scores or on ratings of social behaviors and potential for community living completed by institutional staff before discharge. However, those women experiencing problems tended to be significantly younger at discharge (mean age of 24) than those without community problems (mean age of 30).

Women having problems were usually the victims of exploitation and did not profit financially from their sexual activities. Several of the women were later able to resolve these problems and to resume a more adequate adjustment, sometimes as a result of marriage. For the total sample of 49 persons, there were ultimately 23 marriages. Only one of the high problem group was married at the time the problems were occurring. Four subjects have had a history of repeated, severe sociosexual problems. Sixty percent of the subjects in the high problem group experienced their initial difficulties within six months of their discharge. Subjects tended to have a constellation of problems simultaneously. Only one member of the high problem group was in a live-in employment situation at the time of her difficulties, while one-fifth of the low problem group were so situated. Many of the subjects were known to receive constructive guidance from a responsible person in the community, hereafter labeled "advocate." Advocates were found among landladies, distant relatives, or work supervisors. Approximately two times more of the low problem group than of the high problem group had advocates. In some cases, boyfriends, many of whom later became husbands of these subjects, also seemed to function as advocates. In general, these boyfriends tended to be those that the women had met during their institutional years. Boyfriends who became exploiters of the subjects were likely to be individuals who were not previously institutionalized.

In order to examine the relationship between sex-related infractions at the institution and the later occurrence of sociosexual community problems, a search of the records was performed. All notations directly or indirectly related to heterosexual or homosexual behavior were tabulated for subjects in each group. Factors such as overt homosexuality, preoccupation with sex, and suspected prenancies were noted. Two-thirds of the high problem group and only 17 percent of the low problem group had records of minor infractions. These included passing notes to men, meeting men secretly, or making unauthorized phone calls to men. Several decades ago punishments for such minor infractions included confinement to a "side room" for varying periods of time or removal of privileges such as attending weekly dances. In one incident that occurred in 1954, punishment included shaving the girl's head. About one-third of the high problem group and only 6 percent of the low problem had notations of suspected pregnancies or sexual intercourse while residing within the institution. There was a significant relationship between a history of institutional infractions and sociosexual community problems.

Subjects with institutional infractions were equally likely to have or not to have community problems. However, females who had community problems were almost certain to have had institutional infractions, while those without institutional infractions were almost certain to avoid sociosexual community problems.

An earlier study at the same institution (Clark, Kivitz, and Rosen, 1968; Rosen et al., 1970) failed to find relationships between ratings of social adjustment at the institution and meaningful criteria of community functioning after discharge. The present study suggests that this may not be the case when dealing with sociosexual problems and when behavioral notations from institutional records are used as an index of social adjustment. Females with severe sociosexual community problems were also likely to have had histories of sex-related infractions in the institution. These often involved minor infractions of institutional rules for behaviors usually considered a part of normal adolescent development outside the institution. Females demonstrating such behaviors may be signalling their need for appropriate counseling, structured learning experiences, and support, rather than repressive strategies more typically employed by institutions. It is noteworthy that these females are easily identified within the institution. Failure to provide this help may result in more severe problems outside of the institution, where help is less available. Furthermore, these problems will develop quite rapidly after discharge. It is paradoxical that such help is often not provided by the institution. All females involved were rated in this study as having relatively high potential for community living during their training program. Therefore, they represented the persons receiving the greatest intensity of vocational habilitation and community-oriented training.

It seems evident that appropriate coeducational and socialization experiences should be an important aspect of the community preparation experience of institutional residents. While many areas of cognitive functioning in the retarded may be relatively unrelated to community adjustment, deficits in sociosexual functioning can be extremely incapacitating and extend their influence well beyond the institutional years.

The issue resolves itself primarily into a moral and value judgment, i.e., whether the purpose of the institution is to protect society from potential social failures or to take the risks of properly preparing an individual for community living. If the institutional staff had refused discharge to all females who were presenting sexual infractions, it would have prevented the occurrence of 87 percent of all severe sociosexual community problems in its graduates. The cost of this prevention would have been the unfairness to the approximately 44 percent of all the females discharged during this time period who did make adequate sociosexual adjustments in the community. It is significant that this analysis reflects training and discharge policies at a time when sex education and heterosexual experience were not important aspects of the institutional program. It is impossible to determine what the figures would have been had more active coeducational programs been applied.

EFFECTS OF INSTITUTIONAL LIVING

The typical handicapped person who represents the focus of this chapter is in his twenties. He has lived at the institution for over half his life, attending school during his earlier years and enrolled in vocational training programs at present. His IQ, between 50 and 80, is within a range judged by staff to be suitable for independent functioning in the community. There is probably little or no family involvement with the student. During these final years at the institution the individual is being prepared for discharge to the community, where he will live independently and usually work at some competitive job in an unskilled service or factory occupation. During his training, the individual receives supervised experience in one of several occupational categories provided at the institution. He also attends evening adult education classes, which consist of didactic instruction at skills judged relevant to community living (use of transportation, banking facilities, making change, etc.). Individual and group counseling, usually geared toward practical problems of living and adaptive behaviors, are also available. Typically the individual spent his adolescence in a large open dormitory with perhaps 20 other persons in one room.

During his years of communal living, it is likely that he has been exposed to or indulged in some homosexual behaviors. If he does not actively engage in homosexual acts, it is probable that he knows those individuals in his dormitory who commonly engage in this behavior. The acts themselves may range from mutual or group masturbation to fellatio and sodomy. In the past he may have been reprimanded or punished for such behavior, but, as is more likely the case, there was little in the way of expressed surprise or reaction by staff who have been conditioned to expect such occurrences. Much more likely, however, over the years, there *have* been reprimands, punishments, even expulsion from the institution for heterosexual acting out. It is also probable that during the individual's adolescent years, masturbation was forbidden, ridiculed, and punished, or associated with sin, illness, or acne.

During his earlier years at the institution it was likely that contacts with members of the opposite sex were extremely limited. Although such contacts currently occur with much greater frequency, they are well chaperoned, closely structured, and supervised. Ballroom and square dancing, picnics, classroom experiences, and community trips are usually conducted with both sexes represented, but less formal social contacts are the exception rather than the rule. Houseparents in female dormitories were women, thereby providing little opportunity for the learning of normal sex roles.

Although we cannot cite research to prove our point, two pieces of anecdotal information serve to illustrate the manner in which institutional living can serve as an unnatural environment with adverse influence upon psychosexual development.

The first concerns a young mentally retarded person discharged to independence after spending most of his life within the institution. This man worked as a custodian at a Veteran's Administration Hospital, a position that he fulfilled with such a degree of skill and enthusiasm that it earned him merit awards and commendations. On one occasion an institutional counselor observed this man leaving the hospital swimming pool when a group of nurses entered the water. When questioned about why he left the water, the man explained that he had no intention of impregnating the nurses.

"Where did you get that silly idea?" the counselor asked.

"Why, you never let boys and girls swim together at the institution. I always thought that was the reason."

The second anecdote occurred when one of the authors was giving a sex education talk to the institutional attendant staff. A young man, new to his role of attendant, raised his hand and stated that he thought the information being offered was very valuable, but he wondered why, in his dormitory, boys were made to "pee" sitting down. When this was investigated, it turned out to be the case that female houseparents required male students to sit down while urinating in order to avoid wetting the toilet seat. In a habilitation setting in which concern exists for teaching males a healthy sexual identification, it is unfortunate that such incidents can occur. Fortunately, it was possible to work with the individuals involved and to remedy the situation.

ALTERNATIVE MODELS OF PSYCHOSEXUAL DEVELOPMENT

A prevalent notion among those concerned with personality problems of the mentally handicapped concerns the stages of psychosexual development. This notion derives from the application of psychoanalytic concepts of oral, anal, and phallic phases of development to the development of the mentally retarded. The general thesis advanced is that a retarded child goes through the normal phases of emotional growth, experiencing, however, greater than normal difficulty in relinquishing one mode for another. Since his maturational process is slower, he tends to cling to more infantile modes of gratification for longer periods of time. For example, a well known textbook dealing with mental retardation (Hutt and Gibby, 1958) reports:

> The mentally retarded child experiences great difficulties in coping with the problems of the anal period. In the first place he tends to be rather strongly fixated at oral levels, and so has less psychic energy available to proceed to this next higher level (p. 59) . . . The retarded child often does not adequately resolve his oedipal conflicts. The boy continues to be dependent upon his mother, and he does not become able to assume an adequate masculine role. The girl, too, retains her primary identification with the mother . . . All of this has significant implications for her later emotional behavior (p. 64) . . . A retarded child's relatively weak ego makes it difficult for him to control or modify id drives in accordance with the demands of reality. Such drives tend to be expressed in an uninhibited manner, and the controls that are established tend to remain infantile and relatively ineffective (p. 80) . . . The mentally retarded child, due to his inadequate perception of such results of his behavior, is unable to develop a mature 'social conscience'—or a mature super ego (p. 82) . . . The retarded adolescent has extreme difficulty in dealing with the increase in sexual drives that occurs during puberty . . . If the infantile aspects of the sexual drives of the child persists, as they are more probable to do in the retarded child, then he is apt to engage in some form of *perverse*

> sexual behavior (p. 182) . . . Mentally retarded children, even when they reveal perversion, are *not* necessarily 'fiends.' Rather their sexual behavior simply reflects their more infantile level of development and their emotional retardation in general (p. 184).

This model is a generally pessimistic one since it offers little hope for training or social habilitation. Emphasis upon weak egos and infantile fixations leaves little room for behavioral change except through developmental or maturational change. Fortunately, this model is based more upon theoretical considerations than upon the results of empirical research. More recently, alternative models for conceptualizing the psychosexual adjustment and potential of the mentally retarded have been proposed. Perske (1973), for example, suggests we put aside our "brutish past" in dealing with the sexual development of the mentally retarded and substitute a more humane approach. Habits of overcontrol of sexual behavior should be replaced by greater willingness to accept the risks associated with opportunities for more normal sexual expression. This model includes the acceptance of assumptions that the mentally retarded have their own unique timetable of development that includes the same milestones as other populations; that each retarded individual has the right to achieve his highest reasonable potential; that hazards and risks are inherent in growing up; that they require a family-like atmosphere for optimal development; and that they require skilled help in learning about sex throughout their lives.

Just as Perske's "humane" model can be distinguished from the more restrictive models of previous generations, it is also possible to define several other models of sexual development of the retarded. Despite our justifiable concern about humane, normalizing, and equal treatment for the retarded, such concern should not obscure an objective view of development derived through empirical research. Cursory review of the present status of understanding of this area leads to a model which, stated most simply, views sexual development of the mentally retarded as an adaptive behavior.

Rather than viewing the psychosexual development of the retarded as a facsimile of infantile modes of adjustment, such behavior appears purposive, learned as a result of the unique experience and specific environmental influences to which the mentally retarded are subjected. These include the extremely unnatural stimuli available in institutional settings, as well as the motivational and emotional consequences of inadequate learning at home and in the community. Viewed from this perspective, the sexual adjustment of mentally handicapped persons is at least as normal for their environment as is the sexual adjustment of intellectually normal persons in a more natural environment. As long as we continue to evaluate such adjustment in terms of preconceived notions of "normal" sexuality (however conservative or liberal the viewpoint), we preclude the possibility of an adequate understanding of the mentally retarded, let alone any intelligent attempts at programing or legislating for them.

Sexual adjustment of the mentally retarded is only one small aspect of a larger area of social and emotional development. This broad area of functioning includes interpersonal relationships, occupational and community coping skills, and a wide range of self-sufficiency behaviors, all of which are likely to demonstrate behavioral deficiencies. Sexual deficiencies are likely to represent only a small component of the social deficiencies in this population. They may actually be relatively inconsequential to the individual in terms of survival value. Viewed in the context of the marginal subsistence levels of many mentally retarded living independently, such subtleties as "unresolved oedipal complexes" seem superfluous. This is not to minimize the importance of teaching appropriate sexual behaviors to the mentally retarded, but to anchor such teaching in a total program of social habilitation.

As pertains to remediation or treatment, behavioral deficiencies, rather than behavioral excesses, are the primary target of concern for the majority of the mentally retarded population. Specifically, these deficiencies take the form of informational gaps, attitudinal distortions, and emotional immaturity. Thus, the teaching of new behavior, rather than the control or inhibition of sexual behavior, should be the prime focus. The most successful programs are not likely to be those that provide "sex education" but those that undertake the increase of the sexual repertoire of the mentally retarded. Maximum success should also accrue to those programs structured to undo rather than to promote anxiety and inhibition in relation to sexual responsiveness. It is also apparent that to achieve these goals it will be necessary to change the attitudes of those administrators and teachers of the mentally retarded who have perpetuated the present systems of education and training.

REMEDIAL PROGRAMS

Rosen (1970, 1972) has suggested a two-pronged approach to the training of appropriate sexual behaviors in the mentally retarded. The first approach consists of the application of behavior therapy techniques that have been developed for nonretarded populations and their adaptation for the mentally subnormal. The second involves the training of persons who work with the retarded, particularly within institutional settings where cloistering may be most extreme.

Programs for social learning in the area of heterosexual activities are applicable to all but the very lowest levels of mental retardation. However, the most predominant needs are those of educable, mildly retarded persons with potential for independent community functioning. These persons fall into two categories with regard to sexual adjustment: 1) those with social learning deficits but no overt behavioral deviation; and 2) those who also manifest perverted or inappropriate sexual behavior. Persons falling into the first category require programing for appropriate sexual response. Persons falling into the second category may also need to learn inhibitory responses for inappropriate behavior. Both conditions may result from the absence of opportunity for normal heterosexual learning experiences after years of sheltered institutional living or because of overly repressive or protective family situations. In both conditions the treatment plan is to promote a greater level of social competence through a structured hierarchy of social learning experiences.

Desensitization

The absence of opportunities for constructive learning experiences with members of the opposite sex often makes the prospect of heterosexual contacts extremely fearful. Consequently, techniques of systematic desensitization, described by Wolpe (1958) and evaluated in numerous studies (Geer, 1964; Lang and Lazovik, 1963; Paul, 1966), are often the method of choice for reducing anxiety and initiating approach responses. A graduated fear hierarchy is constructed, beginning with experiences that are without fear-producing qualities for the client, and increasing in gradual steps to more frightening situations. The client is instructed and practiced in methods of deep muscle relaxation, and treatment proceeds by the presentation of structured fantasies representing each level of the fear hierarchy. Each subsequent step in the hierarchy is presented only after the client reports the absence of a fear reaction to the preceding fantasy. In the area of heterosexual relationships, hierarchies can be started with group activity situation (dances, parties) before progressing to individual dating relationships. Depending upon the needs and experience, as well as the prospects for community placement of the individual, this hierarchy can progress to more mature relationships, including sexual intercourse. The method reduces anxiety in the real situation and also provides the client with information and suggestions for behavior.

Programed Heterosexual Experience

After successful completion of desensitization procedures, the individual can practice actual experiences with members of the opposite sex. A procedure of gradually shaping responses to females was suggested by Ferster (1965). He argues that it is desirable to start with a response that is relatively likely to be reinforced, such as simply speaking to females, and then to proceed up the hierarchy of responses that are increasingly less likely to be reinforced, not advancing to the next item in the hierarchy until the preceding one has been well established. Feldman (1966) reports that it may take as long as six months before sexual approach responses to females are well learned, particularly in those persons who report no sexual attraction to females. We have found it useful to use female psychologists and teachers to structure a series of exercises for the male client with social deficits. The client is instructed to report his momentary tension using a simple five-point scale, and these reports determine the rate at which new tasks are presented. The female confederate serves as co-therapist and is practiced in a supportive, yet realistic, feminine role with the client. Typical situations can progress from merely seeing a female at a distance, approaching and entering her office, maintaining eye contact, engaging in a pre-programed conversation, spontaneous conversation, taking a walk with her, and taking her to the coffee shop.

Once the limits of this technique are exhausted, the client is instructed to simulate the same graded series of behaviors in real situations. More freedom exists in halfway houses or outpatient settings than in institutions, but the technique is the same.

Role Playing

There is a great deal of clinical evidence that role playing can be a powerful technique for initiating behavior for which there is a strong inhibitory response (Salter, 1949; Wolpe, 1958). The use of this technique involves the practice of behaviors that are low in the response repertoire of the client in a controlled and supportive manner. Wolpe and Lazarus (1967) have elaborated on the use of role playing techniques, as well as encouragement and reinforcement for such behavior in the real situation as part of more general procedures of assertive training. In this context, their use is viewed as the overcoming of anxiety responses in interpersonal situations. "The counterconditioning of anxiety is thus intertwined on each occasion with the operant conditioning of the instrumental response (acts of assertion) and each facilitates the other." The role playing of anxiety-evoking behaviors is sufficient to elicit timidity and defensive behavior resembling that which occurs in the actual situation, but repetition and practice can result in marked improvement, both in the imaginary and real situations. Modeling of the desired response is accomplished after demonstration by the therapist and reinforcement of the client's attempt at imitation. This technique is especially helpful when inhibition is severe, and is used in teaching conversation skills, telephone behavior, asking for a date, social etiquette, as well as general assertive behavior associated with the sexual role. Role playing can be used in conjunction with programed heterosexual experience.

Sex-related Talk

Davison (1968) has referred to the information value of sex-related "locker room" talk in adolescents. Although this activity is probably the source of misconceptions and distortions in the sex knowledge available to many adolescents, it may be the only source of information available. Within institutions, the lack of adequate sources of authoritative information or opportunities for self-correcting, validating experiences makes sexual knowledge markedly deficient. Because of language deficits, even slang expressions for genitals and sex behavior are misunderstood or entirely absent from the verbal repertoire. Frank sexual talk with a therapist explaining the meaning of slang terms for genital organs, masturbation, and intercourse serves to reduce anxiety related to these topics.

Suggestions to Masturbate

Among boys with deviant sexual behaviors we have found a surprising absence of masturbation. In three out of four cases of boys who were not masturbating, direct suggestion was sufficient to elicit this behavior. Assurances that such behavior was quite prevalent and generally healthy when no other outlet is available serve to dispel notions leading to guilt and fear. We have found it useful to provide clients with 3 × 5 index cards to make daily records of the frequency of successful masturbation and sexually inappropriate responses, such as homosexual contacts. Weekly graphs prepared by the therapist in the client's presence show progress in the substitution of masturbation (in private) for inappropriate behavior.

Aversive Conditioning

When clients have developed inappropriate, bizarre, or perverted sexual behaviors, aversive conditioning techniques may also be useful in teaching inhibitory responses. Feldman (1966) has pointed out that most of the operant responses involved in homosexual behavior cannot be reproduced in a treatment setting and so are not available for manipulation. This also holds true for other forms of deviant sexual behavior. The majority of therapists using aversive procedures have, therefore, utilized a classical conditioning model to associate fear or another strong negative emotion with the previously attractive sexual stimulus. There is some evidence

(Cautela, 1966; Davison, 1968) that this association can also be accomplished in a fantasy situation. Davison successfully applied this method to a college student preoccupied with sadistic fantasies. The initial phase of this treatment involved the counterconditioning of more appropriate sexual fantasies to sexual arousal. The client was instructed to use his sadistic fantasy to masturbate, but to interrupt this fantasy to stare at a photograph of a nude female as long as possible without losing his erection. As orgasm was approaching, he was "at all costs" to focus on the photograph. After the client began to report that images of nude females were sexually arousing, an imaginal aversive conditioning ("covert sensitization") method was applied to the sadistic fantasy. An extremely disgusting scene was paired in imagination with the client's sadistic fantasy until the fantasy was no longer sexually arousing.

While case reports describing the use of imaginal aversive techniques are rare, the method holds promise because of its flexibility with regard to a wide variety of sexual stimuli and behaviors, and because of its ease of application in an office setting. Instructions to the client can be tape recorded and presented during repeated therapy sessions without loss of effectiveness.

IN-SERVICE TRAINING

A crucial aspect of improving sexual adjustment within institutions centers on the instructions given to attendants concerning sexual behaviors when they occur in living units. It is important that houseparents understand that homosexual behaviors should not be condoned, and that they are expected to discourage, prevent, and vocally disapprove of such activity. Furthermore, they must be made to understand that such behaviors are reversible. Houseparents should be encouraged and helped in developing a counseling relationship with the student. They should communicate a genuine interest that the student does change and that such change is expected. This must be followed up by a rather close watch on the student's behavior and confrontation with instances of homosexual encounters when necessary. It is best to help both of the partners engaged in homosexual encounters if possible. In such situations, disappointment should be expressed along with encouragement to do better next time. Evidence that the student is trying to change should be acknowledged. Punishment, restriction, and deprivation for homosexual behavior probably will not work. Normal coeducational activities should be encouraged as much as possible. Appropriate sexual behavior in males should be associated with a masculine image, i.e., "Men don't behave that way." Books such as Gordon's *Facts about Sex for Exceptional Youth* (1969) should be used in correcting misconceptions and providing basic information. Houseparents may need to speak the student's language to make themselves understood (e.g., "bed hopping," "pimping," "taking a walk"). Masturbation should not be punished. Public masturbation, however, should be interrupted and discouraged. Students should be encouraged to use a private latrine.

INSTITUTIONAL RESTRUCTURING

As is true for the general population, some retarded persons are capable of satisfactory sexual and marital relationships; some are not. Some are able to provide for their children; some are not. The only thing that we can be sure of is that they *do* marry and they *do* have children. In light of the dearth of knowledge about this whole area, those of us working in institutions have only one recourse. Bigger and better sex education programs will not suffice. If we are to perpetuate our belief in an habilitation model for large proportions of institutionalized retarded, then we must be willing to structure the institution as nearly as possible for community preparation.

Programs of social learning must be introduced at as early an age as possible. It may very well be impossible, at age twenty, to undo social deficiencies reinforced from early or middle childhood. Institutional staff must be conditioned to perceive retarded persons through eyes that have absolutely no knowledge of retardation or handicap, because it is with just such vision that people will evaluate and react to the handicapped after discharge. Behaviors "tolerated" within institutional confines may be judged illegal, immoral, ludicrous, or weird in the community. They therefore necessitate correction before, rather than after, community release. For many institutional behaviors, remedial education, counseling, or psychotherapy techniques are just not powerful enough to effect meaningful behavior change. In such instances, nothing short of a major revamping of institutional structure and practice will suffice. As pertains to homosexual behaviors, institutional staff are in need of preventative and coping techniques as strenuous as the zeal exerted in preventing pregnancies among the female population. Parents referring children must be told that institutions are learning environments, not cloisters, and that some risk-taking is necessary for promoting growth and responsibility. Most important, though, is our need to continually remind ourselves that inappropriate sexual behavior, like all other behaviors, represents conditioned reactions to environmental stimuli, and not the natural unfolding of predetermined sluggish timetables. The mentally retarded are not eternal children. Rather, their unique educational and living experiences may serve to condition a system of sexual behaviors, attitudes, vocabulary, and feelings that are completely alien to "normal" children and adults.

The effects of social learning techniques on sexual responses are yet to be adequately demonstrated. Experimental studies are needed to evaluate specific types of behavioral intervention upon criteria of behavioral changes, object choices, and other pertinent indices of psychosexual adjustment. Long-term follow-up studies are essential to evaluate properly the procedures described earlier. Therapeutic efforts must be more closely linked to experimental research and theory than previous habilitative efforts have been in other areas of training. Future studies may indicate that sexual deviations, occurring as a result of the absence of opportunity to learn appropriate behavior, as in institutional settings, are more amenable to change than similar behaviors derived from more complex family situations or personality dynamics. Our experience has been that significant change occurs with an amount of effort that seems relatively minor when compared to the very severe aversive conditioning techniques (using electric shock and chemotherapy), which have been used with homosexuals and sexual fetishists. The most successful efforts will probably be those utililizing skillful learning techniques for teaching new behaviors, rather than those relying on aversive conditioning for deviant responses. Whether or not aversive techniques will still be needed when more sophisticated methods for teaching appropriate social behaviors become available is a question for future research. Whatever the methodology, it is clear that the time for fear and superstition, which is associated with social learning in sexual areas, has long passed, and the problem deserves the rigor and enthusiasm of creative experimental approaches.

Resolution of many emotionally laden arguments about sex and the retarded comes not from endless meetings and obsessional concern over outcomes but from social engineering designed to produce good husbands, wives, and parents. Until we have honestly attempted to develop residential institutions as bona fide learning environments for marriage and parenthood, we are certainly in no position to prejudge what retarded persons are or are not capable of performing. Much of the methodology for producing suitable marriage partners is already available if we are willing to apply it.

LITERATURE CITED

Andron, L., and Strum, M. L. 1973. Is "I DO" in the repertoire of the retarded? A study of the functioning of married retarded couples. Ment. Retard. 11:31–34.

Baller, W. R. 1936. A study of the present social status of a group of adults who, when they were in elementary schools, were classified as mentally deficient. Genet. Psychol. Monogr. 18:165–244.

Baller, W. R., Charles, D. C., and Miller, E. L. 1967. Mid-life attainment of the mentally retarded: A longitudinal study. Genet. Psychol. Monogr. 75:235–329.

Bass, M. S. 1963. Marriage, parenthood, and prevention of pregnancy. Amer. J. Ment. Defic. 68:318–333.

Bass, M. S. 1964. Marriage for the mentally deficient. Ment. Retard. 2:198–202.

Bowden, J., Spitz, H. H., and Winters, J. J., Jr. 1971. Follow-up of one retarded couple's marriage. Ment. Retard. 9:42–43.

Brown, B. S., and Courtless, T. F. 1969. The mentally retarded offender. *In* R. C. Allen (ed.), Readings in Law and Psychiatry. Johns Hopkins University Press, Baltimore.

Cautela, J. R. 1966. Treatment of compulsive behavior by covert sensitization. Psychol. Rec. 16:33–41.

Charles, D. C. 1953. Ability and accomplishment of persons earlier judged mentally deficient. Genet. Psychol. Monogr. 47:3–71.

Clark, G. R., Kivitz, M., and Rosen, M. 1968. A transitional program for institutionalized adult retarded. Research and Demonstration Project No. 1275P, Vocational Rehabilitation Administration, U.S. Department of Health, Education, and Welfare, Washington, D.C.

Davies, S. P. 1930. Social Control of the Mentally Deficient. Thomas Y. Crowell Company, New York.

Davison, G. C. 1968. Elimination of a sadistic fantasy by a client-controlled counterconditioning technique: A case study. J. Abnorm. Psychol. 73:84–89.

de la Cruz, F. F., and LaVeck, G. D. 1973. Human Sexuality and the Mentally Retarded: Physiological and Biological Aspects. Brunner/Mazel, New York.

Edgerton, R. B. 1973. Some socio-cultural research considerations. *In* F. F. de la Cruz and G. D. LaVeck (eds.), Human Sexuality and the Mentally Retarded. Brunner/Mazel, New York.

Feldman, M. P. 1966. Aversion therapy for sexual deviations: A critical review. Psychol. Bull. 65:65–79.

Ferster, C. B. 1965. Reinforcement and punishment in the control of homosexual behaviour by social agencies. *In* H. J. Eysenck (ed.), Experiments in Behavior Therapy, pp. 189–207. Pergamon Press Ltd., London.

Floor, L., Baxter, D., Rosen, M., and Zisfein, L. 1975. A survey of marriages among previously institutionalized retardates. Ment. Retard. 13:33–37.

Flory, C. D. 1936. The physical growth of mentally deficient boys. Monograph of the Society for Research and Child Development 1 (16).

Geer, J. H. 1964. Phobia treated by reciprocal inhibition. J. Abnorm. Psychol. 69:642–645.

Glueck, B. 1918. Concerning prisoners. Ment. Hyg. 2:177–218.

Goodman, L., Budner, S., and Lesh, B. 1971. The parent's role in sex education for the retarded. Ment. Retard. 9:43–46.

Gordon, S. 1969. Facts about Sex for Exceptional Youth. New Jersey Association for Brain Damaged Children, East Orange, New Jersey.

Gordon, S. 1972. Missing in special education: Sex. J. Spec. Ed. 5:351–354.

Gordon, S. 1973. Facts about Sex for Today's Youth. John Day, New York.

Hall, J. 1974. Sexual behavior. *In* J. Wortis (ed.), Mental Retardation and Developmental Disabilities, VI. Brunner/Mazel, New York.

Hall, J., Morris, H. L., and Barker, H. R. 1973. Sexual knowledge and attitudes of mentally retarded adolescents. Amer. J. Ment. Defic. 77:706–709.

Hammar, S. L., Wright, L. S., and Jensen, D. L. 1967. Sex education for the retarded adolescent: A survey of parental attitudes and methods of management in 50 adolescent retardates. Clin. Pediatr. 6:621–627.

Hathaway, S. B. 1947. Planned parenthood and metnal deficiency. Amer. J. Ment. Defic. 52:182–186.

Hutt, M. L., and Gibby, R. G. 1958. The Mentally Retarded Child: Development, Education and Guidance. Allyn & Bacon, Boston.

Kempton, W. 1975. A Teacher's Guide to Sex Education for Persons with Learning Disabilities. Duxbury Press, North Scituate, Mass.

Kempton, W., and Foreman, R. 1976. Guidelines for Training in Sexuality and the Mentally Handicapped. Planned Parenthood Association of Southeastern Pennsylvania, Philadelphia.

Kennedy, R. J. R. 1948. The Social Adjustment of Morons in a Connecticut City. Commission to Survey Resources in Connecticut, Hartford, Willport, Conn.

Kennedy, R. J. R. 1966. A Connecticut community revisited: A study of the social adjustment of a group of mentally deficient adults in 1948 and 1960. Project No. 655, Office of Vocational Rehabilitation. U.S. Department of Health, Education, and Welfare, Washington, D.C.

Kugel, R. B., and Mohr, J. 1963. Mental retardation and physical growth. Amer. J. Ment. Defic. 68:41–48.

Lang, P. J., and Lazovik, A. D. 1963. Experimental disensitization of a phobia. J. Abnorm. Psychol. 66:519–525.

Mattinson, J. 1970. Marriage and Mental Handicaps. University of Pittsburgh Press, Pittsburgh.

Meyen, E. L., and Retish, P. M. 1971. Sex education for the mentally retarded: Influencing teachers' attitudes. Ment. Retard. 9:46–49.

Miller, E. L. 1965. Ability and social adjustment at mid-life of persons earlier judged mentally deficient. Genet. Psychol. Monogr. 72:139–198.

Mosier, H. D., Grossman, H. J., and Dingman, H. F. 1962. Secondary sex development in mentally deficient individuals. Child Dev. 33:273–286.

Paul, G. L. 1966. Insight vs. Desensitization in Psychotherapy: An Experiment in Anxiety Reduction. Stanford University Press, Stanford.

Peck. J. R., and Stephens, W. B. 1965. Marriage of young adult male retardates. Amer. J. Ment. Defic. 69:818–827.

Perske, R. 1973. About sexual development: An attempt to be human with the mentally retarded. Ment. Retard. 11:6–8.

Rosen, M. 1970. Conditioning appropriate heterosexual behavior in mentally and socially handicapped populations. Train. Sch. Bull. 66:172–177.

Rosen, M. 1972. Psychosexual adjustment of the mentally handicapped. *In* M. S. Bass (ed.), Sexual Rights and Responsibilities of the Mentally Retarded. Proceedings of the Conference of the American Association on Mental Deficiency, Region IX, October 12–14. University of Delaware, Newark, Delaware.

Rosen, M., Kivitz, M., Clark, G. R., and Floor, L. 1970. Prediction of postinstitutional adjustment of mentally retarded adults. Amer. J. Ment. Defic. 74:726–734.

Salter, A. 1949. Conditioned Reflex Therapy. Creative Age Press, New York.

Ullmann, L. P., and Krasner, L. 1966. Case Studies in Behavior Modification. Holt, Rinehart & Winston, New York.

Wallin, J. E. W. 1956. Mental deficiency. J. Clin. Psychol. Brandon, Vermont.

Wolpe, J. 1958. Psychotherapy by Reciprocal Inhibition. Stanford University Press, Stanford.

Wolpe, J., and Lazarus, A. A. 1967. Behavior Therapy Techniques. Pergamon Press Ltd., London.

Chapter 17

Social Competence, Inappropriate Behavior, and Habilitation

The efforts of those who have been responsible for social habilitation of the mentally retarded have typically been concentrated upon two goals: the first is the training of vocational skills appropriate for functioning in competitive or sheltered employment situations in the community, and the second is the teaching of sufficient academic and social skills to allow the individual to cope with the demands of the community (Gunzburg, 1968). The training of social skills is often limited to job-related or community-related competencies, such as the use of public transportation facilities. In most instances, habilitation programs do not deal with equally critical deficiencies that, if not actually detrimental to survival in the community, may, nevertheless, mark the individual as atypical, deviant, or retarded. Yet social adjustment in the community requires not only the mastery of numerous skills and proficiencies but also the ability to blend into the general population in a manner judged acceptable by society.

This chapter reviews the assessment and teaching of social competencies and examines the question of whether socially inappropriate behaviors occurring in community-bound persons can also be remediated.

SOCIAL COMPETENCE

Measuring Social Skills

By now the assessment and teaching of social knowledge and social skills is a recognized component of social habilitation programs. Doll (1948) was among the earliest to recognize the importance of social competence as a criterion of social adjustment. The Vineland Social Maturity Scale (Doll, 1953) is an age-referenced developmental scale that is still probably the most widely used index of the social functioning of the mentally retarded.

In a more recent formulation, Gunzburg (1968) describes three types of information that are essential to the teacher confronted with the problem of training social competence in the mentally retarded. The first is a knowledge of the individual's ability, the second is a knowledge of his social skills, and the third is a knowledge of what can be expected of persons of his mental ability level. In addition to the traditional academic skills of reading, writing, and numerical knowledge, Gunzburg suggests that social knowledge must include the proper assessment and teaching of time concepts, the handling of financial concepts such as payroll deductions and budgeting, and a knowledge of public services, including the post office, transportation facilities, medical resources, and communication skills. Gunzburg has developed a Progress Assessment Chart (PAC) for measuring social competence in mentally retarded populations and for designing remedial procedures. Like the Vineland, the PAC is based on direct observation of the individual, or on information supplied by a reliable informant. The skills evaluated by the PAC are arranged in a sequence of development according to age levels and are grouped under the four categories of self-help, communication, socialization, and occupation. Each category is further divided into subsections dealing with particular areas of social competence (e.g., self-help includes appropriate dressing, grooming, table habits, budgeting, and health care). Gunzburg provides norms and standards based on large-scale surveys of mentally subnormal persons in Birmingham training centers.

The Adaptive Behavior Scale (Nihira et al., 1969) was designed to evaluate the coping behavior of the mental retardate in relation to the demands and requirements of his environment. The original scale was developed by Leland et al. (1967), and numerous item analysis and validity studies have been conducted (Foster and Nihira, 1969; Nihira, 1969*a*, 1969*b;* Nihira and Shelhaas, 1970).

The classification system provided by the Adaptive Behavior Scale ranges from Level I, mild negative deviation from population norms, to

Level V, the extreme lower limit of adaptive behavior. Part I of the Adaptive Behavior Scale is designed to measure the client's skills and abilities in the following behavior areas: independent functioning, physical development, economic activities, language development, number and time concepts, occupation (domestic), occupation (general), self-direction, responsibility, and socialization.

Clark, Kivitz, and Rosen (1968) developed a Social Achievement Test that assesses ten areas of social functioning: social sight vocabulary, monetary knowledge, measurement, time concepts, letter writing and post office skills, newspaper usage, job application procedure, telephone skills, public transportation knowledge, and banking knowledge. Norms for two alternative forms of the test were collected for 260 mildly retarded institutionalized adults enrolled in vocational habilitation programs at Elwyn Institute. Split half-reliability for the two forms of the test was .99. As might be expected from the verbal nature of many of the items, the test correlates highly with IQ.

A similar effort was made by Halpern et al. (1975), who developed a Social and Prevocational Information Battery for secondary educable mentally retarded pupils enrolled in work-study programs in Oregon. The battery consists of nine subtests (job-search skills, job-related behavior, banking, budgeting, purchasing, home management, physical health care, hygiene and grooming, and functional signs) related to five long-range goals of work-study programs (employability, economic self-sufficiency, family living, personal habits, and communication). Reported reliabilities for the batteries and their modest predictive validity with a criterion of habilitation counselor ratings of community adjustment (.51) one year after graduation from high school suggest that the battery has potential for the evaluation of social competence in this type of population.

The Fundamental Achievement Series (Bennett and Doppelt, 1968) was developed to assess social skills of educationally and socially deprived populations. It consists of a verbal and a numerical test, each of which can be administered within thirty minutes by a cassette tape recording. The verbal test assesses areas such as the recognition of signs and the understanding of transportation, menus, addresses, and phone numbers. The numerical test measures the understanding of numerical and monetary values, calendars, bills, checks and timetelling. Rosen and Hoffman (1975*a*) administered the FAS to 100 residential students with IQs varying between 60 and 101. They report it to be a reliable measure with a mentally retarded population. However, its high correlation with verbal IQ indicates that the test does not measure social functioning uncontaminated by other cognitive factors. Furthermore, test performance did not relate to age or length of institutionalization and has not been evaluated as a predictor of community functioning.

A test of Basic Achievement and Common Knowledge and Skills (BACKS) was developed at the Georgia Rehabilitation Center to assess knowledge of basic educational skills required for daily living, both on the job and off the job (Deshpande and Anderson, 1969). It is designed for adolescents and adults of lower ability and education levels for the purpose of providing remedial instruction. The BACKS test consists of seven short subtests in the areas of basic arithmetic, making change, telling time, using a ruler, measurements, common knowledge, and traffic rules and signs. The BACKS are paper and pencil tests that include a total of 44 items and require 15 to 25 minutes for completion. The standardization and norms were derived from a sample of 717 trainees in pre–vocational training programs. Unfortunately, most of this sample consisted of Black females, so generalization from the test to other populations may be limited. Percentile norms and approximate grade levels for total score only are obtained from the manual. Factor analysis of the BACKS suggests that several of the subtests are factorially pure.

Once the individual has graduated from habilitation training programs, the evaluation of social competence is complex because value judgments invariably influence the choice of criteria of adjustment. Follow-up studies have placed primary emphasis on vocational and economic functioning or have evaluated social functioning in relation to comparison groups. As described in Chapter 9, such studies have reported percentages of persons married, the size of the families, the incidence of church affiliations, and incomes and savings. An innovative approach by Edmonson (1974) has gone beyond the use of categorical data by using indices of social participation as a demonstration of social competence. Two instruments—a questionnaire and a daily diary kept by the subject—were used to sample participation in a variety of activities. Questionnaire items were answered verbally by the subjects and included at-home activities such as meal preparation, leisure time pursuits, and use of the telephone, as well as community activities such as dining in restaurants, visits, attendance at meetings, and use of transportation. The diary utilized pictographic symbols so that even nonreaders could keep running accounts of their daily activities. Social participation scores derived from these instruments proved to be consistent over time and correlated significantly with ratings of overall social competence made by habilitation counselors. The unavailability of such behavioral measures of social competence in the past has hampered an adequate understanding of the social adjustment process of the mentally retarded. Hopefully, the Edmonson techniques will be employed by other investigators to supplement information derived solely from social knowledge types of procedures.

INAPPROPRIATE BEHAVIOR

The literature dealing specifically with abnormal behavior of the mentally retarded has tended to emphasize the incidence of severe emotional disturbance (e.g., psychosis, autism, antisocial and delinquent behavior) and to focus primarily on the moderately, severely, and profoundly retarded and institutionalized populations. Thus, Garfield (1963) concludes that psychotic behavior occurs in a relatively small percentage of mentally retarded, institutionalized persons, and that most mental retardates do not give evidence of serious emotional disturbance, nor do they manifest a particular stereotyped personality. Garfield concludes that the mentally retarded differ among themselves as much as normal groups differ and that they are equally influenced by environmental experiences and interpersonal relationships. The same point has been made by O'Connor and Tizard (1956) and by Sarason and Gladwin (1958). While all of these excellent reviews call for further research and the application of current theoretical constructs of personality development, few writers have dealt with the specific problem of idiosyncratic behaviors of the mentally retarded, particularly the mildly retarded.

The issue of maladaptive and inappropriate behavior is particularly salient within institutions. After spending much of their lives within the artificial and often socially sterile and impoverished environment of a residential institution, it is not surprising that many mentally retarded persons appear different, idiosyncratic, or even bizarre. It is our thesis that much of this behavior bears little direct relation to their intellectual deficiency although it may be commonly learned as a secondary phenomenon in environments that often seem ideally structured to produce such behavior. An article (Bouliew, 1971) asks the question, "Do institutions maintain retarded behavior?" Our experience suggests that the answer to this question is a resounding "Yes," and that the situation may not be limited to institutions.

Jenny is a 40-year-old retarded female living within the institution. She does an adequate job at her housekeeping assignment. Several years ago she was placed in a halfway house program before discharge from the institution but was quickly removed for an incident of sexual indiscretion. It was clear that she showed little sound judgment in her behavior and had no appreciation of the consequences of her acts. Within the institution

Jenny appears a happy, talkative, pleasant personality—perhaps too pleasant. Each time she encounters a staff member her conversation follows the following lines: "Hello, Dr. R., isn't it a beautiful day today? I got my hair set this morning. Wasn't it a beautiful weekend? My girlfriend, S., sends her regards to you." These comments, on the surface, appear friendly and harmless. The behavior is problematic because Jenny repeats the same dialogue again and again with each staff member she encounters, perhaps a dozen times each morning and every day each week. It is not difficult to understand how this behavior develops in a woman with impoverished thinking and a paucity of daily experiences within the institution. Yet such behavior would distinguish her as a somewhat "kooky," dull, boring, and mildly aversive individual in the community. At the institution, however, the behavior is tolerated and consistently reinforced by staff members. In the service of kind, humanitarian, understanding, tolerant, and "enlightened" treatment of the retarded, each staff member in turn repeats the ritual with Jenny, adding his own unique "uh-huhs," nodding approval, and interjecting social amenities ("That's nice. . . ." "Yes, it is. . . ." "Thank you. . . ."). Would it not be more benevolent, kind, and constructive for Jenny if each staff member would ignore her comments, point out their inappropriate quality, and perhaps teach her more meaningful ways of relating to people? The friendliness of staff members toward students of the institution may be a seemingly innocuous phenomenon. Yet, for girls, the unqualified approach to strangers that is sometimes observed in the community may have its roots in the trust they learn to place in adults while living at the institution. Reinforcement of inappropriate behavior occurs in many ways. Usually the reinforcement is inadvertent, innocent, and subtle. It takes the form of attention given to students for tantrums, stealing, dependence, hypochondriacal behavior, hallucinations, bizarre speech, and other undesirable behavior. These factors are not minor. Considerably more training of retarded persons takes place through casual, social contacts with staff than through formal education and training situations.

Spradlin and Girardeau (1966) allude to such learning in a review of the behavior of retarded persons:

> There is some maladaptive behavior which is typically found in institutions. This behavior is developed and maintained by the institutional environment.
>
> For example, the institutional environment provides very little adult attention for the child. However, when the child has a tantrum, is aggressive with others, breaks a window, or exhibits self-destructive behavior, he usually receives a great deal of attention from the attendant and professional personnel. . . .

> Clinging or hugging of both friends and strangers is a behavior which is exhibited in high frequency in institutions for retarded persons. Yet this kind of behavior is generally unacceptable in a community and might even reduce the probability of weekend visits home if the child embarrasses the parents by clinging to neighbors or visitors. This behavior is not an innate characteristic of retarded persons but is generated by the social reinforcements of an institutional environment. The persons in an institutional environment are apt to overlook a retarded person if the person is playing with blocks, drawing or merely talking to them in a conversational voice. However, it is most difficult to overlook a patient who is clinging to you (pp. 290–291).

Unacceptable and inappropriate behavior has been well studied in the severely and profoundly retarded. A series of investigations by Berkson and his colleagues (Berkson, 1964; Berkson and Davenport, 1962; Berkson and Mason, 1963, 1964; Davenport and Berkson, 1963) have supplied a great deal of information about the incidence and parameters of stereotyped movements in the severely retarded. Behaviors such as rocking, eye poking, limb posturing, twirling, thumb sucking, and complex hand movements were studied. Berkson has pointed out that such behaviors are prominent in the repertoire of the severely and profoundly retarded and that they occur in the absence of interactions with the physical and social environment that are more typical of higher intelligence groups. Stereotypy is much more pronounced in restricted environments and is less likely to occur in environments like the playground, which evokes alternative activities. Berkson believes that sterotyped behaviors represent a type of self-stimulation, possibly involving tactual, kinesthetic, and vestibular feedback systems. Such behaviors have a functional similarity to behaviors observed in chimpanzees reared in isolation. Further studies (Kaufman, 1967; Kaufman and Levitt, 1965) relate stereotyped behavior differences to age, sex, time of day, and institutionalization.

The relationship between inappropriate or antisocial behavior and intellectual level has also been studied. In a 1967 census study of 19 public institutions for the mentally retarded (Johnson, 1970), data for over 23,000 individuals were obtained. In addition to intelligence and Vineland Social Quotient scores, information about the residents' self-help skills and antisocial behavior was obtained. The correlations between the test scores and self-help skills, competence and independent functioning were moderately high suggesting the utility of IQs and SQs as useful predictors of these behaviors. The correlations between these scores and "problem behaviors" involving disturbed relations with peers or authority figures were significantly better than chance but were too low to be of practical significance. Severe social and emotional behaviors (screaming, throwing objects, aggressive and destructive behaviors) have also been reported to be independent of intellectual level by Vogel, Kun, and Meshorer (1968), of self-care (Nihira, 1969*b;* Spivack and Spotts, 1966) and of behavioral competence on an adaptive behavior checklist (Gardner and Giampa, 1970). While this finding is contradictory to the results obtained by Rosen and Hoffman (1974), less severe antisocial behaviors were being rated in the Elwyn study. Thus, it would seem that the occurrence of antisocial, emotional, aggressive, and destructive behaviors may be relatively independent of intellectual level. However, less extreme behaviors that would label the individual as different in the community may be more closely related to intellectual level.

It has been repeatedly demonstrated that a wide variety of self-help and social behaviors can be ''shaped'' in severely and profoundly retarded persons using operant conditioning techniques (Bensberg, Colwell, and Cassell, 1965; Blackwood, 1962; Girardeau and Spradlin, 1964; Gorton and Hollis, 1965; Watson, 1967, 1968). Numerous investigators have shown that it is also possible to control self-destructuve behaviors such as scratching, head-banging, and self-hitting (Ragain and Anson, 1976; Thomas and Howard, 1971) by the differential reinforcement of behaviors other than the inappropriate behavior. It seems likely that less extreme, but equally ubiquitous, inappropriate behaviors in the mildly retarded individual can be similarly treated by operant conditioning methods, but there are few reported cases in the literature.

Measurement of Inappropriate Behavior

Despite the acknowledgment of the importance of social adjustment as a criterion for diagnosis of mental retardation that dates back over thirty years, there has been surprisingly little effort to measure socially inappropriate behavior. Part II of the AAMD Adaptive Behavior Scale includes items assessing the frequency of violent and destructive behavior, antisocial behavior, rebellious behavior, untrustworthy behavior, withdrawal, stereotyped behavior, inappropriate interpersonal manners, unacceptable vocal habits, eccentric habits, self-abusive behavior, hyperactive tendencies, sexually aberrant behavior, and psychological disturbances.

Rosen and Hoffman (1974) described an Inventory of Inappropriate Behavior (IIB) for identifying inappropriate social behaviors characterizing a retarded population. The goal was to create a screening tool that could be used by relatively untrained attendant staff as part of a referral process for behavioral treatment. The IIB is intended to provide a rough index of the degree and type of bizarre behavior. It was developed within the context of a residential school and habilitation center for the mentally handicapped and is probably most relevant to measuring inappropriate behavior associated with institutionalization.

The IIB was designed to assess the frequency of stereotyped, bizarre behavior. An initial pool of behavioral items was suggested by vocational training staff of the institution, who listed the bizarre and socially inappropriate behaviors that they judged typical of the more bizarre student population. Each item included in the scale was refined to avoid redundancy and ambiguity. Forty were selected and were categorized into six broad behavioral areas: over-friendliness, bizarre speech and actions, socially awkward behavior, poor personal appearance, belligerence, and childishness.

The scale distinguished three separate populations of students at the institution who differed in competence levels of vocational assignment—an adjustment training group of the severely limited students, a sheltered workshop group, representing a middle level of vocational competence, and a trade training group of students in the final phases of a community preparation program.

POTENTIAL FOR CHANGE: THEORETICAL AND RESEARCH CONSIDERATIONS

This chapter has thus far considered the broad question of social adjustment of the mentally retarded from the broad perspective of social competence and potential for socially acceptable behavior. We have reviewed the measurement and training of social skills and have considered the problem of inappropriate and socially undesirable behaviors that may characterize the mentally retarded, particularly those who have grown up within institutional settings. We have suggested that, while a great deal of attention has been devoted to the teaching of community-oriented skills and knowledge and to the treatment of self-destructive, aggressive, and stereotyped behaviors in the severely retarded, little attention has been devoted to the training of more mildly subnormal individuals to be more socially appropriate. Because there are few empirical studies to draw upon, this problem is examined largely on the basis of inferences from theoretical considerations and basic laboratory research. The major issue here is whether socially inappropriate behaviors in the mildly retarded are amenable to change in programs that are practicable in the typical habilitation setting.

Baumeister (1968) offers a thought-provoking theoretical and empirical analysis of retarded behavior based upon the greater intra-individual variability in performance of the mentally retarded. Pointing out that most theoretical explanations for mentally retarded behavior stem from a defect position based on invariants in behavior (e.g., inferior short-term memory, high distractibility, etc.), he states that the performance of mentally retarded individuals is characterized by its high variability. Baumeister offers evidence that the mentally retarded as a group are more heterogeneous in their behavior than normal intelligence groups, and that this finding may be based on greater intrasubject variability reflecting spontaneous changes over time. Unreliability in measurement of retarded behavior may be due not so much to error in measurement as to real changes within the organism, presumably on a motivational, attentional, or arousal basis. If Baumeister is correct, this fact would account for the inability of the mentally retarded to adapt appropriately to changing environmental exigencies and might also account for their seeming inappropriate or bizarre. It may offer special problems to the habilitation counselor, since more variable behavior is also more difficult to modify.

One requisite for changing inappropriate behavior is that the individual be capable of responding to the behavior of others. Social sensitivity and conformity to pressure by other persons who are perceived as reference groups is the essence of social adjustment. Despite an enormous amount of literature dealing with the effect of group pressure on social conformity within the nonretarded population, the issue has received scanty attention in studies of mental retardation. A study by Zachofsky, Reardon, and O'Conner (1974) investigated whether or not retarded subjects would ''yield'' to group responses that conflicted with what they actually saw in a color-naming task. Yielding was most prevalent in lower IQ subjects but occurred in both groups. The subjects' responses did not vary signifcantly with differences in peer pressure or the presence of an adult authority figure in the group. Retarded adults appeared to approach the task with an initial ''response set'' as either a yielder or non-yielder. Generalization from this study to other social conformity situations is limited. Conformity in the experiment meant responding in an incorrect manner because the experimenter surreptitiously changed the stimulus after the group response and before the subject's response. Our concern is whether or not a mentally retarded person will respond to social pressure in order to behave in a manner that is considered socially correct. Nevertheless, the study does indicate that mentally retarded adults are capable of perceiving peer pressure and that even lower intelligence level persons have this ability.

Another approach to the social responsiveness of the mentally retarded is to investigate their responsiveness to social stimuli. Rosenberg, Spradlin, and Mabel (1961) found a high level of verbal and gestural interaction when two ''high level'' retardates were brought together. The same finding occurred with two ''low level'' retardates. However, there was little interaction between a high level and a low level retardate in a two-person situation. Spradlin, Girardeau, and Corte (1967, 1969) further investigated the parameters of social stimulus control of mentally retarded adolescents. One experiment questioned whether a child would give a candy reinforcement to another when it did not cost him to do so. Three-fourths of the subjects did so and were thus considered to be under social control of the other child in the situation. Since the children were not trained to give the candy and received their own candy regardless of their response, such control must have been developed outside of the experimental situation. A second experiment required a more specific communication response by the "receiver" of the candy to the giver in order for both children to receive their reward. The receiver's response served as a discriminative stimulus to the giver. The investigators interpreted the results of both studies as being indicative of the fact that mentally retarded persons, even relatively low level retardates, can provide social cues sufficient to control the behavior of other retarded persons.

In a series of studies, Affleck (1975*a*, 1975*b*, 1976) has demonstrated a significant positive relationship between role-taking ability in mildly retarded young adult males and the ability to recognize the feelings, motives, and intents of others in social encounters. The role-taking task requires that the individual be able to retell a story from the point of view of each of the characters in the story. The degree to which a mentally retarded person can change his perspective in meeting this task requirement is predictive of his success in role-playing common interpersonal conflict situations that require some problem-solving behavior in order to resolve the conflict. The role-taking task is also related to a measure of interpersonal competence in two-person games requiring reciprocal exchange strategies and to the ability to devise tactics to control the behavior of others. Although generalization from Affleck's results is limited by the constraints of his experimental situations, his efforts to operationalize interpersonal competencies appear to have utility as clinical assessment procedures. The use of role-taking and role-playing procedures as assessment and therapeutic strategies with the retarded is still largely unexplored. It seems reasonable to assume that the ability to perceive the feelings and motives of others would be a prime requisite for the motivation to alter one's own behavior to conform to the expectations of others.

SOCIALIZATION PROGRAMS

A number of attempts to engineer socialization programs geared toward the remediation of inappropriate behavior patterns have been published. Roos

(1968) structured a Hospital Improvement Program at the Austin State School to deal with the socially undesirable behaviors of a group of mildly retarded adolescents. Recognizing that institutional habilitation programs often fail to consider the predominant community subculture of its residents, project staff attempted to shape each resident's behavior to conform to the subculture to which he was likely to be discharged. Training programs focused on outward mobility of the residents rather than compliance to institutional settings. The specific techniques included: counseling and psychotherapy; educational procedures emphasizing small group discussions: role-playing and field trips; exposure to social situations and activities (such as camping) that are designed to build self-confidence and self-reliance; pre-vocational training and placement in employment situations; and a community education program to establish good working relationships with strategic community agencies. Despite the reported success of this program, Roos indicates that project methods and staff were often poorly received by regular institutional staff and concludes that greater success would have been met had the project been implemented relatively independently of the institution.

A socialization program for mildly retarded young adults attending a community mental health/mental retardation center in Philadelphia (Boruchow and Espenshade, 1976) attempted to teach independence and social skills by structured community activities. Clients were taught travel skills using public transportation facilities. Group activities were designed to improve the self-care skills of meal preparation, grooming, shopping, and eating at restaurants. Periodic home visits and family meetings were necessary to gain family support and to overcome fears and dependence-fostering behaviors.

While such programs may be successful in attaining the general goals of increasing social competence and interpersonal skills, they do not deal directly with the remediation of inappropriate behaviors. Socialization and community training programs are necessary, but they are not sufficient conditions for habilitation when clients have learned more severe patterns of inappropriate behavior. This need is particularly salient where institutional behavior patterns of passivity, dependency, submissiveness, low self-esteem, attention-seeking, and inertia prevail. It is for such behaviors that more powerful and more individually tailored procedures must be used to supplement group socialization programs. Unfortunately, there is a dearth of well-validated therapeutic or behavior modification strategies available for this purpose.

Altman and Talkington (1971) reviewed the literature dealing with modeling as a behavior modification procedure and conclude that modeling procedures should be well suited as a training strategy for the mentally retarded. Their reasoning is based upon the efficacy of this procedure with other deviant populations as well as upon theoretical considerations. Since the mentally retarded are described as being outer-directed (Turnure and Zigler, 1964), highly dependent upon external cues for direction of their behavior, and may have intrinsic echolalic and echopraxic tendencies (O'Connor and Hermelin, 1963), the authors conclude that modeling procedures should have utility for providing the mentally retarded with the opportunity for observing and rehearsing socially acceptable behaviors.

Rosen and Hoffman (1975*b*) have developed a group counseling curriculum for teaching appropriate behavior that makes extensive use of modeling procedures. The program attempts to teach acceptable behaviors by making clients more aware of their unacceptable mannerisms. The identification and labeling of such behaviors, in terminology that is understandable and meaningful to mentally retarded clients, is crucial to the success of the program. Modeling by the therapist and the use of videotape recordings of acceptable and unacceptable behavior are heavily relied upon as teaching techniques. Students learn to label inappropriate behavior as "weird" and appropriate behavior as "O.K." Whether the behavior would be considered acceptable in the community or would serve to identify the individual as deviant or abnormal is used as a criterion of acceptability of the behavior. Peer pressure is manipulated within the group to approve or disapprove of unacceptable behaviors when they occur. Such pressure is designated to generalize from the counseling sessions to the dormitory, school, and work settings. The curriculum deals specifically with self-awareness and social image, speech and language mannerisms, social interaction, expression of anger, and the appropriate expression of sexual impulses. Although the use of modeling and videotape techniques seems to have potential for teaching appropriate behaviors to the mentally retarded, investigations of the effectiveness of the approach have not been performed. It must be noted that the types of unacceptable behaviors being considered often represent lifelong adjustments of many retarded persons and are, therefore, extremely impervious to training attempts. It is likely that successful approaches require a 24-hour training regime in a facility that allows total control of the individual's living environment. Few such situations exist.

Several years ago the senior author of this text was able to structure a behavior modification regime for a twelve-year-old child who spoke in a high-pitched falsetto voice. Residence supervisors expressed concern about the child since he was entering puberty and seemed to be manifesting a feminine identification. Medical examinations suggested that there was no physical reason for his squeaky voice. An examination of records and background information revealed that the child had been raised entirely by his mother and an aunt and there had been no available masculine models. Whatever the origin of the behavior, it afforded the boy a great deal of attention. His peers enjoyed his behavior, and he was regarded by both staff and students as the building clown.

A college student working at the institution[1] for the summer was trained to work individually with the child. During the beginning training sessions, it was clear that the child was capable of altering his voice to speak in a lower register although his initial efforts sounded just as artificial as his high-pitched voice. Utilizing a tape recorder, a training regime was initiated. The boy was taught to repeat a series of sentences in a low-pitched voice while receiving food and social reinforcement for his approximations to a standard modeled for him by the therapist. With practice the boy's "new" voice sounded more normal. However, although he was able to perform well within the training sessions, there had been no carry-over to his residence hall.

A staff meeting was held at the dormitory with all houseparents present. Tape recordings of the boy's speech were played to demonstrate that he was capable of appropriate speech. Many of the staff members expressed surprise that such change had been possible. The child was then asked to speak to the group in his new voice. A discussion resulted in a group decision to accept no other voice from the child. Attendants agreed that they were to ignore the boy unless he spoke to them in a masculine voice. A similar meeting was held with the other children in the dormitory.

The program produced immediate and lasting results. Several weeks later the author received a confused phone call from the boy's mother who had not been informed of the program. She expressed concern that her son had suffered some damage to his vocal chords since he was no longer speaking "normally." A parent counseling meeting was arranged to explain the program and enlist the mother's support.

CONCLUSIONS

This chapter has emphasized a distinction between social knowledge and skills and socially appropriate behavior. While many programs, assessment techniques, and curricula have recognized the first area of social adjustment, relatively little attention has been devoted to the second. The availability of numerous adult education curricula for teaching work and

[1]Ms. Judith Horowitz served as therapist for this project.

community survival skills to the mentally retarded has not, unfortunately, led also to evaluative studies for choosing among such curricula. Nor is it known which skills are really critical to independent or semi-independent living. Must the mentally retarded person really understand how to tell time, for example, when radio and telephone provide such services? Must he be able to complete a job application blank when few jobs at levels typically filled by mentally retarded persons require such a procedure? The decision to include or exclude a specific community coping skill in teaching mentally retarded persons still rests on educated guesses rather than on empirical information.

The teaching of socially acceptable behaviors (and the extinction of socially inacceptable behaviors) is probably a more difficult social engineering endeavor than the teaching of community awareness and coping skills. Despite a great deal of effort to make severely retarded populations more socially acceptable, there is little research data to draw upon for dealing with the mildly retarded. Yet these are the persons who would most likely be placed in independent living situations, the persons most likely to be identified as inappropriate because of their greater public exposure, and probably the group most likely to experience hurt and to be sensitive to public criticism, ridicule, or censure.

Despite the lack of empirical studies, there is theoretical reason to believe that mildly retarded persons can learn socially appropriate behaviors and are sensitive to social feedback and social control. The potential of role-playing and modeling procedures for assessment and remediation of inappropriate social behaviors appears high. Habilitation efforts of the future would do well to explore the use of such procedures and to emphasize the training of social skills at least to the same degree that vocational training has been stressed to date.

LITERATURE CITED

Affleck, G. G. 1975*a*. Role-taking ability and interpersonal conflict resolution among retarded young adults. Amer. J. Ment. Defic. 80:233–236.

Affleck, G. G. 1975*b*. Role-taking ability and the interpersonal tactics of retarded children. Amer. J. Ment. Defic. 80:312–316.

Affleck, G. G. 1976. Role-taking ability and the interpersonal tactics of retarded children. Amer. J. Ment. Defic. 80:667–670.

Altman, R., and Talkington, L. W. 1971. Modeling: An alternative behavior modification approach for retardates. Ment. Retard. 9:20–23.

Baumeister, A. A. 1968. Behavioral inadequacy and variability of performance. Amer. J. Ment. Defic. 73:477–483.

Bennett, G. K., and Doppelt, J. E. 1968. Fundamental Achievement Series Manual. The Psychological Corporation, New York.

Bensberg, G. J., Colwell, C. N., and Cassel, R. H. 1965. Teaching the profoundly retarded self-help skill activities by behavior shaping techniques. Amer. J. Ment. Defic. 69:674–679.

Berkson, G. 1964. Stereotyped movements of mental defectives. V. Ward behavior and its relation to an experimental task. Amer. J. Ment. Defic. 69:253–264.

Berkson, G. R., and Davenport, R. K., Jr. 1962. Stereotyped movements of mental defectives. I. Initial Survey. Amer. J. Ment. Defic. 66:849–852.

Berkson, G., and Mason, W. A. 1963. Stereotyped movements of mental defectives. III. Situational effects. Amer. J. Ment. Defic. 68:409–412.

Berkson, G., and Mason, W. A. 1964. Stereotyped movements of mental defectives. IV. The effects of toys and the character of the acts. Amer. J. Ment. Defic. 68:511–524.

Blackwood, R. O. 1962. Operant conditioning as a method of training the mentally retarded. Unpublished doctoral dissertation, Ohio State University.

Boruchow, A. W., and Espenshade, M. E. 1976. A socialization program for mentally retarded young adults. Ment. Retard. 14:40–42.

Bouliew, D. 1971. Do institutions maintain retarded behavior? Ment. Retard. 9:36–38.

Clark, G. R., Kivitz, M. S., and Rosen, M. 1968. A transitional program for institutionalized adult retarded. Research and Demonstration Project No. 1275P, Vocational Rehabilitation Administration, U.S. Department of Health, Education, and Welfare, Washington, D.C.

Davenport, R. K., Jr., and Berkson, C. 1963. Stereotyped movements of mental defectives. II. Effects of novel objects. Amer. J. Ment. Defic. 67:879–882.

Deshpande, A. S., and Anderson, H. E., Jr. 1969. Users and technical manual for the BACKS: A test of basic achievement and common knowledge skills. Telesis Corporation, Athens, Georgia.

Doll, E. A. 1948. Relation of social competence to social adjustment. *In* M. Rosen, G. R. Clark, and M. S. Kivitz (eds.), The History of Mental Retardation: Collected Papers, pp. 267–275. Vol. II. University Park Press, Baltimore, 1976.

Doll, E. A. 1953. The measurement of social competence. Educational Test Bureau, Washington.

Edmonson, B. 1974. Measurement of social participation of retarded adults. Amer. J. Ment. Defic. 78:494–501.

Foster, R., and Nihira, K. 1969. Adaptive behavior as a measure of psychiatric impairment. Amer. J. Ment. Defic. 74:401–404.

Gardner, J. M., and Giampa, F. L. 1970. Behavioral competence and social and emotional behavior in mental retardates. Amer. J. Ment. Defic. 75:168–169.

Garfield, S. L. 1963. Abnormal behavior and mental deficiency. *In* N. R. Ellis (ed.), Handbook of Mental Deficiency: Psychological Theory and Research, pp. 574–601. McGraw-Hill Book Company, New York.

Girardeau, F. L., and Spradlin, J. E. 1964. Token rewards on a cottage program. Ment. Retard. 2:345–351.

Gorton, C. E., and Hollis, J. H. 1965. Redesigning a cottage unit for better programming and research for the severely retarded. Ment. Retard. 3:16–21.

Gunzburg, H. C. 1968. Social competence and mental handicap: An introduction to social education. Bailliére, Tindall & Cox Ltd., London.

Halpern, A. S., Raffeld, P., Irvin, L., and Link, R. 1975. Measuring social and prevocational awareness in mildly retarded adolescents. Amer. J. Ment. Defic. 80:81–89.

Johnson, R. C. 1970. Prediction of independent functioning and problem behavior from measures of IQ and SQ. Amer. J. Ment. Defic. 74:591–593.

Kaufman, M. E. 1967. The effects of institutionalization on development of stereotyped and social behaviors in mental defectives. Amer. J. Ment. Defic. 71:581–585.

Kaufman, M. E., and Levitt, H. 1965. A study of three stereotyped behaviors in institutionalized mental defectives. Amer. J. Ment. Defic. 69:467–473.

Leland, H., Shellhaas, M., Nihara, K., and Foster, R. 1967. Adaptive behavior: A new dimension in the classification of the mentally retarded. Ment. Retard. (Abstr.) 4:359–387.

Nihira, K. 1969*a*. Factorial dimensions of adaptive behavior in mentally retarded children and adolescents. Amer. J. Ment. Defic. 74:130–141.

Nihira, K. 1969*b*. Three factors of adaptive behavior in mentally retarded children, adolescents, and adults. Project News of the Parsons State Hospital and Training Center 4:1–5.

Nihira, K., Foster, R., Shellhaas, M., and Leland, H. 1969. Adaptive Behavior Scales. American Association on Mental Deficiency, Washington, D.C.

Nihira, K., and Shellhaas, M. 1970. Study of adaptive behavior: Its rationale, method and implication in rehabilitation programs. Ment. Retard. 8:11–16.

O'Connor, N., and Hermelin, B. 1963. Speech and thought in severe subnormality. The Macmillan Company, New York.

O'Connor, N., and Tizard, J. 1956. The social problem of mental deficiency. Pergamon Press, New York.

Ragain, R. D., and Anson, J. E. 1976. The control of self-mutilating behavior with positive reinforcement. Ment. Retard. 14:22–25.

Roos, P. 1968. Initiating socialization programs for socially inept adolescents. Ment. Retard. 6:13–17.

Rosen, M., and Hoffman, M. 1974. An inventory of inappropriate behavior. Train. Sch. Bull. 71:179–187.

Rosen, M., and Hoffman, M. 1975*a*. Personal adjustment training, Vol. III. Appropriate behavior training: A group counseling manual for the mentally handicapped. Elwyn Institute, Elwyn, Pa.

Rosen, M., and Hoffman, M. 1975*b*. Use of the fundamental achievement series with a mentally retarded population. The Journal for Special Educators of the Mentally Retarded 11:87–93.

Rosenberg, S., Spradlin, J. E., and Mabel, S. 1961. Interaction among retarded children as a function of their relative language skills. J. Abnorm. Soc. Psychol. 63:402–410.

Sarason, S. B., and Gladwin, T. 1958. Psychological and cultural problems in mental subnormality: A review of research. Genet. Psychol. Monogr. 57:3–289.

Spivack, G., and Spotts, J. 1966. The Devereux child behavior rating scale: Manual. The Devereux Foundation, Devon, Pa.

Spradlin, J. E., and Girardeau, F. L. 1966. The behavior of moderately and severely retarded persons. *In* N. R. Ellis (ed.), International Review of Research in Mental Retardation, pp. 257–298. Vol. I. Academic Press, New York.

Spradlin, J. E., Girardeau, F. L., and Corte, E. 1967. Social and communication behavior of retarded adolescents in a two-person situation. Amer. J. Ment. Defic. 72:473–481.

Spradlin, J. E., Girardeau, F. L., and Corte, E. 1969. Social and communication behavior of retarded adolescents in a two-person situation: II. Amer. J. Ment. Defic. 73:572–577.

Thomas, R. L., and Howard, G. A. 1971. A treatment program for a self-destructive child. Ment. Retard. 9:16–18.

Turnure, J., and Zigler, E. 1964. Outer-directedness in the problem-solving of normal and retarded children. J. Abnorm. Soc. Psychol. 69:427–436.

Vogel, W., Kun, K., and Meshorer, E. 1968. Changes in adaptive behavior in institutionalized retardates in response to environmental enrichment or deprivation. J. Consult. Clin. Psychol. 32:76–82.

Watson, L. S., Jr. 1967. Application of operant conditioning techniques to institutionalized severely and profoundly retarded children. Ment. Retard. (Abstr.) 4:1–18.

Watson, L. S., Jr. 1968. Application of behavior-shaping devices to training severely and profoundly mentally retarded children in an institutional setting. Ment. Retard. 6:21–23.

Zachofsky, T., Reardon, D., and O'Conner, G. 1974. Response of institutionalized retarded adults to social pressure in small groups. Amer. J. Ment. Defic. 79:10–15.

Section VI

The Remediation of Social and Emotional Deficits

Chapter 18

Psychotherapy, Counseling, and/or Behavior Modification

A Treatment Choice Strategy

In previous chapters the importance of emotional and personality factors in influencing the adjustment of the mentally retarded has been indicated. The effects of institutionalization upon personality development were discussed and the suggestion was made that over-sheltering and protection within the home may be as devastating upon the mentally retarded as sequestering them within institutions. The research literature dealing with the emotional development of the mentally retarded has been reviewed, and the conclusion was drawn that even severely retarded individuals are capable of the type of social perception necessary for social control of interpersonal behaviors. Finally, it was suggested that several personality dimensions (acquiescence, helplessness, self-concept, sociosexual development, and inappropriate behaviors) appear to be especially pertinent to the overall social adjustment of the mentally retarded.

The implications of these arguments lead naturally to the area of remediation of emotional, personality, and social deficits. Such treatment has traditionally been found outside the area of habilitation, in which training, education, and counseling efforts are usually closely directed toward vocational adjustment, and in which counseling typically follows a social competence model rather than a personality change model. Psychotherapy has traditionally been considered the realm of the psychiatrist and psychologist, who would at best be used as adjuncts to an habilitation department but not be considered central to the program. The area of counseling has occupied a position midway between psychotherapy and education. Although improved personal adjustment is accepted as a goal of counseling, techniques are usually limited to supportive and information-giving efforts rather than the ''deeper'' personality reorganization usually associated with psychotherapy. In recent years the area of behavior modification has been added to the armamentarium of psychologists, teachers, and counselors working with the retarded. For the most part this has involved the use of operant conditioning procedures for teaching self-help and vocational skills. Gold (1972, 1973), for example, has demonstrated that the use of task analysis procedures within the sheltered workshop can often bring the retarded worker to a productivity level equal to that of a nonretarded worker.

There have been a number of excellent reviews (Chidester and Menninger, 1936; Cowen and Trippe, 1963; Demartino, 1957; Glass, 1957; Leland and Smith, 1962; Stacey and Demartino, 1957) of the literature demonstrating the effectiveness of psychotherapy and counseling with mentally retarded populations. Despite the reservations of many that the mentally retarded are lacking the verbal, abstract thinking, and problem-solving skills judged necessary for psychotherapeutic progress (Rogers, 1951), such reviews are unanimous in concluding that the mentally retarded are capable of improved adjustment according to many criteria, including IQ gains (Gunzburg, 1958; Sarason, 1949; Sternlicht, 1966). Nor is there a paucity of techniques to use in performing counseling and therapy. Sternlicht (1966) describes a variety of novel strategies and procedures that offer promise. Despite such promise, however, all reviewers also agree that the critical research has not yet been done that will demonstrate the effectiveness of therapy, compare the relative effectiveness of psychotherapeutic techniques for various subpopulations of the mentally retarded, or aid in the understanidng of the critical parameters of psychotherapeutic success or failure.

It is the purpose of this chapter to consider the use of therapy, counseling, and behavior change procedures within a habilitation setting and their role as an integral part of the habilitation program. The effectiveness of psychotherapy, counseling, and behavior modification with mentally retarded populations is considered and illustrated. A model is developed that allows a choice of therapeutic counseling or behavior modification strategy according to the desired goal of such remedial procedures. The model should provide guidelines for the habilitation specialist who is choosing a treatment strategy and who is considering implementing the procedure himself or referring the client to a suitable specialist.

ARE THE MENTALLY RETARDED SUITABLE CANDIDATES FOR PSYCHOTHERAPY AND COUNSELING?

Bialer (1967) defines psychotherapy as:

> . . . the systematic utilization of psychological techniques chief of which is a close interpersonal relationship, by a professionally trained therapist in order to help individuals who need or seek his assistance in the amelioration of their emotional or behavioral problems. The procedures involved may include nonverbal as well as verbal techniques and the subjects may or may not be aware of the dynamics of the therapeutic process (p. 139).

A search of the literature over the past thirty years reveals almost no challenge to the conviction that the mentally retarded are capable of improvement, which may be judged by a variety of behavioral criteria, as a result of psychotherapeutic efforts. Weist (1955), for example, challenged the traditional view that the mental retardate does not possess sufficient verbal skills to gain insight into his maladaptive unconscious motivations and is, therefore, not amenable to psychotherapy. Weist argued that insight may not be essential for therapeutic progress:

> They (the mentally retarded) can experience transference, catharsis, definite limits, feelings of acceptance, belongingness, and security. Reality can be made sufficiently appealing that the child automatically gravitates toward it. Will this not aid him along the path from infantile psychosis to a higher level of intellectual and emotional life? In cases where there are structural or physiological limitations or both, will it not lead him at least to a stability which will make him more likeable, more manageable, and consequently more acceptable to someone, his own or another family, outside the hospital? (p. 642).

Sarason (1949) presented several case studies drawn from his experience as an institutional psychologist in which psychotherapy appeared to have positive results. In these cases his perceptions of the clients and his reactions to them were not as "mental defectives" but as immature, childish individuals. His subjects had all experienced inadequate mothering and were deprived of attention and affection within the institution, whatever their primary diagnosis. Sarason concluded that psychotherapy is neither feasible nor indicated for "idiots," "imbeciles," and "some morons (especially the brain-injured type.)" However, he was optimistic about the possibilities of successful therapeutic outcomes with the "garden variety defective" and called for controlled evaluative research studies.

Although the goals of counseling the mentally retarded are often stated more conservatively than the goals of psychotherapy, it is difficult to make clear-cut distinctions between the two. The real differences appear to be in terms of technique rather than objectives. Counselors, as opposed to therapists, are more likely to use group approaches and to rely on more reality-oriented approaches. In both situations a therapeutic relationship is a necessary part of the treatment, and behavior change and better "adjustment" is the objective. Whether a practitioner labels himself a therapist or a counselor depends more upon his training and professional orientation than upon his choice between well differentiated techniques.

Yepsen (1962) discusses various facets of a counseling relationship with the mentally retarded that aim to make the individual capable of adjustment in novel situations. He defines counseling techniques as including supportive and advice-giving practices, emotional support, suggestions and assistance in problem-solving, and the setting of realistic life goals. This counseling is conceptualized as more practical and more reality-oriented than psychotherapy. Seldom do counselors talk of personality reorganization of their clients. Yet psychotherapists also talk of adjustment, express doubt about insight as a relevant criterion of success with most retarded, and are hard pressed to define just what they really mean by personality reorganization. In both counseling and psychotherapy, behavior change becomes the ultimate criterion of improvement, a criterion that is shared with behavior modification approaches.

Thorne (1948) describes the results of counseling and psychotherapy with the mentally retarded within a state institution. The clients he discusses were referred primarily because of their disruptive behavior. The treatment described included institution-wide policies as well as formally structured therapeutic sessions that are not well specified by today's standards for evaluating psychotherapeutic outcome. However, the objectives of the approach are relevant to any contemporary efforts. These include: 1) acceptance of the individual as a worthy person despite his deficits; 2) providing for the expression and clarification of emotional reactions by nondirective methods; 3) training the individual to deal with frustration and to learn emotional controls; 4) clear-cut specification of realistic standards of conduct; 5) building self-confidence and self-respect by the provision of success experiences; and 6) training the individual to seek help from the counselor when he is faced with problems he cannot handle.

Bialer's (1967) review chapter is cautiously optimistic in tone. He tends to suspect earlier research studies on the effectiveness of psychotherapy with the retarded that used IQ increment as a criterion of psychotherapeutic success. Bialer acknowledges that IQ increment may occur as a result of therapy because the individual is freed from emotional constraints and is able to work up to his intellectual potential, rather than because he experienced direct stimulation of intellectual processes.

The confusion about IQ increment as a criterion of therapeutic success stems from the tendency of professionals to invest the IQ with an overabundance of significance as a personality attribute of the mentally retarded. The authors know of no therapy outcome studies with normal populations that used IQ as a criterion of success. Yet, in the field of mental retardation professionals cling to a rigid dichotomy between intellectual and emotional processes, over-interpreting the former and tending to ignore the latter. Despite considerable evidence to the contrary, the IQ tends to be regarded as an index of some distinct process in the brain, sometimes being regarded as the process itself. Accepting this dichotomy, it is sometimes naively assumed that, as a result of training, education, or therapy, underlying organic processes are being manipulated. It is this type of reasoning that leads investigators to use the IQ as an index of therapeutic success.

It is more reasonable to accept the holistic concept of personality that regards both intellectual functioning and emotional expression as unified aspects of the same personality. If psychotherapy has general effectiveness, it is likely that one or both of these dimensions will show change. However, if psychotherapy has specific effects, the nature of personality change will depend closely upon the structure and content of the intervention procedures, namely, the objectives of therapy and the specific techniques and strategies utilized. It makes no more sense to use IQ as a criterion of success in therapy geared toward control of aggressive impulses than it would make to evaluate changes in emotional control after teaching the individual to read.

Bialer's bias in opting for therapy-based techniques to give structure and direction to psychotherapy is relevant to the above point. Only by selecting a therapeutic technique for a specific purpose can we make meaningful predictions about outcomes of psychotherapy and evaluate these outcomes.

The question posed by the subtitle in this chapter is, in reality, a false issue. Rather than ask whether the mentally retarded are suitable for psychotherapy one might better ask whether any specific form of therapy or counseling is suitable for the particular individual, specific problem, and unique setting to which the treatment is to be applied. Similarly, the question of whether or not therapy works is equally meaningless. Sometimes it works and sometimes it doesn't. The reasons for therapeutic failure may vary considerably. A specific technique may be inappropriate to the condition being treated, either for theoretical reasons or because practical considerations made the technique unfeasible. The therapist may be poorly trained in the technique or apply it inconsistently. The client's motivation for cooperation may have been poorly assessed and may have interfered with the efforts of the therapy. The therapy may be sabotaged by other individuals whose interests are antagonistic to the aims or methods of the therapy. Obviously, many extraneous factors can interfere with therapy. This is particularly true within residential situations, where many environmental factors may mitigate the efforts of a therapist.

Of course, therapy works with the retarded . . . sometimes. It is difficult to conceive of a personality structure, even in the severely retarded, so rigid that no amount of therapeutic intervention could effect some change. The crucial issue then is not whether therapy works, but what is the most powerful therapeutic intervention, for whom, under what conditions, and for what purpose?

PLACE OF PSYCHOTHERAPY AND COUNSELING IN AN HABILITATION PROGRAM

The use of psychotherapy or counseling as an adjunct service in an habilitation program derives from a conceptualization of these activities as distinct in goals from the prime mission of an habilitation department. Association of therapy with objectives as abtruse as personality reorganization implies a mystique in the rendering of such services and supports the notion that practitioners of so esoteric an art must indeed be rare. It further implies that the provision of such services should be limited to the very disturbed, those whose emotional problems are so severe that they preclude successful habilitation efforts without drastic personality change. This view is so prevalent that psychotherapy is rarely an integral part of a comprehensive habilitation effort, while counseling, if available, is often limited to practical information-providing or advice-giving efforts.

Gunzburg's (1958) review of psychotherapy with the mentally retarded provides a clarity of thinking that convincingly exposes the error of this logic. He points out that the goal of psychotherapy, like all phases of habilitation treatment, is to deal better with problems of living and working in the community. The authors would extend Gunzburg's reasoning even further by maintaining that the goal of all psychotherapy, not just that administered to mentally retarded populations, is to deal better with the concrete, day-to-day problems of living. With this view in mind, psychotherapy (or counseling) cannot be conceived as disparate from habilitation, but must be viewed as a treatment that shares the basic objectives of any habilitation program and that cannot be treated as anything other than an integral component of the habilitation effort.

Gunzburg points out that the therapist is in a position to supply the warmth and affection of which a mentally retarded individual has often been deprived. Like other habilitation personnel, the therapist can represent the norms and standards of society and guide the individual in effective reality testing. Because of this relationship he is able to introduce and teach new behavior patterns.

Within the institutional setting, psychotherapy and counseling assume special importance. Because of the emotional deprivation frequently associated with institutional living, as well as the effects of separation from families and prior histories leading up to residential placement, it is apparent that client need for therapeutic intervention is high. Gunzburg points out that even when psychotherapy is available within institutions, it is often of very short duration and conducted by poorly trained persons. He expresses doubt that such intervention is helpful and suggests that short-term treatment once terminated does more harm than good.

Another factor mitigating successful therapeutic outcome within institutions can be the institutional environment influencing the individual during the hours when he is not receiving psychotherapy. Even when intensive therapeutic intervention is being applied, an individual is seldom seen more than three or four hours a week. The remainder of time is, of course, spent within whatever educational, training, and residential environment characterizes the institutional program. It seems self-evident that psychotherapeutic treatment would need to be extremely powerful, indeed, for it to be effective in three or four hours when the remainder of the individual's waking hours are spent in an environment antagonistic to therapeutic goals. Gunzburg expresses this best:

> Formal psychotherapy, if carried out in isolation and very often against the deadweight of custodial institutional philosophy, has very little chance of achieving lasting results. . . . Many of the problems, which appear to call urgently for individual or group therapy, are simply the result of unhelpful institutional dealings, have developed there and have a spontaneous remission when the patient is transferred to a new therapeutic hospital environment. Their treatment by formal psychotherapy would be often unnecessary and may be destined to failure in the face of a multitude of adverse environmental factors (p. 391).

For this reason most writers agree that psychotherapy must be carried out on a 24-hour basis within a therapeutic milieu. It is also helpful if the therapist has some administrative responsibility for the 24-hour program or at least is able to influence programmatic decisions made about the client.

Sarason (1949) agrees that the therapist should have administrative authority but believes that he should not be overburdened with routine administrative work. He argues that the client should be allowed to see the therapist whenever he wishes and that it should be made clear to other staff that the therapist does not play a punitive role with the client.

These suggestions are valuable and sound but may represent difficult positions to attain in many settings, particularly in large, multipurpose institutions. In many settings, official attitudes, traditional policies, and interdepartmental rivalries may effectively subvert the best therapeutic intentions. Integration of a psychotherapeutic program into an habilitation program must originate with the highest level of administrative support of that facility and must involve a total commitment to the concept by key administrative staff. To accomplish this end the therapist must often be an accomplished salesman and proselytizer as well as an effective therapist.

With this background in mind, it is necessary to develop guidelines for the implementation of such a therapeutic habilitation program. The approach must be broad enough to deal not only with the individual who draws attention to himself because of his disruptive behavior, but also with those individuals who, though compliant or withdrawn, may be experiencing emotional problems. It is our bias that all persons enrolled within an habilitation setting should be exposed to therapy or counseling and that such counseling should be specifically designed to deal with problems shared by any mentally retarded group, in addition to problems unique to any given individual. It is obvious that a variety of therapeutic strategies, and an overall framework for choosing among such strategies, will be necessary with such an approach. The remainder of this chapter presents a model designed for this purpose. Subsequent chapters apply this model in two areas—group counseling of community-bound mentally retarded persons, and individually applied behavior modification regimes for institutional adjustment or return to the community.

A MODEL FOR APPLYING PSYCHOLOGICAL TREATMENT WITHIN HABILITATION SETTINGS

Bialer (1967) describes what he considers to be the common elements of all psychotherapeutic approaches:

1) an individual seeking help
2) a client-therapist relationship and interaction

3) the impact of the therapist's personality
4) a safe opportunity for the expression of feelings
5) systematic employment of a set of techniques by the therapist
6) initiation of positive behavior changes in real life situations

To these the authors would add several other factors that are seen as complementary to, or an integral part of, those listed above, particularly 2 and 3. The term therapist is meant to include the counselor or other behavior change agent.

7) a commitment by the therapist to the client over a period of time sufficiently long to know the client as a person and to be known by him, to develop a positive regard for the client, and to be regarded highly in return
8) a belief by both therapist and client that therapeutic intervention, however defined, will be effective, i.e., that the therapy makes theoretical or practical sense. The therapy is accepted by the client as important or meaningful to him.
9) an aura of competence or power associated with the therapist and his techniques that is strong enough that the client accepts their potential value to him
10) mutual recognition and acceptance by the client and therapist of well defined long- and short-term goals of therapy
11) a therapist with sufficient ego strength to take charge, accept responsibility, and make decisions regarding the client

As is discussed shortly, therapies differ greatly in the degree to which structure is imposed as a part of the therapeutic procedure. The most structured types of therapy involve the rigid control of behavioral consequences. Operant conditioning, involving analysis and differential manipulation of reinforcement or nonreinforcement, places maximal emphasis on therapeutic technique and tends to minimize or even negate the client-therapist relationship. A later chapter discusses and illustrates the use of behavior modification and operant conditioning approaches to treatment. It is our contention that even in operant conditioning the influence of the therapist as a variable affecting outcome is substantial.

If therapies are alike in sharing so many common elements, it might be argued that it matters little what specific technique is applied. Yet therapies also differ along several dimensions, and the differences may be significant in terms of presenting problems, client variables, situational variables, and specific objectives of the treatment. In many instances the application of psychotherapy is haphazard, based not upon specific principles or need, but upon the particular training, background, and orientation of whatever therapists happen to be available. This situation derives from the relatively minor role that psychotherapy and counseling often play within habilitation settings. In the experience of the authors, it is extremely rare that workshops, training centers, and other habilitation programs are staffed with persons skilled in performing counseling or therapeutic functions. When such persons are available, they are often burdened with other functions, such as evaluation or administrative responsibilities.

Because there are important differences among therapies, such services must be considered as a range of possible approaches rather than as a global, unitary entity that can be applied or not applied. By emphasizing differences among therapies rather than similarities, we are implying that a choice exists in dispensing such services. Given such a choice there is a need for simple guidelines for decision-making.

Surprisingly, despite very comprehensive treatment of the subject in recent reviews, few authors have attempted to make some order from the chaos caused by the plethora of psychotherapeutic and counseling techniques that have been offered as potentially helpful with the mentally retarded. One notable exception is Sternlicht's (1964) theoretical model for the use of psychotherapy with the mentally retarded, which is based upon etiological considerations. Recognizing that the primary cause of the retardation may be neurological deficit, cultural deprivation, or emotional maladjustment, Sternlicht suggests that prognosis by means of psychotherapy will be favorable for the goal of elevating IQ only when the etiology is emotional. IQ increments are not likely to be associated with psychotherapy when etiology is neurological or associated with cultural deprivation. However, Sternlicht argues that psychotherapy will be helpful in all cases in dealing with the secondary emotional response to the mental retardation syndrome.

Such a model, based upon etiology, suffers from many limitations. The concern about etiology is relevant only if one accepts a "cure" or amelioration of mental retardation as a legitimate purpose of psychotherapy. The present authors submit that this has never been, nor should it be, the objective of psychotherapy. Furthermore, even if it were, the diagnosis of mental retardation according to Sternlicht's three categories is often extremely difficult and, therefore, of little practical use in making prognostic statements. Rather than a single etiological factor, it is more often the case that clinicians can recognize a multiplicity of determining factors. Nor is it easy to distinguish between primary and secondary emotional factors. Finally, assuming that psychotherapy will be of benefit in treating secondary emotional problems provides no help in making decisions or stating prognoses for specific types of secondary emotional difficulties. It seems apparent that a useful model for psychotherapy with the mentally retarded should be stated not in terms of presumed etiology, but rather in terms of present behaviors, specific behavioral objectives, and other client and situational variables that can be operationally defined. Let us examine the implications of such an approach.

First, it is necessary for the reader to accept several assumptions. These include an implicit belief in the scientific approach to therapy, i.e., in the empirical method as a basis for studying the underlying tenets of therapy and for evaluating outcomes. Second, it is presumed that effective psychotherapies should be based upon logical, theoretically sound principles rather than upon haphazard or random events or factors. It is accepted that such factors may at present be poorly defined or unrecognized, but that they exist and will eventually be discovered. Finally, it is accepted that the successful outcome of a particular psychotherapy may not "prove" the underlying theoretical rationale. Therapies often work for the wrong reasons. Similarly, if a particular therapy does not work it may be for a variety of reasons:

1) The treatment may not have been effective for the particular purpose for which it was selected. It was chosen as a result of faulty analysis of the problem.
2) The treatment was appropriately chosen but was incorrectly or inconsistently applied.
3) The treatment did not consider specific client variables associated with mental retardation.
4) The treatment worked within a limited therapeutic set of circumstances but did not sufficiently generalize to the total living situation to make meaningful differences in adjustment.

Despite the lack of a direct, one-to-one correspondence between therapeutic practice and results, it is accepted that continued application of theoretically based therapeutic practices, honestly applied and assessed, will eventually result in a theoretically sound and empirically demonstrable set of effective psychotherapeutic tactics. This approach rests squarely upon a logical analysis of the dimensions of the therapeutic process. These dimensions include: client factors; condition, symptom, or behavioral factors; situational factors; therapist variables; differences in the objectives or goals of the therapy; and therapy factors.

Client Factors

Mentally retarded persons are not alike. They probably differ as much amongst each other as normal persons differ from each other. Identifying and labeling intellectual deficits may imply some bases of commonality associated with these conditions but this implication does not preclude the existence of a broad range of individual personality differences that exist even in persons of similar intellectual characteristics. For the purpose of psychotherapy, several of these differences assume greater significance. These include the degree of verbal development and expression, the level of abstract ability, the degree and awareness of the individual, spontaneous and internally directed control, and the motivation for behavioral change. Sternlicht has aptly pointed out that psychotherapy need not rely upon verbal processes and insight. Yet, for some goals verbal expression and the capacity for self-awareness or insight are important requisites for, if not essential elements of, therapeutic movement. Rather than assuming, as Sternlicht seems to imply, that all the mentally retarded are deficient in these cognitive areas and, therefore, require alternative methods of psychotherapy, it is more meaningful to consider each case individually and to choose relatively verbal and abstract approaches only for those persons demonstrating such abilities.

Condition, Symptom, or Behavioral Factors

Not only do clients differ, their particular problems may also vary. The choice of psychotherapeutic approach should rest strongly with the type of problem to be treated. Perhaps the first consideration must be whether or not the decision to administer psychotherapy is made because the individual is drawing attention to himself as a disruptive influence. Such situations are most difficult to deal with because external demands for results are most pronounced, thereby creating greater pressure on the therapist. In these cases the therapist is often perceived as a disciplinarian who is to bring about order and control, and the therapeutic purpose of the treatment from the point of view of the client may often be forgotten. In such cases it may be necessary that a therapist choose a treatment strategy maximally geared toward behavior change, using environmental manipulation and control as a primary method. In other cases, in which the client does not identify himself to administrative personnel as a management problem, the therapist may be able to deal more slowly with the client, using less structured and less directive therapeutic or counseling approaches, and allowing him greater opportunity for emotional expression.

Conditions that may be selected for treatment vary according to the degree that they represent objective, measurable behaviors (e.g., nail-biting, temper outbursts) as opposed to the degree that they represent more subjective processes (anxiety, depression, poor self-concept). They differ according to whether the symptoms are situationally determined or are more enduring personality characteristics. They differ in the manner in which the behavior is learned and maintained by environmental conditons. They differ in the frequency of behavior. Some behaviors are serious in terms of consequence to the individual or those around him but occur so infrequently that they are difficult to treat. They differ according to whether treatment involves unlearning inappropriate behaviors or involves learning new behaviors. They differ according to whether the behaviors can be well specified and observed or whether they are vague, ambiguous, or poorly defined.

Situational Factors

As noted previously, Gunzburg has pointed to the futility of psychotherapy within a situation that may have produced the problem or condition and that maintains that condition, when there is no possibility of effecting positive changes within the total environmental situation. We have also mentioned previously the fact that some behaviors requiring psychotherapy are largely situational in nature, thereby implying that most effective control of that behavior must rely upon some degree of environmental change. Another consideration is the generalization of the behavior being changed. Certain behaviors, once learned, generalize readily to new situations. Language development is one example of a set of behaviors that generalize easily. Most children, once having mastered a new vocabulary word, spontaneously use that word in new contexts. Other behaviors may present considerable difficulty in effecting generalization. Toilet training, for example, is often limited to the specific training situation. The author has known several children who were intially trained to use the toilet for urination at home who would not use a toilet outside the home. With many severely retarded persons the operant conditioning of self-help skills often requires the continued application of reinforcement contingencies for the maintenance of learning. Indeed, professional journals reporting research in operant conditioning often require evidence of return to base rate when reinforcement conditions are withdrawn (extinction) as evidence of the effectiveness of those conditions. It is clear, then, that in such situations the control of situational variables is essential to success in psychotherapy.

Situational variables may be controlled within a total habilitation program in such a way that the client is exposed to a graduated sequence of experiences of increasing responsibility. These situations can vary in such a manner as to successively approximate the real world. By structuring vocational assignments in small steps, for example, it is possible to assist the client in adjusting to discrepancies between the protected setting and the community. The availability of a graduated sequence of programs allows maximum flexibility in choosing strategies for environmental manipulation.

Therapist Variables

The effect of the therapist per se upon therapeutic outcome has not been well studied although there is every reason to believe that it is a powerful influence. Therapists differ in their sex, their training and background, their commitment to the treatment, their overall orientation to therapy, their personalities, their regard for the client, their persuasive ability, their appearance, and many other qualities. Many observers of psychotherapy believe that therapist variables may be the most powerful variables affecting therapeutic movement, and that, in comparison with the personal magnetism, charisma, and ego of the therapist, other treatment variables are less important. At least one research investigation (Fiedler, 1953) has indicated that experienced therapists of differing theoretical persuasions are more similar to each other than are experienced and naive practitioners within the same persuasion. Bialer (1967) discusses the impact of pastoral counseling as being closely related to the perception of the minister as a symbol or representative of God and to the enduring relationship the individual has with his pastor. The secular therapist also strives to create a mysticism about himself and is often perceived by the client as omnipotent. This variable may be overtly manipulated by many therapists or may represent an implicit aspect of their relationship with their clients. The various parameters of what would be called the transference relationship have been well described by analytic psychologists but have never been studied with the mentally retarded.

Interaction between the sex of the therapist and sex of the client may be another significant variable that is, as yet, unstudied with mentally retarded populations. Clients requiring appropriate role models for identification may require therapists of the same sex. Rosen (1970) has described the use of female teachers and psychologists in role playing to teach appropriate heterosexual behaviors to young male adults.

Treatment Goals

The selection of a treatment strategy and the evaluation of the effectiveness of treatment rests upon a precise statement of treatment objectives. One reason why psychotherapy is so often regarded as mysterious is that objectives are poorly defined and therefore improvement cannot be adequately evaluated. The chief reason for ambiguity lies in the acceptance by many therapists of criteria of change that cannot be easily observed or measured. This is not to detract from the importance of subjective factors in considering the emotional adjustment of the mentally retarded. However, it does point to the need for specifying concrete, observable and, as much as possible, quantifiable information as criteria of change. Such objectives may include information derivable from verbal reports by the client, therapist observations, changes in the life situation, direct measurement of client reactions in response to specific stimuli, results of psychological tests, and reports from relevant others. The therapist committed to using hard-nosed empirical criteria of change must discard ambiguous criteria. Examples of the latter include global concepts of "insight," "adjustment," "personality reorganization," and "increased ego strength." If a therapist begins treatment with objectives so poorly specified, it is little wonder that therapy may be of indeterminate length, or, in the case of the retarded, regarded as of little potential value.

On the other hand, if concrete, well defined, and practical objectives are stated, it is possible to arrive at clear-cut decisions about the effectiveness of the approach, the time of successful termination, and the need to alter treatment strategies or to discontinue a hopeless venture.

It seems self-evident to those involved in performing psychotherapy that treatment goals vary, and treatment approaches should be selected to match therapeutic objectives. Yet this point is often overlooked by those who refer clients for psychotherapy as if it were a uniform treatment to be dispensed like medication. Therapeutic goals may encompass very specific behaviors, such as the reduction of aggressive outbursts toward other students. They may be phrased in terms of more general changes, such as the learning of emotional controls, which may, in turn, determine specific behaviors, such as the extinction of temper tantrums. They may be stated in very broad or global terms, such as the enhancement of self-concept or increased feelings of security. They may be circumscribed to certain limited behaviors within a specific setting, such as attendance at a specific work assignment, or they may be identical with the overall training mission of the habilitation agency, such as training the individual for greater independence. Therapeutic goals may range from the teaching of specific social skills to more abtruse cognitive changes in attitude. They may involve motivational changes, such as acceptance of a realistic aspiration level, or emotional reconditioning, such as the reduction in fear or anxiety related to using the subway. It is our contention that no one orientation or strategy is equally appropriate for the varying goals necessitating psychotherapeutic intervention but rather that specific approaches are relatively more or less suited to various objectives.

Therapy Factors

Even a cursory glance at Sternlicht's (1966) comprehensive review of therapeutic procedures will convince the reader of the variety of orthodox and novel approaches to psychotherapy and counseling with the mentally retarded. Individual and group approaches, verbal and nonverbal techniques, music and art therapies, the use of projective techniques, toys and psychodrama, relationship therapies, and educational therapies all have their adherents. Nor have therapists of the mentally retarded lacked for creativity in designing novel approaches. Sternlicht lists the uses of hypnosis (McCord, 1956; Spankus and Freeman, 1962; Sternlicht and Wanderer, 1963), shadow therapy (Robertson, 1964) and audiovisual feedback (Ricker, 1964) among some of the novel procedures that have been employed.

Therapies differ in the amount of control, direction, and individual responsibility for behavioral change that is assumed by the therapist. At one end of the spectrum are nondirective approaches that rely upon and have faith in the capacity of the individual for growth and maturity. It is perhaps this essential philosophy of nondirective counseling that made Rogers (1951) so pessimistic about the prognosis for the mentally retarded. At the other extreme are the behavior therapies in which direct responsibility for change is assumed by the therapist, and lack of improvement is often interpreted on the basis of faulty analysis of the conditions eliciting and maintaining behavior.

Therapies differ in the degree to which the role of the therapist is defined as active or passive, the degree to which group processes are relied upon, and the extent to which verbal and abstract reasoning processes of the client are necessary for client participation. It is apparent that therapies requiring self-awareness and insight as essential for improvement will demand the more limited selection of only the clients who are capable of such cognitive processes. Therapies also differ in the degree to which they rely upon self-starting, initiative, and self-monitoring by the client. Even among the more behaviorally oriented techniques, differences in this respect are clear. The operant conditioner may rely totally on manipulation of external contingencies of reinforcement, leaving little responsibility with the client for self-monitoring and control. Yet many behavior therapies teach self-control and self-monitoring to clients, and such procedures are heavily relied upon for generalization of training procedures.

Table 1 lists the major factors described above and provides a rough ordering of certain critical dimensions that may vary within these factors. The first three columns are regarded as "givens" in the situation since the therapist has little or no control over these factors. The last three columns represent manipulated variables, i.e., the treatment goal, the treatment approach, and the degree to which the external environment is to be controlled. Column 5 lists broad classifications of therapeutic, counseling, or

Table 1. Therapy choice model

↑ Increasing permissiveness, general acceptance

"Given" Variables			Manipulated Variables		
1 Client Factors	2 Condition Factors	3 Therapist Factors	4 Treatment Goals	5 Therapy Choice	6 Situational Control
Verbal and abstract reasoning relatively intact	General personality and developmental problems	Humanistic orientation	Global personality change	Nondirective counseling	Therapeutic milieu
	Emotional deprivation		Enhancement of self-concept and self-awareness	Pastoral counseling	
				Art/music therapy	
	Broad social learning deficits; interpersonal problems	Psychodynamic orientation	Emotional control	Activities programs	
Deficits in verbal and abstract reasoning processes	Affective problems (anxiety, depression)	Cognitive orientation	Teach social information and skills	Analytic/relationship therapy	
	Inappropriate behavior	Behavioral orientation	Behavior control	Education therapy	Contingency management by parents, houseparents
	Specific disruptive behavior			Occupational therapy	
				Reality therapy	
	Self-help deficits			Behavior therapy	
				Operant conditioning	

Increasing direction, control ↓

behavior management intervention, ranging from the least structured nondirective approaches to more structured and directive therapies. This ordering also corresponds roughly with the degree of external, environmental control that must be a necessary part of the treatment. Although a tight one-to-one correspondence among each of the three given factors and the three therapeutic approaches is not possible, the table outlines a general direction for selecting a treatment strategy on the basis of these factors. For example, the more specific the behavior change accepted as a treatment objective, the more necessary it will be to choose a behavior modification strategy, and the greater the need to effect environmental control to achieve generalization. The more general the personality change objective, the greater the need to select a less structured, nondirective approach and to work intensively with the client on an individualized basis. In such cases a generally therapeutic milieu is required rather than tight control of environmental contingencies.

This model is not perfect. No doubt critics will suggest reordering of therapies. Nevertheless the value of the approach lies in its focus on current factors affecting behavior of the individual rather than on presumed etiological factors that may be little related to current behavior or prognosis. The following two chapters deal with two treatment approaches, both of which have an important role in habilitation programs. The first is the use of directive group counseling as an integral part of the habilitation experience of each client. The second is the selective use of behavior modification and behavior therapy for specific behavioral or adjustment problems.

LITERATURE CITED

Bialer, I. 1967. Psychotherapy and other adjustment techniques with the mentally retarded. *In* A. A. Baumeister (ed.), Mental Retardation: Appraisal, Education, and Rehabilitation. Aldine Publishing Company, Chicago.

Chidester, L., and Menninger, K. 1936. The application of psychoanalytic methods to the study of mental retardation. Amer. J. Orthopsychiatry 6:616–625.

Cowen, E. L., and Trippe, M. J. 1963. Psychotherapy and play techniques with the exceptional child and youth. *In* W. M. Cruickshank (ed.), Psychology of Exceptional Children and Youth, pp. 526–591. 2nd Ed. Prentice-Hall, Englewood Cliffs, N.J.

DeMartino, M. F. 1957. Some observations concerning psychotherapeutic techniques with the mentally retarded. *In* C. L. Stacey and M. F. DeMartino (eds.), Counseling and Psychotherapy with the Mentally Retarded, pp. 461–472. The Free Press, Glencoe, Ill.

Fiedler, F. 1953. Quantitative studies on the role of therapists' feelings toward their patients. *In* O. H. Mowrer (ed.), Psychotherapy Theory and Research, pp. 296–315. Ranald Press Co., New York.

Glass, H. L. 1957. Psychotherapy with the mentally retarded. A case history. Train. Sch. Bull. 54:32–34.

Gold, M. W. 1972. Stimulus factors in skill training of the retarded on a complex assembly task: Acquisition transfer and retention. Amer. J. Ment. Defic. 76:517–526.

Gold, M. W. 1973. Factors affecting production by the retarded: Base rate. Ment. Retard. 11:41–44.

Gunzburg, H. C. 1958. Psychotherapy with the feeble-minded. *In* A. M. Clarke and A. D. B. Clarke (eds.), Mental Deficiency: The Changing Outlook, pp. 365–392. The Free Press, Glencoe, Ill.

Leland, H., and Smith, D. 1962. Unstructured material in play therapy for emotionally disturbed brain-damaged mentally retarded children. Amer. J. Ment. Defic. 66:621–628.

McCord, H. 1956. The hypnotizability of the mongoloid-type child. Int. J. Clin. Exp. Hypn. 4:19–20.

Ricker, L. H. 1964. Three approaches to group counseling involving motion pictures with mentally retarded adults. Progress Report, March. MacDonald Training Center, Tampa, Florida.

Robertson, M. F. 1964. Shadow therapy. Ment. Retard. 2:218–223.

Rogers, C. R. 1951. Client-Centered Therapy. Houghton Mifflin Company, Boston.

Rosen, M. 1970. Conditioning appropriate heterosexual behavior in mentally and socially handicapped populations. Train. Sch. Bull. 66:172–177.

Sarason, S. B. 1949. Psychological Problems in Mental Deficiency. Harper & Brothers, New York.

Spankus, W. H., and Freeman, L. G. 1962. Hypnosis in cerebral palsy. Int. J. Clin. Exp. Hypn. 10:135–139.

Stacey, C. L., and DeMartino, M. F. (eds.), 1957. Counseling and Psychotherapy with the Mentally Retarded. The Free Press, Glencoe, Ill.

Sternlicht, M. 1964. A theoretical model for the psychological treatment of mental retardation. Amer. J. Ment. Defic. 68:618–622.

Sternlicht, M. 1966. Psychotherapeutic procedures with the retarded. *In* N. R. Ellis (ed.), International Review of Research in Mental Retardation, pp. 279–354. Vol. 2. Academic Press, New York.

Sternlicht, M., and Wanderer, Z. W. 1963. Hypnotic susceptibility and mental deficiency. Int. J. Clin. Exp. Hypn. 11:104–111.

Thorne, F. C. 1948. Counseling and psychotherapy with mental defectives. Amer. J. Ment. Defic. 52:263–271.

Weist, G. 1955. Psychotherapy with the mentally retarded. Amer. J. Ment. Defic. 59:640–644.

Yepsen, L. N. 1952. Counseling the mentally retarded. Amer. J. Ment. Defic. 57:205–213.

Chapter 19

Personal Adjustment Training

A Group Counseling Program

With growing recognition of the capability of mentally retarded persons to assume independent living and competitive employment (Charles, 1953; Kennedy, 1966; Miller, 1965; Windle, 1962), the need for "normalizing" remedial programs and treatment has taken on great significance. It has been well established that previously institutionalized, mentally subnormal persons are capable of at least a marginal social and occupational adjustment to community living (Goldstein, 1964). However, adjustment in the community spans a broad range of adaptive and maladaptive behaviors. Even persons judged to be making adequate vocational and social adjustment may be experiencing severe stress. As we have indicated previously, follow-up studies indicate that for this population social and emotional deficits tend to overshadow vocational problems. This finding is perhaps understandable in light of the relative ambiguity of social, emotional and personality training needs and procedures, as compared with those in specific job skills.

Along with his cognitive deficits, the once-institutionalized individual is additionally socially handicapped for at least two reasons. First, sheltered institutional segregation serves effectively to deny him many normal community living experiences. Second, the institution itself reinforces the learning of institutionally adaptive, but community maladaptive, behaviors. Recent studies have documented some of the more detrimental effects of institutions (Butterfield and Zigler, 1965; Kugel and Wolfensberger, 1969), but conclusive experimental evidence is still lacking.

Clearly, procedures are needed to reinforce those behaviors that may be related to independent community living. One approach is through the use of counseling and psychotherapy. As seen in the previous chapter, it is often assumed that the mentally retarded person is incapable of benefiting from a therapeutic relationship, but this assumption is more often based upon theoretical considerations than upon research findings. Notwithstanding its effectiveness, the combination of great numbers and great need within institutions makes individual psychotherapy economically unfeasible (Humphreys, 1938). "The tendency to build state institutions housing from one thousand to several thousand children has pointed up the necessity of employing group psychotherapeutic procedures" (Sarason, 1959). The rationale for group therapy is further supported by the severity of social deficits of the institutionalized retarded and the suitability of group therapy techniques for manipulating interpersonal relationships.

Slavson (1956) has advocated the utility of grouping patients in psychotherapy on the basis of pathological similarities. The possiblity of dealing with specific identifiable personality deficits typical of the institutionalized mental retardate is conceivable within this framework. However, limitations imposed by cognitive and verbal deficits frequently necessitate a structured, programed, and directive group therapy approach.

PERSONAL ADJUSTMENT TRAINING

Rosen and Zisfein (1975*a*) have developed such a program. Personal Adjustment Training (PAT) is a group counseling program designed to deal with those social and personality deficits to which institutionalized retarded are judged to be most vulnerable. The program has three basic ingredients: 1) a structured curriculum derived from results of follow-up studies of persons leaving the institution and living independently in the community (Rosen, Floor, and Baxter, 1972); 2) a group dynamics approach, providing immediate peer support and feedback—this approach, which includes the use of video self-confrontation techniques (Bailey and Souder, 1970; Danet, 1968; Satir, 1964), attempts to use each student as both therapist and client; and 3) a behavior therapy model dealing primarily with observable coping behaviors and making use of such techniques as assertive training and role-playing. Underlying each counseling session is an appreciation of the problems that may exist in the self-concept and identity of mentally retarded persons. The procedures described are designed, in various ways, to foster the growth of self-esteem, as well as to teach specific social competencies seen as requisite for independent community living. Three curricula have been developed for different purposes.

Basic PAT was designed primarily for use within institutions. The procedure touches many areas and is intended to deal with social deficiencies associated with institutionalization as well as the failures, rejections, and degradations associated with intellectual subnormality. Assertive training (Rosen and Zisfein, 1975*b*) is a more specialized procedure utilizing the same PAT group format but designed for mentally handicapped persons who demonstrate patterns of compliance, withdrawal, passivity, and unqualified obedience associated with histories of overprotection or cloistering. Assertive training attempts to teach clients assertive responses necessary to secure the basic rewards and compensations of life without violating the rights of others. A third PAT curriculum, appropriate behavior training (Rosen and Hoffman, 1975), was developed for the lower functioning individual demonstrating bizarre or inappropriate behaviors that would be considered unacceptable in the community.

The three PAT curricula fall midway along the dimension of directiveness and structure outlined in the previous chapter. They retain the nondirective features and lack of control postulated as important in dealing with more general personality changes in self-concept but use more structured and directive approaches for teaching specific social behaviors. The curricula combine features of the classroom with therapeutic approaches, yet are designed to be conducted by counselors without extensive training in psychotherapy. The use of a planned curriculum does not limit the group leader to the material described in the training manuals but, rather, offers a general framework and orientation that may serve as a springboard for other innovative strategies.

Basic PAT

The basic PAT curriculum is organized around five general units and requires approximately 12 sessions of group counseling. The five units, their respective goals, and the methods employed are summarized in Table 1.

The counseling procedures are described as follows:

Self-Evaluation: Identity, Self-Concept —This unit, the core of PAT, is designed to improve the client's general level of self-regard, and to encourage efforts at self-evaluation and awareness of oneself as a social stimulus. The specific procedures utilized are:

Whom am I? —The therapist asks each group member, in turn, to answer the question "Who am I?" The clients are instructed that in addition to their names, they are to tell something about themselves. The

Table 1. Basic PAT outline

Unit number	Title	Purpose	Techniques
1	Self-evaluation: Identity, Self-concept	To improve level of self-regard and achieve more realistic relation between aspirations and abilities. To increase efforts at self-evaluation and awareness of oneself as a social stimulus. To improve appearance, grooming, personality traits.	Self-ratings on bipolar dimensions; "Who am I?" questions; Level of Aspiration board–type techniques; video-tape recordings and playback to students; sociometric techniques.
2	Acquiescence-Exploitation	To reduce tendencies to be acquiescent/submissive to attempts at coercion or exploitation.	Pill-taking; paper signing; financial exploitation; demonstrations and group discussions.
3	Self-assertion	To decondition helplessness, dependency, and passivity by teaching assertive roles.	Role-playing; cassette tape recordings of aggressive and assertive roles.
4	Heterosexual behavior	To increase student's repertoire of heterosexual responses; to decondition anxiety about members of the opposite sex; to increase social awareness and teach coping behaviors for functioning in a bisexual environment.	Modeling; role-playing social situations.
5	Independence-Leadership	To reduce tendencies toward helplessness and dependency in problem-solving situations.	Group problem-solving situations; leadership training.

therapist introduces the essential concept that each group member is an independent person who has a right to like or dislike something, to express preferences or aversions, and to adjust his behavior accordingly.

Self-Ratings —During this session the clients are assisted in making self-ratings along a set of bipolar adjective dimensions. It is emphasized by the therapist that extreme positions do not signify "good" or "bad." Dimensions utilized include physical traits: smart-dumb, outgoing-shy, etc. When it is clear that a client has genuinely underrated himself, the therapist uses these opportunities to inflate his lowered self-estimates and to correct inaccurate self-perceptions.

Level of Aspiration (LA) Procedure —The purpose of this procedure is to display graphically to each group member consistent patterns of under- or over-estimation of his own capabilities. The specific procedure involves repeated estimates of anticipated performance on a simple motor task. The therapist demonstrates a pegboard assembly task. Clients are asked, trial by trial, to estimate their performance on this task. The discrepancy between the client's estimate and his actual performance is graphically illustrated for him and interpreted in terms of self-confidence.

Videotape Self-Confrontation —This procedure allows the client to see and judge for himself his own appearance and behavior and to become aware of himself as a social stimulus. The value of this procedure derives from numerous sources: the multisensory feedback mechanism provided by the video technique, immediate social feedback from other group members, and the opportunity for an isolated self-perception, perhaps for the first time. The therapist leads a general group discussion dealing with such questions as: "What do you like? Do you like how you look? Would you rather look like someone else? Is this how you thought you looked?" Where negative feedback ensues, the therapist provides support and alternative positive behaviors.

Sociometry —A standard sociometric procedure is conducted individually with each client after the first few sessions. Clients are asked to choose one member (exclusive of himself) of the group who best fits each of several dimensions such as: "Who has the best chance of making it on his own? Who looks the nicest? Who would you like to be friends with?" Sociograms, which plot the relative psychological distance between people in the group, are drawn and used in the group counseling session.

Acquiescence-Exploitation —The objective of this session is the reduction of tendencies toward acquiescent, compliant, or submissive behaviors in coercive or exploitative situations. The specific procedures include the use of a set of standard legal forms, which the clients are asked to sign, and the offering of a pill, actually a small sugared candy, that clients

Table 2. Assertive training (AT) outline

Unit number	Topic	Goals	Techniques
	(Introduction and explanation)	(To explain purpose of and overall plan for AT)	
1	Expressing appropriate affect	To teach use of voice, face, and expression as conveyors of feelings and moods (Means of communication)	Videotapes of bland vs. differentiated affect, mirrors to monitor and check self-expression, cassette-taping of voice, index cards of prescribed emotional situations, role-playing
2	Expressing good feelings and positive statements	To teach appropriate expression and receiving of: a. thanks b. compliments c. simple apologies d. elaborate apologies	Role-playing, use of mirror, modeling
3*a*	Expressing needs and desires	To teach appropriate times and effective means of expressing wants and preferences: a. wanting, asking for b. attention-getting c. social assertion d. initiative	Index cards with prescribed situations, modeling, role-playing

3*b*	Expressing needs and desires	To teach appropriate times and effective means of securing that which one ''deserves'' or ''earns'': e. deserving, earning—distinctions among situations where it's ''worth it'' to be assertive f. dealing with rudeness g. expression of anger: 1) how 2) why 3) alternatives	Modeling, cassette tape recorder and feedback, role-playing
4	Saying ''no''	To teach appropriate situations where one must know how to say ''no''	Modeling, video-tapes, role-playing
5	Stating opinions; Contradictions	To decondition fear of stating preference, personal opinions: a. agreeing b. disagreeing c. own opinion	Modeling, role-playing
6	Asserting self to authority figures	To decondition fear of assertion to: employer, landlord, salesman, police	Role-playing, modeling

are told will "make you feel good." It is likely that the clients will sign the forms without reading or understanding them, just as they are likely to take the pill. The therapist criticizes the clients' unquestioning compliance, citing possible ramifications. It is emphasized that not every adult is a friend, counselor, houseparent, or therapist. The necessity for critical and individual evaluation of people and requests is stressed.

Self-Assertion —These sessions are intended to decondition passive, meek, and apathetic behaviors. A secondary and broader goal is the demonstration to clients of the relationship between one's manner of self-expression and the manner in which one is perceived and treated by others. Procedures are directed toward the improvement of the submissive, monotonous, and vulnerable qualities of the voice. Clients are encouraged to use their voices as a vehicle of emotional expression and are reminded of the importance of such expression. Techniques utilized include the use of tape-recorded speech samples, self- and mutual introductions, modeling, and role-playing of angry responses. The therapist explains in various ways that the manner in which the client says his name indicates a great deal about the way he thinks of himself ("If you don't respect yourself, how is anyone else to respect you?") The final step involves the role-playing of situations in which anger is appropriate, using hypothetical, anger-evoking situations. The therapist reinforces the idea that, if he is treated unjustly, the client is obliged to express his anger and assert himself as an individual outside of the therapy situation.

Heterosexual Behavior —The purpose of this procedure is to train appropriate behaviors with members of the opposite sex. This entails the reduction of anxiety in social situations as well as the teaching of the "niceties" demanded of such situations. Once again, procedures involve client role-playing of prescribed social situations immediately following exposure to therapist modeling. Prerecorded videotapes depicting various social situations provide a basis for group discussion. Homework assignments, such as using a dormitory telephone, are also useful.

Independence-Leadership —Independence-leadership training provides practice in decision-making and problem-solving. Implicit in this goal is the encouragement of self-reliant and self-initiated activity. Clients must learn to reverse the tendencies toward helplessness, hesitation, and inhibition usually exhibited in situations demanding independence. The group is presented with a series of hypothetical problem situations. In certain of these, a leader is appointed by the therapist, while in others, a leader emerges naturally. The restructuring of the group that evolves and the patterns of participation during these exercises form the basis for later discussion.

Assertive Training

The basic PAT course may serve to identify persons who require more intensive counseling experiences designed specifically to teach assertive responses. Assertive training was developed for a more homogeneous population of shy, passive, withdrawn, and insecure individuals. Such persons rarely draw attention to themselves as management problems; indeed, they are often perceived by houseparents as compliant, well-behaved individuals and are seldom singled out for special therapeutic services. Yet their diffidence should not be misinterpreted as good adjustment because it may be just as detrimental to community functioning as more overt antisocial behavior.

Assertive training is organized around six general units and requires approximately ten sessions. Each session is approximately one hour in duration. The six units, their respective goals and the methods employed are summarized in Table 2.

APPROPRIATE BEHAVIOR TRAINING

Studies of institutions for the retarded provide ample evidence of the high frequency of socially awkward, inappropriate, or bizarre behavior exhibited in such settings (Roos, 1968; Thormahlen, 1965). These behaviors are not incidental to the mentally retarded, but stem from experiences within the home or institutional setting. The learning of maladaptive behavior syndromes is tolerated, and indeed, sanctioned, through a sympathetic and protective perception of the retarded. Although the exhibition of bizarre behavior is accepted within the institution, it is nevertheless not conformable to integration into community life. While these behaviors appear innocuous, they serve to draw attention and often abuse to the individual. Given current procedures in behavior modification, however, it is possible to reverse these problematic behaviors and teach socially acceptable responses (Ayllon and Haughton, 1962; Girardeau and Spradlin, 1964; Lovaas, 1967).

Appropriate behavior training (ABT) is a highly structured, directive group situation designed for moderately to severely mentally retarded adults. Through the use of learning techniques such as modeling, role-playing, and social reinforcement, clients are taught to identify and structure their own behavior patterns. ABT brings the client's actions in line with social rules and demands and leads him to develop a more socially responsive orientation.

The format was constructed to deal with those areas felt to be most defeating and maladaptive. In order to identify and define such behavior,

Table 3. Appropriate Behavior Training (ABT) outline

Unit number	Title	Purpose	Techniques
	(Introduction)	(Orientation in the concept and terminology of ABT)	(Identification and labeling of behavior)
1	Self-evaluation	To promote self-awareness and social responsiveness; to teach codes of appropriate dress and physical mannerism; to establish a positive self-image	Modeling, labeling, video tape recordings, and playback
2	Speech	To improve quality and content of speech	Modeling, labeling, role-playing
3	Social Interaction	To increase awareness of oneself as a social stimulus; to teach awareness of situational cues and social expectations	Modeling, labeling, role-playing social situations
4	Expression of Anger	To teach clients to express feelings of anger and hostility in an appropriate manner	Modeling, labeling, role-playing social situations, group discussion
5	Sexual Behavior	To impose a structure upon the exhibition of self-stimulating behavior, to teach clients to differentiate behavior according to locale and situation	Modeling, labeling, role-playing social situations, group discussion
	Recapitulation	To integrate and review previous units, to demonstrate gains by students	Identification, labeling, group discussion

an Inventory of Inappropriate Behavior (IIB), described in Chapter 17, was developed. Counseling sessions are structured to deal with the six general areas measured by this inventory: over-friendliness, bizarre speech and actions, socially awkward behavior, poor personal appearance, belligerence, and childishness. 'Over-friendliness' includes behaviors like the indiscriminate approaching of strangers. 'Bizarre speech and actions' refer to stereotypic, idiosyncratic actions such as rambling speech and inappropriate laughter. 'Socially awkward behavior' refers to "clinging vine" mannerisms and persevering use of social pleasantries. 'Poor personal appearance' considers cleanliness, clothing, and posture. 'Belligerence' is reserved for stereotyped responses of anger or destructive behaviors. 'Childishness' refers to tantrums, whining, excessive dependence, extreme attention seeking, and other regressive mannerisms.

Through the use of consistent behavior monitoring and management, such unacceptable behaviors are replaced with socially adaptive skills. Utilizing group counseling procedures, ABT is intended to provide the means and motivation for the clients' adoption of acceptable social skills and behaviors. The identification and labeling of such behaviors in terminology that is meaningful and understandable to clients is of great importance in teaching them to discriminate appropriate from inappropriate actions. It is assumed that once the individual can develop more responsibility for, and control over, his actions, he will be more responsive to social and vocational training efforts.

The curriculum includes five areas relevant to inappropriate behavior: self-evaluation, speech, social interaction, expression of anger, and sexual behavior. Inappropriate behaviors are immediately focused on and given negative connotations. They are defined as childish and socially unacceptable, and labeled "weird," "crazy," "no good," or "silly." More appropriate behavior patterns are then presented as alternatives. Such actions are depicted as normal and adult, and labeled "OK." After clients have learned and mastered the "weird" versus "OK" labels, they are taught to observe and identify bizarre behavior in themselves as well as in others. The primary force behind the changing of behavior patterns rests with the social reinforcement given in the group. The curriculum is outlined in Table 3.

EVALUATING THE EFFECTIVENESS OF BASIC PAT

The effects of PAT were studied (Zisfein and Rosen, 1974) in a group of socially deficient adolescents and young adults in terms of the general goals of the counseling program:

1) The improvement of level of self-regard, achievement of a realistic balance between aspirations and abilities, and the development of a heightened awareness of self as a social stimulus.
2) The reduction of acquiescent or submissive behavior in response to coercive or exploitative attempts by others.
3) The reduction of patterns of helplessness, dependency, and passivity and the learning of the assertive responses.
4) The learning of self-initiated problem-solving behavior.
5) The learning of appropriate heterosexual responses and the reduction of anxiety toward members of the opposite sex.

Evaluation procedures utilized in the study were constructed to reflect the target areas of the curriculum that were judged to be both measureable and responsive to therapeutic efforts. Before and after measures encompassed both subjective reports by the subjects and outwardly discernible behaviors.

Participants chosen were enrolled in vocational habilitation and community preparation programs at the Institute. The group consisted of 25 members, 19 receiving treatment and 6 as a no-treatment control group. Of the 25, 23 were residents at the institution, and 2 were living at home and commuting to school during the day. The treatment population was divided into three counseling groups, each with a different counselor. Table 4 presents chronological age, IQ, and residential or day status data for both the treatment and the control populations.

METHOD

All group members were evaluated using a set of scales and behavioral measures; this evaluation served as a pre-test measurement. The three treatment groups were then enrolled in a twelve-week group counseling situation. The three counselors closely followed counseling guidelines

Table 4. Characteristics of treatment and control groups

	Treatment Group	Control Group
Number of subjects	19	6
Mean CA (S.D.)[a]	23.2(4.8)	22.5(3.3)
Mean IQ (S.D.)[a]	72.9(8.9)	74.9(8.2)
Residential	17	6
Day	2	0

[a]S.D. = standard deviation. CA = chronological age.

specified in the *Personal Adjustment Training Manual* (Zisfein and Rosen, 1972). They met frequently to discuss the training procedures that were sequenced so that the three groups would progress at about the same rate. Counselors also observed each other through observation windows. The control participants received no treatment, and they never met as a group for any purpose. After 12 weeks of therapy, the evaluation procedures were readministered for the entire group. Six weeks after the post-treatment evaluation, one measure (acquiescence) was re-administered.

The following measures were included and used in both pre- and post-counseling evaluations.

Self-Evaluation

The group was presented with a series of 21 bipolar adjectives on which they were asked to rate themselves using a wooden slider along a scale ranging from 1 to 5. Adjectives were selected to reflect physical, social, and competence aspects of self-concept, e.g., leader-follower, scared-confident, talkative-quiet, outgoing-shy. The scale numbers 1 and 5 represented extreme ratings; 5 indicated "always" or "very much," 1 "never" or "not at all." Qualitative definitions were also given for ratings of 2, 3, and 4.

Sociometry

Treatment individuals were asked to make eight different sociometric ratings, including answering such questions as "Who do you think has the best chance of making it on his own?" and "Who do you think stands up for himself the best?" The number of choices each group member received was tabulated, and "stars" and "isolates" for each group were identified.

Video tapes

Each member of the group was administered a two-minute structured interview. The procedure was recorded on video tape. The questions asked dealt with job placement, job competence, and future plans. Questions were selected to reflect aspects of confidence and assurance. Video tapes were scored "blindly" by two raters who were not informed of the purpose of the research efforts or of personal adjustment training. The raters scored each tape on a 5-point scale in response to eight specific questions concerning physical appearance, stance, voice, and self-confidence (e.g., "How neatly is the individual dressed?"). The tapes were shown in random order without regard to treatment-control status or pre/post situation. Pre- and post-comparisons were made from a composite score representing the sum of all questions. An inter-rater reliability check was performed.

The two rates also made separate judgments of the "pre" and "post" video tapes after being informed of the purpose of PAT. The two tapes were shown consecutively without regard to the pre- or post-order. On the basis of self-confidence demonstrated on the tapes, raters were asked to judge whether they were viewing the participant before or after treatment.

"What would you do if... ?"

A series of hypothetical situations designed to evoke either passive or assertive responses was presented, e.g., "What would you do if you were in a restaurant and a waiter spilled soup all over you?" or "What would you do if a stranger stopped and asked you for money?" These responses were scored for "acquiescence" and "assertion" by two raters and inter-rater reliability was determined.

Behavioral measures

Three behavioral measures of acquiescence were used:

1. Document-signing. Each participant was asked to sign a "legal" document with numerous blank spaces and intricate terminology. No explanation was given for the request to sign the document.
2. Money-lending. Immediately after the presentation of the document the experimenter asked: "Do you have a quarter I can have?"
3. Petition-signing. All subjects were approached in an informal setting and asked to sign a petition. The request was made by an experimenter who was dressed so as not to resemble a staff member. The subjects were told that signatures were being solicited so that the experimenter could win a TV set. The petition itself was worded so that it said nothing meaningful.

With the exception of petition-signing, all measures were obtained at single interview sessions conducted immediately before and after treatment. Petition-signing was accomplished on only one occasion, six weeks after the termination of treatment.

RESULTS

Self-evaluation

Mean scores for the 21-item total increased from pre- to post-test conditions for both treatment and control groups. The difference in change between the two groups failed to reach statistical significance. Item-by-item analysis was also unproductive of group differences.

Sociometry

Pre- and post-test totals for individual and composite groups were categorized around intervals equal to the average number of expected votes. There was a small tendency for "isolate" and "star" extremes to fall more closely to the mean interval in the post-therapy test.

Video tapes

Scores for each treatment and control participant were tabulated independently for each rater. Means for inter-rater reliabilities (Spearman rho) for pre- and post-therapy ratings of all four groups combined were .78 for pre-therapy test ($p < .01$), and .54 for post-therapy test ($p < .01$). Totals for subjects on pre- and post-therapy tapes were compared (t-test) and were not significant. No significant differences could be demonstrated between pre- and post-ratings for either rater. The blind comparison of pre- and post-video tapes failed to produce accurate discrimination of treatment conditons for either therapy subjects or controls. Raters were only about 50 percent accurate in their judgment and showed only 40 percent agreement in their ratings.

"What would you do if... ?"

Acquiescence and assertion scores were tabulated pre- and post-treatment. Inter-rater reliability (Spearman r_s) was .98 for acquiescence and .88 for assertion. Changes in a positive or negative direction from pre- to post-test were evaluated. Nonsignificant results were obtained for both acquiescence and assertive measures for treatment groups. Changes in controls were also nonsignificant. Acquiescence scores, however, even on the pre-test, were close to the maximum in a nonacquiescent direction.

Behavioral measures

Every treatment subject ($N = 19$) and control group member ($N = 6$) signed the "legal document" before treatment. Of the treatment group, 4 signed and 15 refused to sign after treatment. The change in pre- to post-condition for the treatment group was evaluated by the McNemarr Test and was significant at $p < .001$. Of the control group, four signed and two refused to sign in the post-measure. In a follow-up six weeks later, only 16 of the original 19 treatment members could be reached. Of these, nine signed the petition and seven refused to sign. All original control group subjects signed the paper.

In the pre-treatment request for money, 12 treatment individuals complied ($N = 19$), as did three control members ($N = 6$). In the post-treatment replication, only two treatment subjects complied ($N = 19$) and no controls ($N = 6$) complied. The change in the treatment group from pre- to post-therapy test was significant at $p < .001$.

Despite clinical impressions and anecdotal reports of therapeutic changes following PAT, objective indices failed, for the most part, to demonstrate greater change in persons receiving PAT than in a no-treatment control group. The explanation lies either in sufficient sensitivity or unreliability of the specific measures employed. While positive changes occurred with self-evaluation, changes of equal magnitude occurred with the control individuals. The "What would you do if. . . ?" measure yielded reliable ratings but failed to demonstrate change in either group. Video tape ratings were far too unreliable to be of any value.

In contrast to verbal measures, however, PAT-specific changes may have been reflected in the behavioral measures, particularly the document- and petition-signing measures. Although they could not be statistically evaluated because of the small number, significant trends in a nonacquiescent direction were suggested by the data. Had all evaluative measures been of a behavioral nature, other differences might also have been demonstrated. Adequate precision in measurement remains to be developed.

On the post-test measure, two of the controls who had originally signed the document now refused, and three who gave money later refused. That all controls reverted back to signing when approached by a confederate out of an office setting seems to indicate their failure to generalize the lesson they had heard of only second-hand. Some treatment members, on the other hand, who had active lessons concerning the dangers of indiscriminate document-signing, seemed to have internalized the lesson. These results are tabulated in Table 5.

In response to the "What would you do if. . . ?" scale, the participants, for the most part, seemed to know the right things to say. Most verbally claimed that they would refuse to sign things or give money or things away indiscriminately. A few minutes later, however, every one ($N = 25$) signed a document, and 15 offered money. This seems to confirm the importance of behavioral, active-learning models for mentally handicapped individuals. The fact that a characteristic feature of retardation is concreteness and difficulty in transferring from one modality to another or one context to another is well established. It is logical then, for teaching to be most effective in student-participant simulated situations.

Finally, there have been anecdotal and subjective reports from various staff members throughout the institution of noticeable changes in former PAT students. One boy, previously a reliable source of disruption, was reported now to behave appropriately in class, to volunteer information,

Table 5. Response to acquiescence measures[a]

Group	Pre-therapy test (N=19) Document-signing	Pre-therapy test (N=19) Money-lending	Post-therapy test (N=19) Document-signing	Post-therapy test (N=19) Money-lending	Follow-up test (N=16) Petition-signing
Treatment groups	100	63	21	10	56
Control group	100	50	67	0	100

[a]Expressed as percent who responded with acquiescence.

and to listen while others spoke. Other feedback has indicated that students demonstrated much improved interactions in the dormitories and that far better care was demonstrated about appearance and grooming. One girl, formerly afraid to talk in more than a whisper, was overheard shouting in the dormitory.

It is unfortunate that such changes were not more amenable to measurement. It may have been unrealistic to expect that mentally handicapped persons would be able to make the subtle self-rating discriminations demanded by this study. Until evaluators are able to measure objectively change in so abstract a concept as self-esteem, evaluation efforts should focus on demonstrable behavioral changes.

LITERATURE CITED

Ayllon, T., and Haughton, E. 1962. Control of the behavior of schizophrenic patients by food. J. Exp. Anal. Behav. 5:343–352.

Bailey, K. G., and Souder, W. T., Jr. 1970. Audiotape and videotape self-confrontation in psychotherapy. Psychol. Bull. 74:127–137.

Butterfield, E. C., and Zigler, E. 1965. The influence of differing institutional social climates on the effectiveness of social reinforcement in the mentally retarded. Amer. J. Ment. Defic. 70:48–56.

Charles, D. C. 1953. Ability and accomplishment of persons earlier judged mentally deficient. Genet. Psychol. Monogr. 47:3–71.

Danet, B. N. 1968. Self-confrontation in psychotherapy reviewed. Amer. J. Psychother. 22:245–258.

Girardeau, F. L., and Spradlin, J. E. 1964. Token rewards in a cottage program. Ment. Retard. 2:345–351.

Goldstein, H. 1964. Social and occupational adjustment. *In* H. A. Stevens and R. Heber (eds.), Mental Retardation. University of Chicago Press, Chicago.

Humphreys, E. J. 1938. The field of psychiatry in relation to the work of the state school. Proc. Amer. Ass. Ment. Defic. 43:80–89.

Kennedy, R. J. 1966. A Connecticut community revisited: A study of the social adjustment of a group of mentally deficient adults in 1948 and 1960. Project No.

655, Office of Vocational Rehabilitation, U.S. Department of Health, Education, and Welfare, Washington, D.C.

Kugel, R., and Wolfensberger, W. (eds.). 1969. Changing patterns in residential services for the mentally retarded. President's Committee on Mental Retardation, Washington, D.C.

Lovaas, O. I. 1967. Behavior Therapy Approach to Treatment of Childhood Schizophrenia. Minnesota Symposium on Child Development. University of Minnesota Press, Minnesota.

Miller, E. L. 1965. Ability and social adjustment at mid-life of persons earlier judged mentally deficient. Genet. Psychol. Monogr. 72:139–198.

Roos, P. 1968. Initiating socialization programs for socially inept adolescents. Ment. Retard. 6:13–17.

Rosen, M., Floor, L., and Baxter, D. 1972. The institutional personality. Brit. J. Ment. Subnormal. 17:125–131.

Rosen, M., and Hoffman, M. 1975. Personal Adjustment Training: A Group Counseling Manual for the Mentally Handicapped. Vol. III. Appropriate Behavior Training. Elwyn Institute, Elwyn, Pennsylvania.

Rosen, M., and Zisfein, L. 1975*a*. Personal Adjustment Training: A Group Counseling Manual for the Mentally Handicapped. Vol. I. Basic Course. Elwyn Institute, Elwyn, Pennsylvania.

Rosen, M., and Zisfein, L. 1975*b*. Personal Adjustment Training: A Group Counseling Manual for the Mentally Handicapped. Vol. II. Assertive Training. Elwyn Institute, Elwyn, Pennsylvania.

Sarason, S. B. 1959. Psychological Problems in Mental Deficiency. Harper & Row, New York.

Satir, V. 1964. Conjoint Family Therapy. Science and Behavior Books, Palo Alto, California.

Slavson, S. R. 1956. The Fields of Group Psychotherapy. John Wiley & Sons Inc., New York.

Thormahlen, P. W. 1965. A study of on-the-ward training of trainable mentally retarded children in a state institution. California Mental Health Research Monograph, No. 4, California Department of Mental Hygiene, Bureau of Research and Statistics.

Windle, C. 1962. Prognosis of mental subnormals. Amer. J. Ment. Defic. 66.

Zisfein, L. S., and Rosen, M. 1972. Personal Adjustment Training: A Manual of Group Counseling Procedures for Use within Institutions for the Handicapped. Elwyn Institute, Elwyn, Pennsylvania.

Zisfein, L., and Rosen, M. 1974. Effects of a personal adjustment training group counseling program. Ment. Retard. 12:50–53.

Chapter 20

Dealing with Severe Emotional Problems

Preceding chapters dealing with personality and emotional functioning of the mentally retarded have suggested problems that are shared by large numbers of mentally retarded adults. These problems may be secondary to intellectual deficits and a consequence of histories of oversheltering, failure, rejection, labeling, and exclusion from experiences available to the ordinary citizen. The group counseling models described in the previous chapter were designed to deal with learned behavioral patterns and low self-esteem postulated as characteristic of mentally retarded persons in general.

Yet, many mentally retarded persons may also demonstrate emotional and behavioral problems that distinguish them from other handicapped clients. These problems may be severe enough to prevent them from participating in habilitation programs. It is not uncommon for higher functioning mentally retarded clients to be excluded from ongoing programs because of their emotional problems, or to be treated as more severely limited individuals than would be justifiable solely on the basis of their intellectual or vocational skills. In some cases, such individuals must be removed from the habilitation setting to a more structured psychiatric facility. When this occurs, it represents a failure of the habilitation program because the individual is usually lost as an habilitation candidate, perhaps permanently.

In Chapter 18 the use of psychotherapy for such problems is discussed, and a general scheme for choosing among psychotherapy or counseling strategies on the basis of a number of client, therapist, and situational factors is presented. It was suggested that insight, relationship, dynamically oriented psychotherapists were most suitable for clients demonstrating verbal and abstract ability, while behavior modification techniques might be more appropriate for less verbal and more cognitively impaired persons.

This chapter explores means of dealing with the more severe emotional problems, considering both administrative and strategic factors.

With greater acceptance of deinstitutionalization and normalization principles, the need to deal with more severe behavioral problems becomes increasingly salient. This is true within the residential institution, as well as within community settings. No longer can the habilitation program afford the luxury of dealing exclusively with the mildly retarded, easily manageable client, for whom the sole objective of habilitation is the provision of a marketable vocational skill and the rudiments of social acceptability. If habilitation programs remain blind to the methodologies that may be effective with the severely disturbed, problem client, they may well find themselves out of business.

The methods discussed here are those that should be applied within the habilitation setting. The chapter discusses how that setting may be restructured to deal with more severe emotional or psychiatric problems without destroying the overall teaching and training character of that setting.

TYPES OF PROBLEMS ENCOUNTERED

The emotional problems encountered within a population enrolled in community-oriented vocational habilitation programs may vary as widely as emotional problems encountered in normal populations. They include problems like anxiety and fears relating to community living; problems with authority figures, such as work supervisors; social deficits or inappropriate behaviors that would draw attention to the individual, labeling him as deviant, or that would in other ways be unacceptable in the community; aggressive, destructive or antisocial behaviors that might bring the individual to the attention of legal authorities; excessive withdrawal; sexual disturbances, including homosexual problems; psychotic reactions involving thinking disturbances or severe affective disorders; and more long-term personality traits or characterological disorders.

TREATMENT OF EXCESSIVE FEARS OR ANXIETY WITHIN A MENTALLY RETARDED POPULATION

The fact that many mentally retarded adults have never had the opportunity to engage in normal activities is sufficient reason to expect a certain degree of apprehension about these activities. This is particularly true when cloistering has been extreme, and the problem is frequently encountered within residential programs attempting to teach a repertoire of new social behaviors to the mentally retarded. For an individual who has spent most of his life within the institution, the prospect of independence can be frightening. We have seen some mentally retarded individuals exposed to a modern-day shopping mall, supermarket, bus terminal, or busy intersection who became overwhelmed by the intensity of the stimulation in such settings. In other cases there has been a history of traumatic occurrences associated with specific community resources. Rosen, Zisfein, and Hardy (1972) describe the use of "in vivo desensitization" to deal with a variety of community and separation fears in a mildly retarded female adult being trained for discharge from the institution.

A Case Study

The subject, Margaret, was a 37-year-old, mildly retarded woman who had lived at a large residential institution for the mentally retarded for 16 of her 37 years. Margaret was treated for a general fear of separation from the institution and specific fears of community situations like crowds, department stores, trolley cars, and escalators. The treatment was initiated in the context of a vocational and social habilitation program, described in Chapter 5, geared to prepare Margaret for transition from the institution to independent living. The ongoing program in which Margaret was enrolled seemed insufficient to help her overcome her fears, which were incapacitating to the extent that they acted as a deterrent to the final planning for discharge to a community-based halfway house facility. Although more severe than those of other students undergoing similar habilitation treatment, the fears that Margaret demonstrated represented an exaggerated form of concern shared by most of the clients enrolled in this program.

Margaret was admitted to the institution in 1955 upon referral from a social agency after the break-up of her family and a series of foster home placements. Margaret is diagnosed as having mild mental retardation associated with cerebral palsy. She has a left hemiplegia with almost no function or sensation in her left arm and hand and walks with a noticeable limp. It is believed that Margaret's fear of crowds relates to her sensitivity to, and embarrassment at, being observed because of her physical disability. For the first two years following admission, Margaret experienced seizures, but these are now controlled by medication. Margaret was assigned to and performed satisfactorily at various work areas within the institution for her first seven years in residence at the institution. With the development of habilitative programs and philosophy at the institution (Wilkie et al., 1968), Margaret's training became more intensive. Margaret was given training in housekeeping skills and worked at the institution hospital and laundry. She also attended adult education classes, which provided instruction in community socialization skills and included periodic community excursions for exposure to and familiarization with community resources. Not until the latter stages of this program did the intensity of Margaret's separation fears become apparent.

At the time of her referral, Margaret was enrolled in what was to be one of the final phases of her training. While residing at the institution, she worked daily as a housekeeping aide at a local hospital in the community. She experienced extreme tension during her daily trip to work on the trolley, fearing seizures or "blackouts." At other times she felt a "tension" in her affected arm and, despite her self-consciousness, felt obliged to hold it down to prevent a tremor. The farther from the door she sat, the greater the tension, presumably because of increased difficulty in escaping. A persistent premonition was that the trolley would never reach its destination.

In addition, Margaret described a general fear of crowds; crowded department stores, escalators, and restaurants elicited sweating, a rapid heart beat, and a feeling that she would pass out.

Because Margaret's fears had not responded to group habilitative efforts, an individual therapeutic approach was chosen. Margaret's verbal limitations and the urgency of her symptoms seemed to preclude a traditional counseling approach. Instead, a desensitization strategy was chosen, done in vivo, however, rather than by traditional use of fantasy procedure (Wolpe and Lazarus, 1966).

It was assumed that Margaret's fear of specific crowd situations had been learned and that institutional cloistering had effectively served to maintain this fear by sheltering her sufficiently to prevent extinction. The overall strategy was to decondition this fear by gradually exposing Margaret to increasingly higher levels of fearful stimulation. As she gained experience and confidence at one level of stimulation, the next more intense level was introduced. Margaret was never pressured to accomplish more than she believed herself able to handle at any one time.

Margaret was initially questioned about her fears and the situations that elicited them. She was told that she had learned these fears and could learn to overcome them as well. She was taught a simple muscle relaxing technique similar to that described by Jacobson (1938) adapted to the comprehension of a mildly retarded woman. Margaret was instructed to communicate the intensity of her fears by means of a ten-point scale ranging from complete calm to acute anxiety. The scale served throughout therapy as an effective communicative tool.

Ensuing therapy sessions were held in a community suburban shopping center. Margaret was asked to relax until she reached a level of zero on her subjective fear scale. With continued relaxation instructions, she was gradually led into a department store. At any rise in her subjective fear level, Margaret was allowed to walk out of the store and relax before reentering. After three or four trials she was able to enter and remain in the store for several minutes with a therapist by her side. Gradually, as she moved increasingly larger distances from the therapist, she browsed around the store looking at things that interested her. If any fear arose, Margaret was instructed to walk immediately towards the therapist, who was always within her sight. In this manner it was possible to teach Margaret to separate greater distances from the therapist. After approximately one hour at the shopping center, Margaret was able both to enter the store and to browse alone for five- to ten-minute periods. In subsequent sessions in other stores, Margaret learned to interact with clerks and to make purchases without tension. Opposed to her initial need to be accompanied by a therapist, Margaret was later able to transact her business independently.

Several therapy sessions were devoted to approach and inspection of trolley cars without actually boarding the car. Eventually Margaret was encouraged to make short trolley trips accompanied by the therapist. These were unlike her usual trips to work in that Margaret was required to get off immediately upon feeling tense. By the third month of treatment Margaret reported no adverse reaction to her daily trolley ride.

One session was designed to help Margaret overcome her fear of riding escalators. Because of her physical problems, getting on and off the escalator was a most frightening prospect. Margaret traced the onset of her fear to an early experience of having caught her foot in an escalator. Initially Margaret was helped onto an escalator and held by two therapists, one on either side of her. On subsequent trials Margaret used only one therapist and grasped the handrail with her good arm. By the fifth trial she was able to negotiate both the up and down escalator independently.

Approximately six months after the initiation of therapy, Margaret was taken to visit Chestnut Hall, a community-based halfway house in Philadelphia. The trip involved both a trolley car and an elevated train. She was shown several of the apartments used by students during the transitional phase of the community release program and was taken for a walk around the surrounding neighborhood.

An overnight stay at Chestnut Hall was arranged. Except for an unfortunate incident in which she inadvertently locked herself in her room for a few minutes, the visit was successful. Margaret attended preparation and socialization classes held at the facility. During a second stay a few weeks later Margaret cooked a spaghetti dinner for herself and a staff member. She also left from the facility to go to work on the following morning although she requested that a fellow worker accompany her on the trip. Although Margaret appeared considerably less fearful about the community, she began expressing resistance about leaving the institution. She was specifically concerned about leaving her roommate of many years and the loneliness she anticipated upon entering the halfway house program. Margaret was reassured that she would not be forced to leave the institution against her wishes.

After several overnight visits to the halfway house, Margaret was finally transferred there on a residential basis. At the present time she shares an apartment at Chestnut Hall, commutes alone to her job each day, and participates in counseling and adult education classes in the evening.

TREATING SOCIALLY INAPPROPRIATE BEHAVIOR

Although the precise control of a total behavior modification program is not always feasible within the habilitation setting, there are a number of general principles and strategies that make good psychological sense no matter what the theoretical orientation of staff.

The principles of reinforcement and extinction and the techniques of shaping, fading, and time-out are well described in many sources and need not be overly elaborated here. Nor can we deal at great length with the intricacies of behavior analysis or data collection. The interested reader is referred to one of many fine sources describing the use of behavior modification procedures and their application with the mentally retarded (Ayllon and Azrin, 1968; Bandura, 1969; Bensberg, 1965; Gardner, 1971; Watson, 1967, 1968). Rather, this chapter describes how behavioral principles can be applied in working with severe emotional disturbance, *even in programs that are not strictly organized as operant conditioning regimes and are administered by persons who are not experts in behavior analysis and behavior shaping*.

A behavior that consistently leads to gratification will tend to recur—any stimulus or stimulus situation that is pleasing or satisfying to the individual will increase the likelihood of a behavior when it consistently follows that behavior. This is the principle of reinforcement; the stimulus situation is termed the reinforcement. Conversely, a previously reinforced behavior will become less probable when it no longer leads to that reinforcement. This situation is labeled extinction. The essence of behavior modification approaches to training and education is the systematic application of the contingencies of reinforcement to increase or decrease the likelihood of occurrence of a given behavior. In some cases it is desirable that a learned behavior be eliminated from the individual's repertoire. Behavior modification requires that the reinforcement for that behavior be identified. Since behavior does not occur in a vacuum, it is assumed that a reinforcer exists in the environment that was probably responsible for the learning of that behavior and that is responsible for maintaining the behavior. In other cases it is desirable that the individual learn a new behavior. In most cases where the elimination of a behavior is the desired goal, it is usually advantageous not only to remove the reinforcement for that behavior (extinction) but also to teach an alternate behavior by applying appropriate reinforcement. Behavior that is learned on the basis of its consequences is termed operant behavior. Most overt behavior encountered within an habilitation facility would fall in this category.

The habilitation worker encounters many situations in which it is possible to use simple behavioral interventions, to manipulate contingencies of reinforcement, and to reverse or to manage better severe behavioral problems of clients.

A Case Study

The senior author of this text was asked to work with a severely retarded man whose behavior was so unmanageable that he had spent many years living within the hospital of the institution, where he was unable to participate in regular educational or work programs, rather than in a residential dormitory. The student was physically aggressive and also had learned to tear his clothes off when he became upset. Nurses and hospital aides, largely female, were unable to control his behavior and expressed fear of his aggressive outbursts. Other nurses learned to short circuit or prevent his tantrums by infantilizing him and plying him with food rewards when it appeared that he would lose control.

It was apparent that much of the unmanageable behavior was purposive in that it evoked attention and other forms of reinforcement. Meetings with hospital staff and support from medical authorities made it possible to reverse these conditons. A reward system was initiated for appropriate behaviors on the ward, using Cokes as the reinforcement every hour. In a very short period of time it was possible to allow the student to attend an activities program on the grounds for a few hours a day. The Cokes were still used as a reinforcement. The frequency of temper outbursts decreased dramatically, and it was possible to maintain the progress for many months without regression. When regressions did occur, it was always found that the regime was not being followed, and it was necessary to impose more direct supervision of the prescribed behavioral regime. The student continues to be a long-term resident of the institution. He probably will never be able to be maintained without special attention to behavioral continegencies. It is recognized that his behavior will periodically break down and that he represents a lifetime behavior management problem with limited prognosis for marked improvement in adaptive behavior. Yet, even this severely disturbed individual can be helped to function at a level affording him some dignity within an habilitation setting geared toward higher functioning students.

Despite the obvious good sense of reinforcement regimes and the wealth of empirical evidence that such programs work, it is difficult to teach work supervisors, attendant staff, and teachers to ignore inappropriate behavior rather than reinforce it, and to attend to appropriate behavior when it occurs. A case study described by Rosen and Wesner (1973) illustrates the influence of reinforcement in maintaining a disruptive behavior and the complexities of environmental control. Although the subject was a teenager, the issues involved are equally pertinent to habilitation goals with adult clients.

[In 1885, Gilles de la Tourette described a "nervous affliction characterized by motor incoordination, accompanied by echolalia and coprolalia." This condition typically begins in childhood, with tics that progress to involve the upper limbs, trunk, or the entire body. Later, vocal tics, such as frequent coughing, clearing the throat, grunting, and then coprolalia (the compulsive speaking or shouting of obscene words) become consistent symptoms. Although patients have been known to be relatively free of the symptoms for months or even years, the condition is considered resistant to nearly all forms of treatment (Gilles de la Tourette, 1885). Some authors believe an organic disturbance of the brain underlies the symptoms, but consistent neuropathologic evidence is lacking. Other authors attribute the symptoms to psychological factors, perhaps acting on an organic substratum (Challas, Chapel, and Jenkins, 1967). An excellent review of the literature is provided by Kellman (1965).]

A Case Study

The subject exhibited bizarre twirling, obscene gesturing with finger and tongue, and repeated verbalizations of obscene four-letter words at inopportune times. He was diagnosed as a case of Tourette's syndrome. The boy was living in a special therapeutic milieu administered along rather permissive lines. The unit supervisors, psychiatric consultants, and the boy's peers had learned to tolerate his behavior. However, he presented serious management problems in school, where the effects of his symptoms were disruptive in class and kept him from any serious involvement in the teaching situation. The obscene nature of the child's verbal outburst served both to upset his teacher and to entertain the other children in the class. The boy was sent to the principal's office several times each day, where he was observed to manifest a high frequency of verbal and gestural responses for all passersby.

The operant nature of the child's behavior was demonstrated by tabulating the frequency of obscene speech or barking and obscene gestures in the classroom, first when the boy did not know he was being observed and then immediately after the experimenter entered the room. The average frequency of response increased from approximately one per minute to four responses per minute. Motor gestures, mostly of an obscene nature, also increased to a frequency of 5.7 per minute. The figures suggest how strongly the response was manipulated by social reinforcement once the child was aware that he was being observed.

An individual therapy session was initiated. The subject was reinforced by an electric light in a small box that turned on for every 30-second period without vocal or gross motor response, following a procedure described by Patterson (1965). He was instructed that the number of times the light appeared would be counted and that he would be rewarded at the end of the therapy session with a piece of candy for each light. Concurrently, he was verbally reinforced for making tongue gestures. The purpose of this strategy was to substitute tongue movements for the vocal response, since they would be less maladaptive. Both vocal and gross motor responses decreased under this regime, while tongue movements first increased, then decreased.

The same regime was maintained for several brief therapy sessions on consecutive days. By the fourth day of therapy, the data suggested that the subject was able to control both vocal and motor responses without obvious increase in tension for short periods of time. Tongue movements persisted and were encouraged, but they tended to decrease as the subject achieved more control over vocal and gross motor responses. The reinforcement regime was continued during the third session, with the added manipulation of teaching the subject to relax. A relaxation procedure similar to that described for use in desensitization (Jacobson, 1938; Wolpe and Lazarus, 1966) was used. During the session the subject maintained a record free of gross motor and vocal responses for seven consecutive minutes. Again, tongue movements also tended to diminish, although the subject was encouraged to use them if necessary. It did not appear that the subject required a substitute response in order to maintain symptom-free behavior.

The program was then introduced into the classroom. The entire class was rewarded at the end of the time period with candy for each of the subject's symptom-free 30-second time intervals. The purpose of this procedure was to use peers as reinforcers for behavior control rather than as reinforcers for the coprolalic response, as had been previously occurring. During the first 15-minute classroom session, the class received only four reinforcements. Although it was not possible to record tongue movements, they were observed to be high.

During the second classroom session the class received 18 reinforcements. During the third classroom session the class received 27 out of 30 possible reinforcements. However, monitoring of the subject's vocal response, on the same day the reinforcement schedule was not being maintained, indicated the same base-rate level of response of about one per minute. The subject was instructed that there would be periodic and frequent monitoring of his response through the intercom but that he would not know when this was to happen. For a period of several weeks the therapist was able to maintain relatively symptom-free intervals.

Eventually, the therapist weaned the child from the program by training his teacher to maintain a regime of praise and reward for behavioral control and by avoiding special treatment or emotional response to the vocal or motor behavior. Trips to the principal's office for classroom outbursts were specifically forbidden. Interestingly, however, the symptoms the child presented remained a problem in his residence unit, where no program was maintained beyond the drug therapy.

The data presented are consistent with the conclusion of Browning and Stover (1971) that, at least to a large degree, Tourette's syndrome responses are operant in nature. The subject in the present study showed a marked increment in the frequency of response when he was being directly observed. His response in class was markedly increased in frequency with a female teacher, particularly one who was upset by the nature of his vocal and motor responses. The lack of generalization of the behavior beyond the classroom setting further supports this conclusion. Presumably, reinforcement contingencies supporting the behavior first observed in school were still maintained in his dormitory.

While pharmaceutical treatment of Tourette's syndrome is proving to be the treatment of choice (Healy, 1970; Lucas, 1967; Shapiro and Shapiro, 1968), it is likely that even persons receiving medication still need psychological help and special management.

INTENSIVE TREATMENT AND THERAPEUTIC MILIEU PROGRAMS

It is not uncommon for the habilitation facility to encounter clients with emotional problems so severe that they preclude meaningful participation in the programs or services of that facility. In some cases these problems are so severe that they require that the client be referred to a self-contained psychiatric behavior modification unit. Often this necessitates referral to another facility, such as a mental hospital. It is extremely rare that an habilitation facility for the mentally retarded individual is also equipped to deal with severely disturbed individuals while still maintaining overall habilitation goals. Within institutions the locked sideroom and closed ward for aggressive and destructive persons are still very much in evidence. Yet within the institutional setting it is possible to structure a therapeutic situation for such individuals that is geared toward overall habilitation objectives and integrated within the context of the overall habilitation programs. Although it is the authors' bias that behavior modification provides the most appropriate model for structuring such a situation, other more psychiatrically oriented approaches are also possible. Some basic principles and guidelines for expanding the institutional habilitation facility to deal with severe behavioral and emotional problems are presented below.

First, it is necessary to designate a residential facility where more seriously disturbed persons may be temporarily housed while they are receiving intensive treatment. The facility may be part of a larger hospital unit, although in the authors' experience it is best to remove the medical flavor of the intensive treatment setting.

Once a physical setting is selected it is necessary to educate habilitation staff concerning the capabilities of the unit, its objectives, means of referral, suitable clients for referral, discharge and follow-up procedures, and the overall philosophy of the unit. In facilities that have long histories of discharging persons because of psychiatric problems, a considerable amount of re-educating may be required. It is necessary to instill the attitude that the intensive unit serves as a treatment function and should not be viewed as a long-term custodial situation. Nor should it be viewed as a means of discharge from the institution or habilitation program. In one institution for the retarded a psychiatric unit was added to deal with severe behavioral problems, but it was used as a referral source only for clients who had already been written off as habilitation prospects and as a means of expediting eventual discharge. It is absolutely essential that habilitation personnel, in making referrals to an intensive treatment unit, maintain an active involvement in the programing for that client while he resides in the unit. They should be apprised of his progress at all times and should be willing to accept the client back into regular programs when he has shown sufficient behavioral change to warrant it.

In training staff for operation of an intensive treatment unit for the severely disturbed, it is necessary to instill a basic belief in human dignity no matter how severe the behavioral disturbance. Behaviorally disturbed and mentally retarded persons with severe intellectual deficits may be grossly unattractive to attendant staff. Training personnel must be made to realize before accepting employment in such a setting that they will be dealing with persons who may not be toilet trained, who may be difficult to keep clothed, who may have no language, and who may be aggressive or destructive. Not to be prepared to deal with such behaviors will predispose the individual to failure. On the other hand it is necessary to look beyond the overt behavior and to observe the patient in order to understand his motivations. The importance of maintaining cleanliness and appropriate physical appearance lies not only in the effects upon the client but also in its effects upon the overall morale of staff. The attendant and other line personnel in a therapeutic unit must be trained to question the meaning to the client of any disruptive behavior in terms of its consequences. Behavior modification techniques provide a system for determining both the instigating conditions for disruptive behavior, as well as the conditions of reinforcement that maintain that behavior.

The term therapeutic milieu is frequently invoked to describe psychiatric treatment programs that include residential and total life treatment. While many diverse programs have been included under the same general rubric, the essence of the term lies in the intention of structuring an environment that will promote psychological growth. This includes elements that encompass not only acceptance and "tender loving care," but also a sufficient degree of structure to ensure that the individual can learn to differentiate between behaviors that are appropriate, acceptable, and productive for him from those that are inappropriate, socially deviant, and generally self-defeating. A therapeutic environment is neither a return to the womb nor a "brave new world." Although the authors are in general sympathy with the aims and many methods of behavior modification, it is not our belief that treatment for emotional disturbance must be limited strictly to the strategies of operant conditioning. The therapeutic environment must allow choice among alternative ways of responding and must lead to differential consequences according to standards that are generally accepted in our culture for behavior. The individual, no matter how disagreeable his behavior, must be accepted as a person and afforded the basic dignity he deserves as a human being. But not every aspect of his behavior need be accepted, and the environment must be such that expectations for appropriate and productive behavior are clearly defined. While the therapeutic milieu serves in many ways to approximate the outside world, it may be in many ways markedly dissimilar from a natural environment. Unfortunately, the real world is not always structured in such a way that it teaches and supports behaviors we judge to be psychologically healthy. It is a common phenomenon of psychiatric programs that persons who progress within the controlled hospital setting may regress shortly after return to the community. In such cases the individual may be returning to the very set of environmental conditions that brought on his emotional problems. The use of halfway houses and outpatient clinics to provide follow-up services is one way mental health professionals attempt to change not only the individual, but also his family's involvement in the therapeutic process. It is clear then that a therapeutic environment may not be a natural environment.

BLUEPRINT FOR A BEHAVIOR MANAGER

The competent behavior manager within a therapeutic milieu should be able to be accepting of the individual, despite his behavior, but strong enough to react differentially to him on the basis of the appropriateness of his behavior. He should be sensitive enough to the individual to recognize what is appropriate and acceptable and should have developed conceptions of healthy and unhealthy, mature and immature, and appropriate and inappropriate behavior. He should care enough for people that he will take the trouble to monitor the client's behavior and to question his own responses to the client. He should be strong enough to implement constructive behavioral approaches, skilled enough to have a repertoire of strategies for specific behavioral problems, flexible enough to change a regime that doesn't work, and humble enough to admit when he is wrong and to seek help. He should be sufficiently well trained and integrated into a treatment system to view himself as a therapeutic behavior change agent and an important (perhaps the most important) cog in the treatment team.

THE TOTAL HABILITATION PROGRAM

Every habilitation program has its failures—those clients who not only fail to benefit from the program, but also are unable to participate in it. The psychiatric hospital and the residential school for the mentally retarded have traditionally played a game of hot potato with the emotionally or behaviorally disturbed mentally retarded individual. The residential school disclaims responsibility because the individual's severe behavioral disturbance makes him too difficult a management problem, and he cannot be contained in their regular school or vocational training program. "Treat his emotional problems and make him more amenable for rehabilitation" is a frequently heard referral plea. The psychiatric setting, on the other hand, may also deny responsibility for such persons because their intellectual limitations connote the taint of irreversibility. The argument about which disability is primary, mental retardation or emotional disturbance, often becomes a nonproductive and hair-splitting dialogue of little value to the client.

Recent attacks upon institutions and calls for total normalization (Wolfensberger, 1971*a*, 1971*b*) have questioned the future need for institutions. Despite their previous failures, residential institutions can play an important role in the development of resources for the total habilitation process, including the behavioral and psychological support required by the emotionally disturbed mentally retarded. The existence of a therapeutic milieu situation as an integrated component of the overall habilitation program is within the realm of possibility for residential instituions. Rather than prophesying the demise of institutions, we call for a new role for such facilities. This role should combine vocational and social habilitation services with intensive treatment of more severely disturbed mentally retarded clients.

LITERATURE CITED

Ayllon, T., and Azrin, N. H. 1968. The Token Economy: A Motivational System for Therapy and Rehabilitation. Appleton-Century-Crofts, New York.

Bandura, A. 1969. Principles of Behavior Modification. Holt, Rinehart & Winston, New York.

Bensberg, G. J. 1965. Teaching the mentally retarded. Southern Regional Education Board, Atlanta, Georgia.

Browning, R. M., and Stover, D. O. 1971. Behavior Modification in Child Treatment: An Experimental and Clinical Approach. Aldine-Atherton, Chicago.

Challas, G., Chapel, J., and Jenkins, R. L. 1967. Tourette's disease: Control of symptoms and its clinical course. Int. J. Neuropsychiatry 3:95–109.

Gardner, W. I. 1971. Behavior Modification in Mental Retardation: The Education and Rehabilitation of the Mentally Retarded Adolescent and Adult. Aldine Publishing Company, Chicago.

Gilles de la Tourette, G. 1885. Étude sur une affection nerveuse charactérisée par de l'incoordination motrice accompagnée d'echolalie et de coprolalie. Arch. Neurol. (Paris) 7:158.

Healy, C. E. 1970. Gilles de la Tourette's syndrome (Maladie des Tics): Successful treatment with haloperidol. Amer. J. Dis. Child. 120:62–63.

Jacobson, E. 1938. Progressive Relaxation. University of Chicago Press, Chicago.

Kellman, D. H. 1965. Gilles de la Tourette's disease in children: A review of the literature. J. Child Psychol. Psychiatry 6:219–226.

Lucas, A. R. 1967. Gilles de la Tourette's disease in children: Treatment with haloperidol. Amer. J. Psychiatry 124:243–245.

Patterson, G. R. 1965. An application of conditioning techniques to the control of a hyperactive child. *In* L. P. Ullman and L. Krasner (eds.), Case Studies in Behavior Modification. Holt, Rinehart & Winston, New York.

Rosen, M., and Wesner, C. 1973. A behavioral approach to Tourette's syndrome. J. Consult. Clin. Psychol. 41:308–312.

Rosen, M., Zisfein, L., and Hardy, M. 1972. The clinical application of behavior modification techniques: Three case studies. Brit. J. Ment. Subnormal. Vol. XVIII, No. 35:1–8.

Shapiro, A. K., and Shapiro, E. 1968. Treatment of Gilles de la Tourette's syndrome with haloperidol. Brit. J. Psychiatry 114:345–350.

Watson, L. S. 1967. Application of operant conditioning techniques to institutionalized severely and profoundly retarded children. Ment. Retard. (Abstr.) 4:1–18.

Watson, L. S. 1968. Application of behavior-shaping devices to training severely and profoundly retarded children in an institutional setting. Ment. Retard. 6:21–23.

Wilkie, E. A., Kivitz, M. S., Clark, G. R., Byer, M. J., and Cohen, J. S. 1968. Developing a comprehensive rehabilitation program with an institutional setting. Ment. Retard. 6:35–39.

Wolfensberger, W. 1971*a*. Will there always be an institution? I: The impact of epidemiological trends. Ment. Retard. 9:14–20.

Wolfensberger, W. 1971*b*. Will there always be an institution? II: The impact of new service models. Ment. Retard. 9:31–38.

Wolpe, J., and Lazarus, A. A. 1966. Behavior Therapy Techniques. Pergamon Press, New York.

Section VII

Summary and Conclusions

Chapter 21

New Challenges for Habilitation

IMPACT OF NEW LEGISLATION

Early in this decade, federal and state courts began to apply constitutional concepts, such as due process, protection from cruel and unusual punishment, and equal protection under the law, to mentally retarded citizens. In Alabama (*Wyatt* v. *Stickney,* 1972) the courts declared habilitative services at the state's institutions and hospitals to be inadequate and ordered an improvement in services, a reduction in institutionalized populations, and the return of many mentally retarded residents to community settings. A similar effort in New York State (*New York State Association for Retarded Children* v. *Rockefeller*) resulted in increased effort and expense by that state to improve conditions at the Willowbrook State School.

One principle that is increasingly applied is that of the "least restrictive alternative." The Constitution of the United States guarantees that Americans will be provided the freedom to live as they please, with government intervention only when absolutely necessary and with intervention being the least restrictive possible. This is currently being interpreted as a mandate for habilitation of the individual within the community as often as possible, as opposed to more restrictive institutional settings.

The principle of normalization, first applied in Scandinavian countries (Nirje, 1970), emphasized the value of providing the mentally retarded with opportunities for lives structured as closely as possible to those enjoyed by other members of society. Concerns about safeguarding the liberty of mentally handicapped citizens within institutions turned the attention of the courts to the practice of using institutional residents as workers without monetary compensation. Such "institutional peonage," as it was termed, was interpreted as involuntary servitude and a violation of the thirteenth amendment (*Sauder* v. *Brannan; Wyatt* v. *Stickney; Dale* v. *New York*).

Exclusionary policies of public school that served to deny many mentally retarded children an education were first successfully attacked in Pennsylvania. In 1971, a federal district court, in *Pennsylvania Association for Retarded Children* v. *Commonwealth of Pennsylvania,* entered a consent decree mandating that Pennsylvania's public schools must cease the exclusion of mentally retarded children on the basis of their retardation. Furthermore, parents must be notified of placement in a special class or school and are entitled to an independent assessment with a formal hearing for their child to determine whether that class is appropriate for him according to his abilities. Parents now have the right to be represented by legal counsel at this hearing, as well as by other professionals, and to examine all of their child's school records. Similar "right to education" laws modeled after the Pennsylvania decision have been enacted in many states.

Other fundamental rights of the mentally retarded, i.e., to marry, to have children, to vote, and to enter into a legal contract, are currently being fought for in the courts, although these rights are still denied the mentally retarded in many states. The issues are by no means simple. There is little question that many mentally retarded citizens will not be capable of assuming privileges and responsibilities considered to be their legal rights. However, the burden of responsibility is shifting to those administrators or public officials who would deny these rights to the mentally retarded to provide sufficient reason for restrictive or exclusionary practices rather than being upon the mentally retarded citizen or his family to secure the rights. For the first time in over a century and a quarter of concern for the mentally retarded in this country, public awareness is directed toward providing the mentally retarded citizen with the opportunities for life, liberty, and the pursuit of happiness, available to ordinary citizens, and to safeguard his basic human rights. In 1939, the official journal of the American Association on Mental Deficiency listed among its stated objectives:

> The construction of institutions for the feebleminded; a complete census and registration of all mentally deficient children of school age; the segregation of mentally deficient persons in institutional care and training with a permanent segregation of those who cannot make satisfactory social adjustments in the

community; parole for all suitable institutionally trained mentally defective persons; extra-institutional supervision of all defectives in the community.

Rights of Mentally Retarded Persons, published as an official policy statement of that same organization in 1975, includes specific rights to exert freedom of choice in making decisions, to live in the least restrictive environment, to seek gainful employment and fair pay, to be part of a family, to marry and have a family, to be free to move without deprivation of liberty by institutionalization, to speak openly, to maintain privacy, to practice a religion, to interact with peers, and to receive publicly supported education, vocational training, and habilitative programs.

These changes have had significant repercussions upon the administrative policies of institutions for the mentally retarded and public school programs. They have directly affected the lives of thousands of mentally retarded citizens. However, the extent to which these philosophies have changed the thinking and practice of persons directly involved in providing habilitative services is open to question. It is one thing to agree that many mentally retarded citizens are capable of and entitled to freedoms and opportunities available to the rest of society. However, it is quite another to accept the challenge of preparing these persons so that they are capable of using new opportunities. Schools, hospitals, habilitation centers, and other agencies providing services to the mentally retarded have made advances in reversing attitudes and policies of generations and in meeting the letter and spirit of current legislation. Yet, the task of teaching mentally retarded citizens to be husbands and wives and parents, to be good citizens, to enjoy their new-found liberties, and to be adequate, happy, fulfilled persons presents so formidable a challenge that few professionals have attempted to deal with it. The provision of community information and training in the rudiments of social competency to handle banking, paychecks, ''the world of work'' budgeting, and transportation, while important, represents only the most meager portion of what habilitative training is capable of providing.

As professionals who have accepted the responsibility for training the mentally retarded, we now bear a moral responsibility to go beyond the obvious, the commonplace, and the relatively simple educational problems in habilitation in order to find ways of teaching essential life-enriching behaviors and skills. If we do not accept this aspect of our role, we may be faced with a backlash to normalization and deinstitutionalization policies far worse than the conditions that originally generated progress. Such backlash would be difficult to deal with because it would come from the mentally retarded themselves and from their families if we fail to fulfill our promises to them for better lives. It will also come from the general public when it no longer wishes to provide the financial support or take the risks for persons who fail to become integrated into the mainstream as "ordinary citizens."

RECAPITULATION

This book began with a history of the concept and practice of habilitation in this country. It traced how the mid-nineteenth century optimism about training the mentally retarded gave way to a period of alarm, pessimism, segregation, and control. It described how schools became institutions, and restrictive laws were enacted reflecting prevalent perceptions of the mentally handicapped individual as sick, dangerous, deviant, or subhuman. It described the gradual change toward more optimistic attitudes and acceptance of moral and financial responsibility for the mentally disabled, culminating in current deinstitutionalization and normalization policies.

Next we described the emerging concept of mental retardation as a differentiated diagnostic category closely related to evaluation strategies affecting habilitative treatment. The results of intellectual testing of the mentally retarded increased disillusionment about the effectiveness of education upon mental growth. More sophisticated understanding of the limitations of the IQ measure as an infallible index of intellectual capacity was accompanied by greater emphasis upon social function and coping behavior in diagnosis and evaluation of the mentally retarded. The development of vocational evaluation procedures in the post–World War II era provided assessment strategies for the mentally retarded when habilitation goals were finally accepted for this population. Recent emphasis placed upon criterion-referenced rather than norm-referenced tests is again having repercussions in the development of evaluation instruments for the retarded that are free of cultural bias and more directly suitable for assessing competency rather than intellect. We suggested the need for evaluation and habilitation to go beyond normalization in finding ways to assess more meaningful "quality of life" dimensions of behavior.

To set the stage for our later discussion of needed changes in habilitation goals and programs, we outlined a research utilization philosophy for habilitation facilities. We argued that behavioral research should be a part of any treatment program and that such research should be directly concerned with the important programmatic and administrative decision-making of that facility. We illustrated the application of this model at one institution for the retarded where program evaluation, program development, and dissemination efforts were closely related to progressive changes in institutional structure over a twelve-year period.

Next we examined more thoroughly the habilitative process as it is traditionally defined, beginning with the enactment of Public Law 333 in 1965. Chapter 4 outlined the entire sequence of habilitation training, beginning with prevocational and vocational evaluation and proceeding through the exploratory work situation, and the utilizing of various training programs to implement a vocational plan for the client. The use of the sheltered workshop, job training stations, transitional experiences, counseling, and job placement was described. The importance of social habilitation was emphasized, and various approaches to this type of training were discussed. Concern was expressed that mentally retarded persons exhibit severe social deficiencies that cannot be corrected through legislation or minimized solely by humanitarian motivations. The need to develop more powerful social learning procedures is a far more difficult task than teaching saleable job skills.

The implementation of such an habilitation program was illustrated by an historical account of a major residential institution for the mentally retarded. The beginnings of the institution as one of the first American schools for the mentally handicapped, its gradual evolution as a custodial institution in the post–Civil War era, and its transformation into an education and habilitation center in the early 1960s were described. The manner in which traditional attitudes and methods of operation gave way to more modern habilitation programing was depicted. The concept of a "continuum of services" was illustrated with the extension of institutional services to the community in the form of halfway house, group home, and follow-up programs. An extension of this concept to a cerebral palsied population was also considered.

The detailed inspection of changes in one institution led us to a consideration of the effects of institutions in general upon the development of intelligence and personality. The call of some for an end to institutions is contrasted with a more moderate position seeking a new role for residential institutions with less distinct demarcation between institution and community. This discussion was continued in Chapter 8, where the principle of normalization was discussed. We attempted to clarify confusion in the meaning of the concept by describing normalization as a legal and humanitarian idea but not as a psychological principle. The most serious criticism of normalization lies in what it omits from what we consider to be desirable and feasible goals for training the mentally retarded for community living. Concepts of adjustment and psychological health were examined as criteria of evaluating the mentally retarded.

In Section IV we shifted our attention from the institution to the community. We considered the implications of follow-up studies of persons previously identified in institutions or public schools and living in the community. The concept of adjustment was again examined in light of these studies, and the need for continuing follow-up research was outlined. The development of realistic training programs for community living can proceed logically only from more detailed information about the life styles of mentally retarded persons presently living in the community. Despite the fact that voluminous data have already been collected, present knowledge of the factors affecting community adjustment is limited to only the most broadly defined and basic dimensions of community living. A detailed description of a follow-up study conducted at Elwyn Institute was included to provide a more vivid illustration of follow-up research, including brief vignettes of individual retarded citizens in the community. The lack of information concerning factors determining community adjustment is evident in the failure of the prognostic studies reviewed in Chapter 11. This chapter also continued the presentation of research utilization and set the stage for our consideration of emotional and personality variables in the habilitation process.

Next we considered the significance of personality and emotional factors in the overall functioning of the mentally retarded. Earlier conceptions such as "instinctual weakness" and "moral imbecility" gave way to more ambitious attempts to study empirically the psychology of mentally retarded persons. We saw how theoretical formulations that were first developed for normal populations were applied to the mentally handicapped. Four such formulations were considered: Rotter's social learning theory, Piaget's theory of moral development of the child, Freudian psychoanalytic theory, and Zigler's motivational-cognitive position.

The relevance of such theorizing and research to the day-to-day functioning of the habilitation worker has not been well defined. We conclude that the field of mental retardation does not include an integrated and comprehensive understanding of personality development of the mentally handicapped that can be easily applied by clinicians, teachers, and habilitation workers. The elements of a personality model were suggested.

Subsequent chapters in Section V suggested several dimensions of personality that may characterize mentally retarded populations more than they do other groups. Our pilot attempts to study empirically these dimensions were presented. Overcompliance or acquiescence to persuasion by others was seen as related to problems of exploitation. Patterns of inertia, passivity, or helplessness may develop from histories of oversheltering and overprotection. The self-concept held by the mentally retarded individual, as measured by the manner in which he evaluates his capacity to achieve important goals, may be the most central personality construct affecting his inappropriate behavior. Simple laboratory procedures of assessing self-esteem appear to have great potential for clinical application. Despite the misgivings of many concerned professionals, normalization of the mentally retarded necessitates preparation for heterosexual living. The marriage and child-rearing experiences of mentally retarded persons in the community provide guidelines for structuring social learning programs for persons presently enrolled in training programs. Psychosexual development of the retarded is best understood not as a facsimile of infantile modes of adjustment, but as purposive behavior learned as a result of unique and sometimes idiosyncratic environmental experiences. The importance of behavioral training rather than sex education was stressed. The significance and measurement of social competence was next considered, with particular emphasis upon the learning and perpetuation of inappropriate behaviors by mentally handicapped populations.

In describing the mentally retarded as characterized by certain personality variables, we have not intended to imply that such variables are limited to the mentally retarded or that they exhaust the number of ways the mentally retarded may vary from each other. Acquiescence, helplessness, and the other dimensions discussed previously are areas of personality functioning that can be attributed to some persons of normal intelligence as well as to the mentally retarded. Once psychologists and habilitation specialists are ready to acknowledge that personality dimensions are important considerations in the mentally retarded, it may open the door for a better understanding of these same personality dimensions in nonhandicapped populations as well.

We do not regard our pilot investigations as proven fact. Rather, we offer these variables as speculative. We recognize that our constructs may invite criticism, but we hope that they will also stimulate thinking and research. The behaviors we have described are debilitating to many mentally handicapped persons we have studied. Even if they prove to hold for the mentally retarded in general, it will always be necessary to study each individual reference to these specific dimensions. We have emphasized the need for idiographic approaches to evaluation as well as the need for new assessment techniques to carry out such studies.

Finally, we examined methods of treatment of emotional and social learning problems. Chapter 18 considered the suitability of the mentally retarded for psychotherapeutic intervention, given their cognitive and verbal deficits. Sternlicht's etiological model for the use of psychotherapy with mentally retarded populations was examined and rejected in favor of one based upon current behavior, specific behavioral objectives, and other operationally defined client and situational variables. A group counseling program was presented for dealing with the basic emotional, behavioral and personality characteristics of the mentally retarded described earlier. This curriculum is viewed by the authors as a beginning and a springboard for habilitation counselors to plan remedial programs, rather than as an inflexible curriculum for counseling. The preceding chapter deals with the treatment of more severely disturbed individuals who are typically excluded from habilitation programs because of the difficulties in behavior management of such persons. It suggests that habilitation workers will be increasingly called upon to deal with such behaviors and that a therapeutic milieu unit for the severely disturbed should be a part of a comprehensive habilitation program.

We are approaching the end of our journey. One task remains undone. We have examined where we have been, but we have not, as yet, indicated where we should be headed. The remainder of this chapter points to some new, uncharted areas. First, we will explore a construct that we label freedom and constraint and that seems to beckon to us because of continued needs of the mentally retarded for greater independence in community settings. Next, we wish to describe the type of person we believe is needed to implement future habilitation programs for the mentally retarded. Finally, we will outline a course of action and research that we believe is demanded in our field.

FREEDOM AND CONSTRAINT WITHIN RESIDENTIAL SETTINGS

The background for the implementation of the concept of ''least restrictive environment'' for training the mentally retarded (Public Law 94-103) lay in the abuses within state and private institutions that had, in many instances, gone unchecked for generations. Application of this concept has been in the form of deinstitutionalization programs designed with the aim of providing normalizing experiences to thousands of mentally retarded citizens previously denied adequate training, education, and treatment and often living in situations of neglect and degradation.

Despite the unanimous endorsement of these principles by professionals working with the mentally retarded, the implementation of deinstitutionalization and normalization programs has aroused a great deal of criticism. The confusion and controversy over normalization and deinstitutionalization efforts stem from the very extreme positions about the future demise of institutions taken by some writers (Wolfensberger, 1971*a*, 1971*b*), and the tacit assumption made by others that institutions represent the most restrictive residential settings, while community living in the form of group homes, foster homes, nursing homes, and independent living represents less restrictive alternatives.

The position taken here, on the other hand, is that normalization and deinstitutionalization solutions to the problems of the mentally retarded have been overly simplistic. It is assumed, instead, that degrees of freedom or restriction represent multidimensional variables determined by many complex factors within any social setting. Thus, for some individuals the institution may allow greater freedom than the community.

The desire to provide protection, shelter, and special care for the handicapped, though well intended, has often been abused and has acted to impose greater handicaps. Growing up within a residential institution may exert more influence upon the personality and behavior of the mentally retarded than his original intellectual limitations. Sometimes these restraints have been based upon false information, invalid research findings, or value judgments that may change over time. It would be desirable to develop adequate criteria for evaluating the restrictions placed upon individuals in relation to their needs and the greatest good for the individual.

In properly evaluating residential situations with regard to constraint, it is necessary to consider that complete freedom is neither available nor desirable for any ctitizen. Laws, rules, and regulations based on societal needs dictate constraints that must be imposed in any society. Nor is freedom always most beneficial to the individual. In many cases individual needs dictate some form of restriction or constraint in the form of supervision, training, and safety requirements.

What often appears to be a constraint on a superficial basis may, in reality, be a means for greater mobility or freedom. A wheelchair for a physically handicapped individual is a form of constraint dictated by his motor deficits but allows greater freedom of movement. An automobile vastly increaes mobility but imposes restrictions in the form of driving licenses and traffic laws. Similarly, it may be that intellectual capacities and educational deficits may require restrictions that allow ultimately for greater degrees of freedom. A mentally retarded youngster, for example, may require the teaching methods of a special class to maximize his educational opportunities. Legal, financial, and physical constraints may sometimes have similar value. Thus, it is impossible to evaluate properly external constraints placed upon the individual without also considering the reason for the constraints, their effectiveness and their relation to the individual's need.

Many different types of constraint may limit the freedom of any individual. These include: physical constraints, such as tranquilizers, strait jackets and time-out rooms; geographic constraints; time constraints, such as appointments and dinner times; social constraints imposed by convention and training; economic and financial constraints; legal constraints, such as laws, rules, customs, and norms; and personal constraints imposed by individual characteristics and limitations, such as intellectual, physical, educational, and vocational skills.

Such constraints should be subject to observation and measurement. It should be possible to develop meaningful and reliable measures of constraints that may be imposed by residential living situations upon mentally retarded persons and to evaluate a broad range of such situations in terms of these criteria. The evaluation should be general enough and sufficiently well defined to allow application within institutions, group homes, halfway houses, foster homes, nursing homes, and independent living arrangements. Such things as social interactions and geographic mobility of persons within various settings should be studied. The physical settings themselves can be evaluated using scales such as that developed by Gunzburg (1973). Subjective feelings of constraint should also be assessed.

It is anticipated that such research may lead to a more realistic appreciation of the advantages and limitations of many social climates for the mentally handicapped. It may demonstrate ways of improving these climates. It may provide new dimensions and concepts with which to evaluate the needs of the individual mentally retarded citizen and the resources of various environmental options for meeting these needs. Finally it may reveal a new and more meaningful role that institutions may assume in serving the handicapped.

THE NEW HABILITATION SPECIALIST

Of the three authors of this book, only one was ever a student at a bona fide habilitation department and can legitimately call himself an habilitation psychologist. Even his credentials were later "contaminated" by doctoral training in clinical psychology. The other two authors are a clinical psychologist with training and interests in research and a psychiatrist with a background in public health. Thus, it is with some degree of hesitation that we venture to outline our ideas about the training of habilitation specialists. Nevertheless, the implications of all we have suggested in this book lead logically toward changing concepts concerning the training and competence of professionals who must implement habilitation services.

In describing this hypothetical professional, we have drawn heavily upon a model that has served for the past three decades in the training of clinical psychologists and that has generally been labeled the scientist-professional model. The most recent, and one of the most eloquent, expositions of this model (Shakow, 1976) describes such training as combining the values of the scientist and the values of the humanist in actual practice:

> A clearer definition of the scientist-professional perhaps comes from a deeper examination of the value systems that characterize such a person. The value systems include a self-image of a psychologist identified with both his or her field and its history, and beyond that with science, whose major value Bronowski calls the 'habit of truth.' This habit is manifested in the constant effort to guide one's actions through inquiry into what is fact and verifiable, rather than to act on the basis of faith, wish, or precipitateness. Underlying and combined with this 'hardheadedness' lies a sensitive, humanistic approach to the problems of persons and their societies. The scientist-professional recognizes, in the context of our overwhelming ignorance, the primacy of the need to build for the future well-being of persons and groups on a solid base of knowledge. Thus, integral to this attitude is an implicit modesty, the acceptance of the need for experiment, and the long-term view. (p. 554).

It is not our wish to suggest that all habilitation specialists must also be psychologists or scientists. Rather, we envision a wedding of scientific values and attitudes with the humanitarian concern for the needs of handicapped persons. The habilitation specialist should see his work as an extension of theoretical knowledge and empirical findings. While perhaps not actively pursuing applied research (although he may), he must place himself in close proximity with such research, both to provide the critical insights in planning investigations and to interpret their findings. He must be flexible enough to modify his habilitation efforts on the basis of empirical findings and honest enough to subject his methods and programs to empirical study. While it goes without saying that he must express sympathy and understanding in a helping relationship, it is equally important that he recognize that sympathy and understanding cannot stand alone in effecting successful habilitative outcomes. The habilitation specialist must, therefore, learn to distrust the intuitive, the traditional, the speculative, and the innovative, at least to the extent of demanding verification. He must possess a capacity for questioning formulations, his own as well as others', when they no longer account for the facts. On the other hand, he must be attuned to developing new formulations and alert to increasing his knowledge and understanding by his critical attitude.

It is our belief that the training of habilitation specialists should include at least two major areas of learning that are not presently a part of master's level training programs. The first is a greater exposure to theoretical formulations of personality and emotional development, including both normal and abnormal manifestations. This can be provided primarily through course work. The second area is more difficult to teach because it reflects more directly an attitudinal state rather than an area of increased knowledge or competency. We suggest that at least one-half of the internship or practicum experience of the habilitation specialist be spent in an apprenticeship position within an habilitation research laboratory. It may be that a second internship year would be required for this purpose. The purpose of this experience, which should also be supported by prior coursework, would not be to produce a research scientist. Rather, it would be intended to familiarize the individual with research philosophy and methods, to sensitize him to empirical attitudes, and to teach him to communicate with researchers on a give-and-take basis. Such exposure would be invaluable in bringing about a state of affairs in which the habilitation specialist could, as Shakow demands of psychologists, practice his profession objectively, and the researcher might practice his science humanistically.

THE TASK REMAINING

Our commitment to a research utilization model, first elaborated in an earlier chapter, and our search for a new breed of habilitation specialist sympathetic to research attitudes and goals rest upon a basic confidence in habilitation as a helping profession for finding ways of coping with mental retardation. The goals of Seguin are no less valid today than they were a century and a quarter ago. But the methods of habilitation have fallen far short of their original promise. It was not more idealistic of Seguin to return the mentally retarded to the mainstream of society in 1850 than it is to pursue normalization goals today. When the physiological training advocated by Seguin failed to produce this desired result, or did not prove feasible, the authorities of the day turned against the underlying philosophy of habilitation. Their energies became diverted toward the protectionistic motivations well known to readers of this book. Yet it was not Seguin's objectives that were at fault, only his manner of implementing them that proved inadequate.

Now that the habilitation path from which we have strayed has been rediscovered, we may be faced with the same unsettling realization—that our methods are suspect. During the past decade many facilities serving the retarded were willing to cast aside the misconceptions of a previous century, both medical and educational. No longer would we call the retarded "sick" or "uneducable" or other labels that served no useful purpose. The introduction of vocational evaluation, sheltered workshops, work samples, and job placement has undoubtedly represented an improvement over medical or custodial treatment of the mentally retarded. The application of behavior modification approaches to work productivity within job training sites has represented another improvement. Yet we have repeatedly pointed out throughout this book that job training is not enough, and the social habilitation techniques presently being used in preparing mentally retarded persons to be socially competent individuals are painfully inadequate. While we may have the technology to teach mentally retarded adults to assemble bicycle brakes, even to normal productivity levels, we have little technology for teaching them to speak and act appropriately, to respond appropriately, or to enjoy life.

Yet the means of developing such technology is within our grasp. A coordinated effort of researchers and service-oriented professionals could develop a data bank of information upon which programs of the future could be based. A division of labor among facilities serving the mentally retarded could be made so that specialization of training objectives is achieved. In defining new roles for residential settings, one option appears most compelling: Social learning objectives in adult retarded will require considerably more than individual and group therapy approaches.

We have already specified a number of areas in which applied research efforts will have direct repercussions on methods and materials for habilitation. In 1958, Tizard called for an end to follow-up studies intended to demonstrate the capability of mentally retarded persons for community functioning because he believed the point had already been well established. If this were the only purpose of follow-up studies, Tizard would be correct. Yet the commitment to total habilitation and community functioning of the mentally retarded is still novel in most communities. Although the concept of employment of the handicapped is generally accepted by industry today, it is doubtful that mentally retarded workers will be completely accepted in industrial and business settings for many years. Integration into community churches and social structures is even further away. The follow-up study is more relevant today than ever before in order to learn of the total adjustment process of these individuals and their interface with community resources and structures. Only through descriptive accounts of the behavior and functioning of mentally retarded persons in a variety of community settings will we be able to make successful decisions regarding selection, community preparation, and community placement.

The development of evaluation techniques for assessing community knowledge and skills of the mentally retarded has only scratched the surface. The few procedures available for assessing community knowledge do not begin to fill the needs for evaluating the individual's suitability to handle a myriad of everyday living demands, some of critical significance, some crucial for survival in the community. Dozens of specific and reliable measurement instruments are required in areas such as time-telling, measurement, social sight vocabulary, banking, money recognition, and calendar knowledge. Nothing can be taken for granted. This assumption pertains not only to whether or not an individual of given intellectual level can handle a specific community skill, but also to the "teachability" of the skill and its relevance to successful community functioning. The development of such criterion-referenced tests, which can be administered even to nonverbal or illiterate persons, is a prerequisite for adequate program development, as well as for individual program decisions for the mentally retarded.

Paralleling the development of assessment procedures, there should be an equivalent number of teaching packages in the same relevant community coping areas. These packages may take the form of teacher-administered and directed "tutorial" programs or self-administered programed instruction materials. This effort must go beyond the stopping point that has characterized most educational materials for the mentally retarded to date, i.e., beyond development without evaluation. Numerous materials are placed upon the market each year with little or no attempt to field test the programs and assess their effectiveness as instructional aids. In discussing limits to the educability of mentally retarded children, Bricker (1970) has written:

> . . . Only the failure of a perfectly valid, perfectly reliable, perfectly efficient program of training will convince me that the identification of the deficit is sufficient reason to stop trying to educate the child. Somehow, I cannot feel that we have reached perfection in the development of training programs (p. 20).

Similarly, in the field of habilitation we have a long history of questioning the validity of assessment techniques but have paid scant attention to the validity of educational materials for achieving specific educational goals. Habilitation counselors and teachers require more than pictures of coins in a book arranged and labeled compulsively according to denomination. They need sophisticated programs, suitable for persons of limited conceptual skills. These programs should be sufficiently researched to instill the confidence that they will accomplish concrete behavioral objectives. The field of education is only just beginning to come to grips with accountability for individual learning, prescriptive teaching, and time-framed behavioral objectives. The field of habilitation may still be light years away from this type of methodology.

Not only should individual materials be evaluated, but entire programs need to be subjected to the scrutiny of controlled experimental study. Walls and Tseng (1976) discuss criteria that have been used in evaluating client outcomes in habilitation. Follow-up studies provide a vital source of information for evaluating the success or failure of habilitation efforts. Unfortunately, outcomes measured in most studies are far removed in time and may be conceptually unrelated to habilitation training. In order for outcome studies to provide information about the adequacy of training, they must be chosen to be specific to particular training goals and should bear some theoretical relationship to the training. To use productivity, absenteeism, employment stability, job satisfaction, and other complex social phenomena as criteria in general vocational and social habilitation efforts is likely to invite the derivation of zero-order correlation coefficients. However, if habilitation specialists can learn to program in terms of simple, clearly stated operational objectives, then evaluation of the training in terms of outcome is simplified. Why accept absenteeism, for example, as a criterion of success, when training never dealt specifically with teaching the individual not to be absent? Why use employment satisfaction as a criterion when little attention was devoted by the program to making the individual happy with his job? Earlier we made the identical criticism of prediction studies in habilitation. Predictability will occur not only with the acceptance of standardized research procedures, as Bolton (1972) suggests, but also with the acceptance of greater accountability in measuring, teaching, and evaluating specific behavioral repertoires. As we have indicated repeatedly in this book, such accountability must also include the area of emotional adjustment and the assessment of the client as part of a community system.

Several years ago one of the authors published a paper in a mental retardation journal summarizing research at Elwyn over a ten-year period. Shortly after the article appeared in print, a letter was received from Dr. Robert Haskall, Superintendent of the Wayne County Training School thirty years ago, and now retired and a resident of the Leeward Islands. Dr. Haskall enclosed a reprint of an article (Haskall, 1944) that he had written during that era that was similar in intent to our own and summarized a fifteen-year period of research. The paper described the work of Strauss and Lehtinen dealing with the brain-injured child; the early environmental stimulation studies of Kephart, and later Kirk; the perceptual investigations of Werner; and the educational studies of Hegge; as well as numerous medical investigations. The research summarized in Haskall's paper is as current today as it was at the time of publication. Dr. Haskall, who was 97 years old at the time he wrote to us, seemed to be saying that there was little new under the sun. It is hard to challenge this argument, because the research studies Haskall described in 1944 were precursors of today's interest in minimal brain damage, learning disability, infant stimulation, and special education programs. The meager beginnings we describe in the present volume pale by contrast. The research conducted at the Wayne County Training School in the 1940s is impressive, not because it filled research journals or built elegant theories, but because it was translated directly into programs and policies. We end this book with the hope that tomorrow's field of habilitation can follow from today's research efforts in as meaningful and direct a manner.

LITERATURE CITED

Bolton, B. 1972. The prediction of rehabilitation outcomes. J. Appl. Rehab. Couns. 3:16–24.

Bricker, W. A. 1970. Identifying and modifying behavioral deficits. Amer. J. Ment. Defic. 75:16–21.

Gunzburg, H. C. 1973. The physical environment of the mentally handicapped. VIII. 39 steps leading towards normalized living practices in living units for the mentally handicapped. Brit. J. Ment. Subnormal. XIX (2):91–99.

Haskall, R. H. 1944. The development of a research program in mental deficiency over a fifteen-year period. Amer. J. Psychiatry 101:73–81.

Nirje, B. 1970. The normalization principle—Implications and comments. J. Ment. Subnormal. XVI(31):62–70.

Shakow, D. 1976. What is clinical psychology? Amer. Psychol. 31:553–560.

Tizard, J. 1958. Longitudinal and follow-up studies. *In* A. Clarke and A. D. B. Clarke (eds.), Mental Deficiency: The Changing Outlook, pp. 422–449. Methuen & Co., London.

Walls, R. T., and Tseng, M. S. 1976. Measurement of client outcomes in rehabilitation. *In* B. Bolton (ed.), Handbook of Measurement and Evaluation in Rehabilitation, pp. 207–225. University Park Press, Baltimore.

Wolfensberger, W. 1971*a*. Will there always be an institution? I: The impact of epidemiological trends. Ment. Retard. 9:14–20.

Wolfensberger, W. 1971*b*. Will there always be an institution? II: The impact of new service models. Ment. Retard. 9:31–38.

Index